Cardiology

For UKMLA and Medical Exams

First and second edition authors

Anjana Siva

Mark Noble

Mohamed K Al-Obaidi

Third edition authors

Ajay Jain

Matthew Ginks

Fourth edition authors

Antonia Churchhouse

Julian Ormerod

Fifth edition

Thomas Foster

Jasmine Shen

6th Edition
CRASH COURSE

SERIES EDITOR

Philip Xiu

MA (Cantab), MB BChir, MRCP, MRCGP, MScClinEd, FHEA, MAcadMEd, RCPathME
Honorary Senior Lecturer
Leeds University School of Medicine
PCN Educational Lead
Medical Examiner
Leeds Teaching Hospital Trust
Leeds, UK

FACULTY ADVISOR

David E. Newby

BA, BSc (Hons), PhD, BM, DM, DSc, MRCP, FRSE, FMedSci, FESC, FACC
Professor, British Heart Foundation Duke of Edinburgh Chair of Cardiology

Cardiology

For UKMLA and Medical Exams

Jasmine Shen

MBChB
Core Trainee, Acute Care Common Stem
NHS Lothian

Thomas Foster

MBChB, BMedSci (Hons), FRCR
Consultant Cardiothoracic Radiologist
NHS Lothian
Honorary Clinical Senior Lecturer
The University of Edinburgh

ELSEVIER

First edition 1999

Second edition 2005

Third edition 2008

Fourth edition 2013

Updated fourth edition 2015

Fifth edition 2019

Sixth edition 2025

Notices

Practitioners and researchers must always rely on their own experience and knowledge in evaluating and using any information, methods, compounds or experiments described herein. Because of rapid advances in the medical sciences, in particular, independent verification of diagnoses and drug dosages should be made. To the fullest extent of the law, no responsibility is assumed by Elsevier, authors, editors or contributors for any injury and/or damage to persons or property as a matter of products liability, negligence or otherwise, or from any use or operation of any methods, products, instructions, or ideas contained in the material herein.

ISBN: 978-0-4431-1534-9

Content Strategist: Trinity Hutton
Content Project Manager: Ayan Dhar
Design: Miles Hitchen
Marketing Manager: Deborah Watkins

Printed in India by Thomson Press (Ltd)

Last digit is the print number: 9 8 7 6 5 4 3 2 1

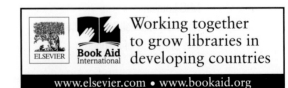

Series editor's foreword

With great honour and pride, we present the latest edition of the *Crash Course* series. This series has traversed a journey of nearly a quarter-century, stemming from the vision of Dr. Dan Horton-Szar, and his legacy continues to walk with us on this pathway of knowledge.

The series has been popular with students worldwide, selling over **1 million copies** and being translated into more than **8 languages**, reinforcing our commitment to global learning.

We remain extremely grateful for your unwavering trust. The series has once again been refreshed and fully upgraded in accordance with the rapidly changing medical guidelines, ensuring the content is comprehensive, accurate and fully up-to-date.

This latest series continues our tradition of integrating clinical practice with basic medical sciences, tailored meticulously for today's medical undergraduate curriculum. A central highlight of this instalment is our emphasis on high-yield exam content designed specifically for the UKMLA curriculum.

The addition of the **Rapid UKMLA Index** at the beginning of the book enhances this offering, serving as a valuable aid to students to track their exam preparation efficiently. We also revised all self-assessment questions to align with the single best answer format in line with the latest UKMLA examination style. We have also added ***High-Yield Association Tables***. These are essential tools designed to aid students in recognizing clinical patterns and acing vignette-style exam questions. By condensing complex medical scenarios into digestible, manageable insights, these tables ensure efficient learning. They connect symptoms, diagnosis, and treatment, bolstering understanding and confidence in tackling the rigorous UKMLA exams. This comprehensive approach makes these tables an indispensable asset in your exam preparations.

Utilizing student feedback, we have strived to maintain the core principles of this series: delivering precise and readable text that brings together depth and clarity. The authors are experienced junior doctors who successfully navigated these exams recently, ensuring practical and tested guidance. A team of expert faculty advisors from across the United Kingdom ensures the content's accuracy, making it resilient and reliable.

As we turn a new chapter with the latest edition, we honour the past, cherish the present, and embrace the promise of the future. We wish you every success in your journey of learning and growth and hope that this series adds value to your life, both as students and as future medical professionals.

Philip Xiu

Authors

"Cardiology is a popular and competitive specialty that combines history taking and clinical examination with a wide range of investigations and interventions. As cardiovascular disease is the leading cause of death in developed countries a sound understanding of cardiology is vital. The specialty is constantly evolving with advances in diagnostic tests and novel treatment options. This is reflected in this fully revised and updated sixth edition, which incorporates both underlying science and its clinical application. This new edition also includes a new vascular disease chapter covering key arterial and venous pathologies.

We are aware that assessments are constantly changing and, as a result, have developed an up-to-date self-assessment section, including Single Best Answer Questions, OSCE cases and ECG cases. We have also added in High Yield Association Tables that should help with last-minute studying.

With this book, our intention is to give quick, clear summaries to save you time during a busy rotation or during exam revision. We aim to provide additional details and tips to add to your insight into clinical practice, gain extra points in exams and become a competent junior doctor. We hope that this book also gives you an opportunity to further your interest and enjoyment of cardiology. We wish you all the best with your studies and future careers!"

Jasmine Shen and Thomas Foster

Faculty advisor

"The excellent Crash Course series summarizes the key learning points for the 'information-overloaded' undergraduate medical student. The series format enhances learning through concise text, comprehension check boxes and hints and tips boxes. The key salient points are presented in a user-friendly and easy-to-read manner that enables the rapid assimilation of core knowledge.

This sixth edition of Crash Course Cardiology provides a comprehensive single text bringing together all the knowledge you need when studying cardiology and cardiovascular medicine, incorporating all the essential basic knowledge that provides an invaluable foundation for application to clinical practice. The book takes the reader through first principles to inform the basis and presentation of cardiovascular disease, ultimately leading to the investigation and management of common cardiovascular disorders. This logical, sequential progression enhances learning and understanding of the cardiovascular system in clinical medicine.

This book is a 'must' for the time-pressed student who needs to use their revision time efficiently and effectively in the modern era of systems-based medical education."

Professor David E. Newby

Acknowledgement

We would first like to thank Professor David Newby once again for all his invaluable help and advice. We also want to acknowledge the whole team at Elsevier and all our clinical teachers over the past few years. Lastly, we would like to thank our families (including our son Leo!) and friends for all their support.

Jasmine Shen and Thomas Foster

Series editor's acknowledgement

We would like to express our sincere gratitude to those who have provided their support and expertise in preparing this sixth edition of the *Crash Course* series. Our junior doctor contributors' participation in crafting the manuscript has been indispensable. Their first-hand experience and current medical knowledge have infused realism and practicality into our content.

Our faculty editors deserve a special note of thanks. They have extensively validated the correctness of the information, ensuring that the content is not just accurate but also contemporaneous, credible, and aligns with the latest medical standards.

We extend our heartfelt thanks to our publisher, Elsevier. Their staff have demonstrated an unwavering commitment to quality, maintaining the high standards set since the first edition. Their insights have routinely enriched the content and process alike.

Our Commissioning Editor, Jeremy Bowes, deserves a special mention for his consistent support and guiding hand throughout the development process. His directions and advice have bettered this edition and spurred us on our quest for excellence.

We are greatly indebted to Alex Mortimer for her wisdom, practical insights and valuable guidance. A big thank you to our Content Strategists, Trinity Hutton and Cloe Holland-Borosh, who need special acknowledgement for meticulously outlining the direction and scope of the content. They've managed to mix details with a strategic plan, keeping our readers in mind.

Lastly, much gratitude is owed to our Content Product Managers, Taranpreet Kaur, Ayan Dhar, Shivani Pal and Tapajyoti Chaudhuri, who have juggled the numerous day-to-day tasks with utmost dedication and perseverance. Despite the ever-approaching deadlines, they have shown remarkable patience and steadfast determination, ensuring that each step of the book's development was accomplished seamlessly.

In conclusion, we sincerely thank each of these wonderful people for their outstanding contributions and support, without which this work wouldn't have been achieved. Their passion, commitment and collaborative effort have helped us bring this edition together.

Philip Xiu

Rapid UKMLA Index

continued

Table 1 UKMLA Conditions and Where to Find Them—cont'd

Priority	UKMLA Conditions	Chapter	Page
2	Pericardial disease	Chapter 6: Chest pain Chapter 16: Diseases of the myocardium and pericardium	60, 64 208
1	Peripheral vascular disease	Chapter 18: Vascular disease	233
1	Pulmonary embolism	Chapter 6: Chest pain Chapter 18: Vascular disease	60 228
3	Pulmonary hypertension	Chapter 17: Congenital heart disease Chapter 18: Vascular disease	214 230
3	Right heart valve disease	Chapter 10: Heart murmurs Chapter 15: Valvular disease	91 190, 192
3	Unstable angina	Chapter 6: Chest pain Chapter 11: Atherosclerosis and its risk factors Chapter 12: Stable angina and acute coronary syndromes	60, 64 104 129
3	Vasovagal syncope	Chapter 2: The cardiac cycle, control of cardiac output and haemodynamic regulation Chapter 9: Syncope	31 83
1	Venous ulcers	Chapter 18: Vascular disease	239

Table 2 UKMLA Presentations and Where to Find Them

UKMLA Presentations	Chapter	Page
Blackouts and faints	Chapter 2: The cardiac cycle, control of cardiac output and haemodynamic regulation Chapter 9: Syncope Chapter 14: Arrhythmias	31 83 151
Breathlessness	Chapter 7: Breathlessness and peripheral oedema Chapter 13: Heart failure Chapter 16: Diseases of the myocardium and pericardium	67 141 203
Cardiorespiratory arrest	Chapter 12: Stable angina and acute coronary syndromes Chapter 14: Arrhythmias	129 171
Chest pain	Chapter 6: Chest pain Chapter 12: Stable angina and acute coronary syndromes Chapter 16: Diseases of the myocardium and pericardium Chapter 18: Vascular disease	59 123 203 227
Cold, painful, pale, pulseless leg/foot	Chapter 18: Vascular disease	234
Cough	Chapter 6: Chest pain Chapter 7: Breathlessness and peripheral oedema Chapter 13: Heart failure	60 67 141
Cyanosis	Chapter 7: Breathlessness and peripheral oedema Chapter 10: Heart murmurs Chapter 17: Congenital heart disease	69 91 214
Dizziness	Chapter 9: Syncope Chapter 14: Arrhythmias	83 165
Driving advice	Chapter 9: Syncope Chapter 14: Arrhythmias	89 156
Erectile dysfunction	Chapter 18: Vascular disease	234

Contents

Section 1

THE BASICS

WHY DO WE NEED A CARDIOVASCULAR SYSTEM?

The cardiovascular system serves to provide rapid transport of nutrients to the body tissues and allows rapid removal of waste products. Smaller, less complex organisms don't need such a system as their needs can be met by simple diffusion. The evolution of the cardiovascular system aided diffusion, allowing the development of larger organisms. The cardiovascular system allows nutrients:

- To diffuse into the system at their source (e.g., oxygen from the alveoli).
- To travel long distances quickly.
- To diffuse into tissues where they are needed (e.g., oxygen to working muscle).

This active process requires a pump, the heart, and relies on a transport medium, the blood. Blood is made up of cells (mainly red and white blood cells) and plasma (water, proteins, electrolytes, etc.).

Functions of the cardiovascular system

The main functions of the cardiovascular system are:

1. Rapid transport of nutrients (oxygen, amino acids, glucose, fatty acids, water, etc.).
2. Removal of waste products of metabolism (carbon dioxide, urea, creatinine, etc.).
3. Hormonal control, by transporting hormones to their target organs and by secreting its own hormones (e.g., atrial natriuretic peptide (ANP)).
4. Temperature regulation, by controlling heat distribution between the body core and the skin.
5. Reproduction, by producing penis erection and providing nutrition to the foetus via a complex system of placental blood flow.
6. Host defence, by transporting immune cells, antigens and other mediators (e.g., antibodies).

ANATOMY OF THE HEART AND GREAT VESSELS

Overview of the heart and circulation

The heart consists of two muscular pumps (left and right ventricles). Each pump has a reservoir (left and right atria). The two pumps each serve a different circulation.

The right ventricle is the pump for the pulmonary circulation. It receives blood from the right atrium, which is then pumped through the pulmonary arteries into the lungs. Here, it is oxygenated and gives up carbon dioxide; blood then returns via the pulmonary veins into the left atrium of the heart and then the left ventricle.

The left ventricle is the pump for the systemic circulation. Blood is pumped from the left ventricle via the aorta to the rest of the body. In the body tissues, nutrients and waste products are exchanged. Blood returns to the right atrium via the superior and inferior vena cavae.

The two circulations operate simultaneously and are arranged in series. Unidirectional flow is ensured by the heart valves, arterial pressure differences and valves in the veins (Fig. 1.1).

CLINICAL NOTES

Failure of an individual pump is possible, e.g., right heart failure as a result of severe lung disease (cor pulmonale).

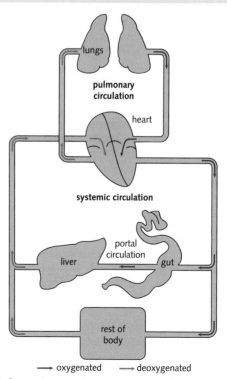

Fig. 1.1 Systemic and pulmonary circulations.

The circulatory system is made up of arteries, veins, capillaries and lymphatic vessels:

1. Arteries transport blood from the heart to the tissues.
2. Capillaries are where the diffusion of nutrients and waste products takes place.
3. Veins return blood from the tissues to the heart. (The mesenteric veins and the hepatic portal vein are exceptions, transporting blood from the bowel to the liver.)
4. Lymphatic vessels return to the blood any excess water and nutrients that have diffused out of capillaries.

HINTS AND TIPS

Arteries carry oxygenated blood and veins carry deoxygenated blood. The two exceptions to this rule are the umbilical and pulmonary vessels where this is reversed.

The volume of blood ejected from one ventricle during 1 minute is called the cardiac output. The cardiac output of each ventricle is equal overall, but there may be occasional beat-by-beat variation. The entire output of the right ventricle passes through the lungs and into the left side of the heart. The output of the left ventricle passes into the aorta and is distributed to various organs and tissues according to their metabolic requirements or particular functions (e.g., the kidney receives 20% of cardiac output so that its excretory function can be maintained). This distribution can be changed to meet changes in demand (e.g., during exercise, the flow to the skeletal muscle is increased considerably).

Blood is driven through vessels by pressure. This pressure, which is produced by the ejection of blood from the ventricles, is highest in the aorta (about 120 mmHg above atmospheric pressure) and lowest in the great veins (almost atmospheric). It is this pressure difference that moves blood through the arteries, capillaries and veins.

The mediastinum

This is the space between the two pleural cavities. It contains all the structures of the chest except the lungs and pleura. The mediastinum extends from the superior thoracic aperture to the diaphragm and from the sternum to the vertebrae and is divided into superior and inferior parts by the plane passing from the sternal angle to the T4/T5 intervertebral disc. The inferior mediastinum is then further subdivided into anterior, middle and posterior parts (Fig. 1.2). The contents of each part are shown in Table 1.1. The structures in the mediastinum are surrounded by loose connective tissue, nerves, blood vessels and lymph vessels. It can accommodate movement and volume changes.

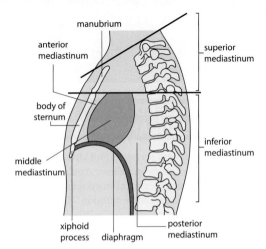

Fig. 1.2 Lateral view of the mediastinum.

Table 1.1 Contents of the mediastinum

Mediastinal compartment	Contents
Superior	Great vessels Thymus Trachea Oesophagus
Anterior	Internal thoracic artery Thymus
Middle	Heart and pericardium Origins of the great vessels
Posterior	Descending aorta Oesophagus Sympathetic chain

The heart is in the middle mediastinum, and it has the following relations:

1. Superiorly, the great vessels and bronchi.
2. Inferiorly, the diaphragm.
3. Laterally, the pleurae and lungs.
4. Anteriorly, the thymus.
5. Posteriorly, the oesophagus.

The structures visible on a normal chest X-ray are shown in Fig. 1.3.

The external structure of the heart

The heart lies obliquely about two-thirds to the left and one-third to the right of the median plane (Figs. 1.4–1.6). It has the following surfaces:

1. The base of the heart is located posteriorly and is formed mainly by the left atrium.

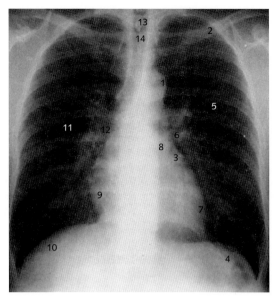

Fig. 1.3 Normal posteroanterior (PA) chest X-ray. *1*, Arch of aorta/aortic knuckle; *2*, clavicle; *3*, left atrial appendage; *4*, left dome of diaphragm; *5*, left lung; *6*, left hilum; *7*, left ventricular border; *8*, pulmonary trunk; *9*, right atrial border; *10*, right dome of diaphragm; *11*, right lung; *12*, right hilum; *13*, spine of vertebrae; *14*, trachea. (Courtesy Professor Dame M. Turner-Warwick, Dr. M. Hodson, Professor B. Corrin and Dr. I. Kerr.)

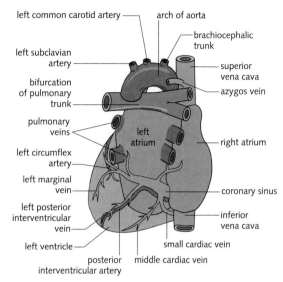

Fig. 1.5 Posteroinferior external view of the heart.

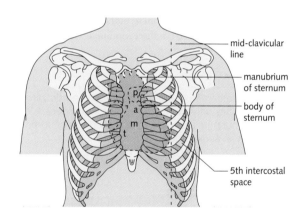

Fig. 1.6 Surface markings of the heart (*a*, aortic valve; *m*, mitral valve; *p*, pulmonary valve; *t*, tricuspid valve). These are anatomical relations – see Fig. 5.5 for auscultatory areas.

2. The apex of the heart is formed by the left ventricle and is posterior to the left fifth intercostal space.
3. The sternocostal surface of the heart is formed mainly by the right ventricle.
4. The diaphragmatic surface is formed mainly by the left ventricle and part of the right ventricle.
5. The pulmonary surface is mainly formed by the left ventricle.

The heart borders of the anterior surface are as follows:

1. Right: right atrium.
2. Left: left ventricle and left auricle.
3. Inferior: right ventricle mainly and part of the left ventricle.
4. Superior: right and left auricles.

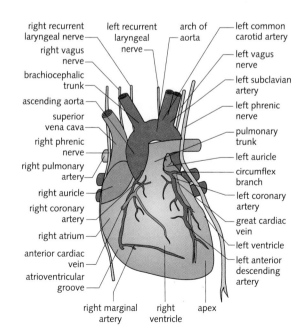

Fig. 1.4 Sternocostal external view of the heart.

5

The internal structure of the heart

The internal structure of the heart is shown in Fig. 1.7. The right atrium contains the orifices of the superior and inferior venae cavae and coronary sinus. The right ventricle is separated from the right atrium by the tricuspid (three cusps) valve. The right ventricle is separated from its outflow tract (the pulmonary trunk) by the pulmonary valve. This has three semilunar valve cusps.

The left atrium has the orifices of four pulmonary veins in its posterior wall and is separated from the left ventricle by the mitral (sometimes referred to as bicuspid, i.e., two cusps) valve. The left ventricle is separated from its outflow tract (the aorta) by the aortic valve, which also has three semilunar valve cusps.

Coronary arteries

The coronary arteries are shown in Figs. 1.8 and 1.9. The left coronary artery arises just distal to the left anterior cusp of the aortic valve. The right coronary artery arises from the right anterior aortic sinus just above the right anterior cusp of the aortic valve. The coronary arteries are the first branches of the aorta; the heart supplies itself with a blood supply before any other organ.

Coronary veins

The coronary veins drain mainly into the coronary sinus, which drains directly into the right atrium (Figs. 1.10 and 1.11). Some small veins drain directly into the heart chambers, generally on the right side.

Great vessels

'Great vessels' is the term used to denote the large arteries and veins that are directly related to the heart. The great arteries include the pulmonary trunk and the aorta (and sometimes its three main branches: the brachiocephalic, left common carotid and left subclavian arteries). The great veins include the pulmonary veins and the superior and inferior venae cavae. The great vessels and their thoracic branches are illustrated in Figs. 1.12–1.14.

Tissue layers of the heart and pericardium

Fig. 1.15 shows the tissue layers of the heart and pericardium.

Pericardium

The pericardium consists of an outer fibrous pericardial sac, enclosing the whole heart, and an inner double layer of flat mesothelial cells, called the serous pericardium. The two layers of serous pericardium are:

- The parietal pericardium – attached to the fibrous sac.
- The visceral pericardium – forms part of the epicardium and covers the heart's outer surface.

The serous pericardium produces approximately 50 mL of pericardial fluid, which sits in the pericardial cavity formed by the parietal and visceral layers. This fluid provides lubrication so the heart can move within the pericardium during the cardiac cycle.

The pericardium is fused with the central tendon of the diaphragm at its base, the sternum by the sternopericardial ligament anteriorly, and the tunica adventitia of the great vessels.

Heart

The heart itself contains three layers:

- Epicardium.
- Myocardium.
- Endocardium.

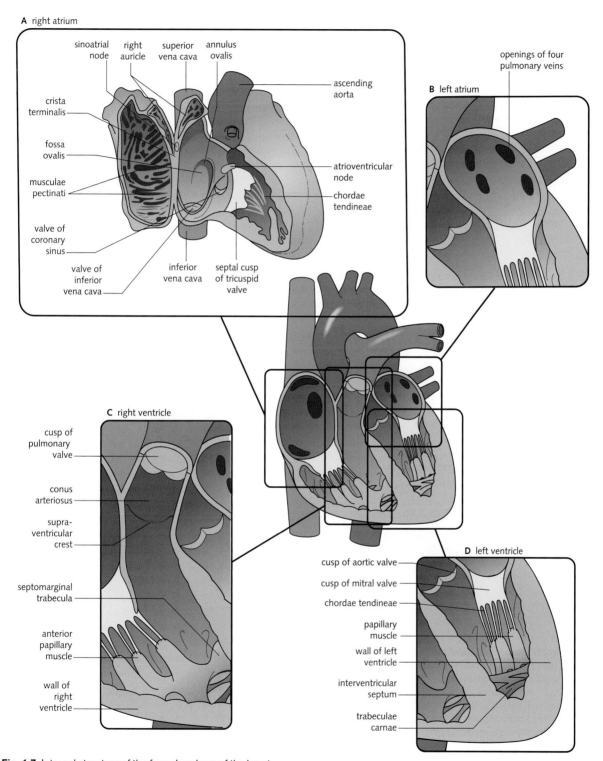

A right atrium

sinoatrial node
right auricle
superior vena cava
annulus ovalis
openings of four pulmonary veins
ascending aorta
B left atrium
crista terminalis
fossa ovalis
atrioventricular node
musculae pectinati
chordae tendineae
valve of coronary sinus
valve of inferior vena cava
inferior vena cava
septal cusp of tricuspid valve

C right ventricle
cusp of pulmonary valve
conus arteriosus
supra-ventricular crest
septomarginal trabecula
anterior papillary muscle
wall of right ventricle

D left ventricle
cusp of aortic valve
cusp of mitral valve
chordae tendineae
papillary muscle
wall of left ventricle
interventricular septum
trabeculae carnae

Fig. 1.7 Internal structure of the four chambers of the heart.

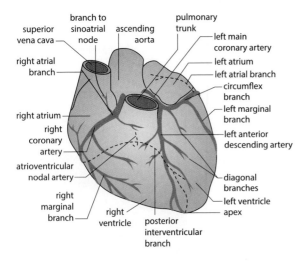

Fig. 1.8 Anterior surface of the heart showing coronary arteries. The left coronary artery has two terminal branches: the left anterior descending artery (also called the anterior interventricular branch, or 'widow's artery') and the left circumflex artery. The left anterior descending artery supplies both ventricles and the interventricular septum. The left circumflex artery supplies the left atrium and the inferior part of the left ventricle. The right coronary artery supplies the sinoatrial node via the right atrial branch in 60% of the population; it is otherwise supplied by the circumflex artery.

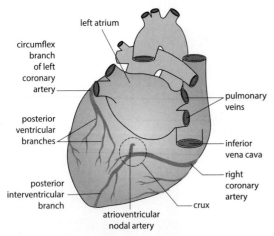

Fig. 1.9 Posteroinferior surface of the heart showing coronary arteries. The right coronary artery usually gives off a right marginal branch and a large posterior interventricular branch. Near the apex, the posterior interventricular branch may anastomose with the left anterior descending artery. The right coronary artery mainly supplies the right atrium, right ventricle and interventricular septum. It may also supply part of the left atrium and left ventricle. The nodal branch supplies the atrioventricular node and arises from the right coronary artery in 90% of the population.

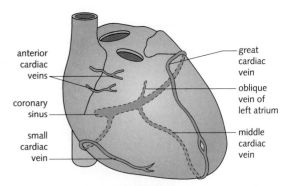

Fig. 1.10 Anterior view of the heart showing coronary veins.

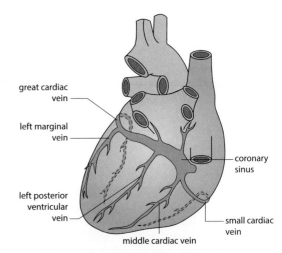

Fig. 1.11 Posteroinferior view of the heart showing coronary veins.

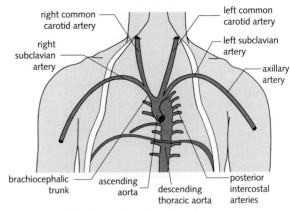

Fig. 1.12 The thoracic aorta and its branches.

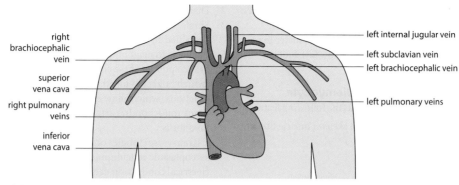

Fig. 1.13 Veins of the thorax.

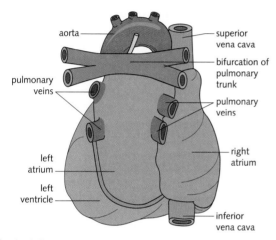

Fig. 1.14 Posterior view of the pulmonary vessels.

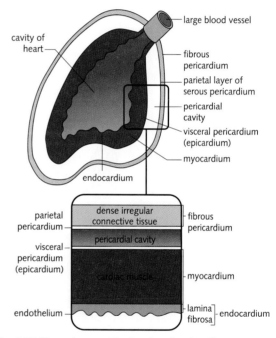

Fig. 1.15 Tissue layers of the heart and pericardium.

Epicardium

The epicardium is a thin layer of connective tissue containing adipose tissue, nerves, coronary arteries and veins.

Myocardium

The myocardium is the thickest layer and is made up of cardiac muscle cells. The myocardium is thickest in the left ventricle and thinnest in the atria. All the muscle layers attach to the fibrocollagenous heart skeleton, which provides a stable base for contraction. The atrial myocardium secretes ANP when stretched, promoting salt and water excretion. The ventricular myocardium secretes brain natriuretic peptide (BNP) when stretched, which seems rather a misnomer. BNP is sometimes used to monitor left ventricular dysfunction in heart failure.

Endocardium

The endocardium has three layers: an outermost connective tissue layer (which contains nerves, veins and Purkinje fibres), a middle layer of connective tissue and a flat endothelial cell layer.

Heart valves

The heart valves are avascular (i.e., they have no blood supply) (Fig. 1.16). This is important if bacteria invade the valves because there is little immune reaction and infective endocarditis may result. Their avascular nature also means that they can be replaced with a porcine (pig) or bovine (cow) tissue valve without immune rejection.

Cardiac myocytes

There are three types of myocytes – contractile myocytes, nodal cells and conduction fibres:

1. Contractile myocytes make up the majority of the myocardium.

2. Nodal cells make up the SA node and AV node, and generate electrical impulses.
3. Conduction (Purkinje) fibres have a greater diameter than contractile myocytes (70–80 μm) and allow fast action potential conduction.

Ultrastructure of the typical cardiomyocyte

The typical cardiac myocyte (Fig. 1.17) has the following features:

1. Length of 50 to 100 μm (shorter than skeletal muscle fibres).

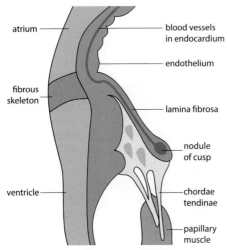

Fig. 1.16 Structure of a heart valve.

2. Diameter of 10 to 20 μm.
3. Single, central nucleus.
4. Branched structure.
5. Attached to neighbouring cells via intercalated disks at branch points. These cell junctions consist of desmosomes (which hold cells together via proteoglycan bridges) and gap junctions (which allow electrical conductivity).
6. Many mitochondria arranged in rows between intracellular myofibrils.
7. T (transverse) tubules organized in diads with cisternae of sarcoplasmic reticulum (Fig. 1.18), which enable rapid electrical conduction deep into the cell, activating the whole contractile apparatus.
8. Extensive sarcoplasmic reticulum, which stores Ca^{2+} ions necessary for electrical activity and contraction.

Each myocyte contains many myofibril-like units (similar to the myofibrils of skeletal muscle) (see Fig. 1.18). These consist of sarcomeres attached end-to-end and collected into a bundle. A sarcomere is the basic contractile unit. It is composed of two bands, the A band and the I band, between two Z lines.

1. The A (anisotropic) band is made of thick myosin filaments and interdigitating actin filaments.
2. The I (isotropic) band is made of thin actin filaments that do not overlap with myosin filaments. Troponin and tropomyosin are also in the thin filaments.
3. The Z line is a dark-staining structure containing α-actinin protein that provides attachment for the thin filaments.

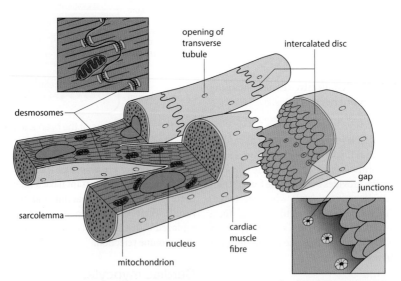

Fig. 1.17 Cardiac myocyte arrangement. Myocytes are branched and attach to each other through desmosomes to form muscle fibres. Gap junctions enable rapid electrical conductivity between cells. There is an extensive sarcoplasmic reticulum, which is the internal Ca^{2+} store. The contractile elements within each cell produce characteristic bands and lines. In between each myofibril unit, there are rows of mitochondria. Accompanying blood vessels and connective tissue lie alongside each muscle fibre. (Redrawn with permission from Tortora, G.J., Grabowski, S.R., 2000. *Principles of anatomy and physiology*, ninth ed. John Wiley & Sons, New York.)

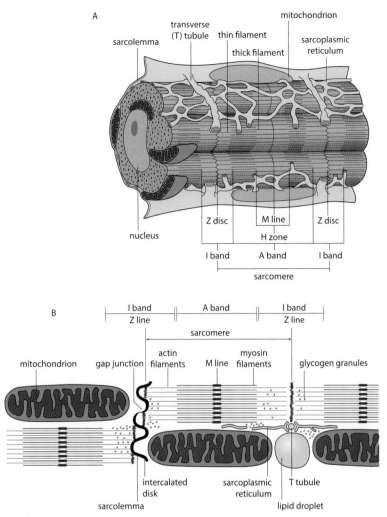

Fig. 1.18 Electron micrographic appearance of cardiac muscle. (A) Each myocyte has rows of mitochondria in between myofibril-like units. There is also an extensive sarcoplasmic reticulum and T tubule system. (B) Close-up of a myofibril-like unit shows the following bands: A band, myosin with some actin; I band, actin; Z line, attachment point for actin; M line, links myosin fibres. (Reproduced with permission from (A) Williams, P.L. (Ed.), 1989. *Gray's anatomy*, thirty-seventh ed. Churchill Livingstone, Edinburgh; (B) Davies, A., Blakeley, A.G.H., Kidd, C., 2001. *Human physiology*. Churchill Livingstone, Edinburgh.)

DEVELOPMENT OF THE HEART AND GREAT VESSELS

The heart develops in the cardiogenic region of the mesoderm from week 3. This region is at the cranial end of the embryonic disc. Angioblastic cords (aggregates of endothelial cell precursors) develop and coalesce to form two lateral endocardial tubes. During week 4, these tubes fuse to form the primitive heart tube and the heart begins to pump (Fig. 1.19).

From weeks 5 to 8, the primitive heart tube folds and remodels to form four chambers. Initially, the primitive heart tube develops a series of expansions separated by shallow sulci (infoldings) (Fig. 1.20).

The primitive atrium will give rise to parts of both future atria. The primitive ventricle will make up most of the left ventricle. The bulbus cordis will form the right ventricle. The truncus arteriosus will form the ascending aorta and pulmonary trunk.

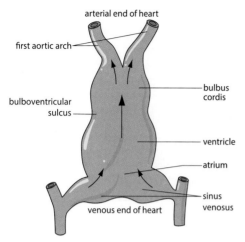

Fig. 1.19 Primitive heart tube at 21 days.

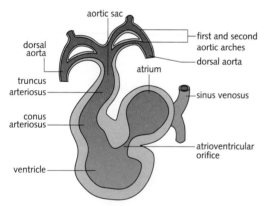

Fig. 1.20 Primitive heart tube as it folds and expands.

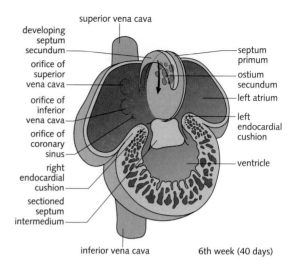

Fig. 1.21 Initial septation of the atria. The septum primum forms at day 33, and eventually leaves a hole (the ostium secundum). The septum secundum develops later, at day 40, and is deficient at the foramen ovale. (Redrawn with permission from Larsen, W.J., 1997. *Human embryology*, second ed. Churchill Livingstone, Edinburgh.)

Venous blood initially enters the sinus horns of the sinus venosus from the cardinal veins (a branch of the umbilical vein). Within the next few weeks, the whole systemic venous return is shifted to the right sinus horn through the newly formed superior and inferior venae cavae. The left sinus horn becomes the coronary sinus, which drains the myocardium.

In weeks 5 to 6, the septum primum and the septum secundum grow to separate the right and left atria (Fig. 1.21). These septa are incomplete and leave two openings (foramina or ostia) that allow blood to move between the atria. The septum primum grows downwards from the superior posterior wall. The foramen (ostium primum) it creates narrows as the septum grows.

While the septum primum is growing, the thicker septum secundum also starts to form. This septum secundum does not meet the septum intermedium, leaving an opening called the foramen ovale near the floor of the right atrium.

Blood now has to shunt from the right to the left atrium through the two staggered openings in the septum, the foramen ovale and the ostium secundum (Fig. 1.22). At birth, the two septa usually fuse to abolish any foramen between the atria.

During weeks 5 to 6, the atrioventricular (tricuspid and mitral) valves develop. The heart undergoes some changes that bring the atria and ventricles into their correct positions and align outflow tracts with the ventricles.

The inferior part of the bulboventricular sulcus grows into the muscular ventricular septum. Growth stops in week 7 to wait for the left outflow tract to develop, leaving an interventricular foramen.

In weeks 7 to 8, the truncus arteriosus (the common outflow tract of the heart) is divided in two by a spiral process of central septation, which results in the formation of the aorta and pulmonary trunk. This septum is called the truncoconal septum. This septum also grows into the ventricles, and it forms the membranous ventricular septum, which joins the muscular ventricular septum. This completes the septation of the ventricles. Swellings develop at the inferior end of the truncus

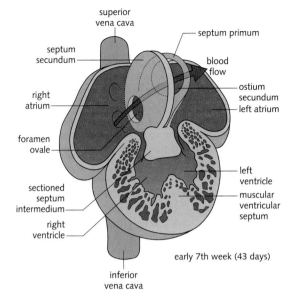

Fig. 1.22 Completed septation of the atria. The septum primum is deficient superiorly at the ostium secundum. The septum secundum is deficient inferiorly at the foramen ovale. Blood shunts from the right atrium through these two holes in the septa to the left atrium. In this way, blood bypasses the lungs in the foetal circulation. As these two openings are staggered, fusion of the septum primum and secundum will abolish any shunt between the atria. (Redrawn with permission from Larsen, W.J., 1997. *Human embryology*, second ed. Churchill Livingstone, Edinburgh.)

arteriosus, and these give rise to the arterial (pulmonary and aortic) valves.

Development of the vasculature

The vasculature develops from the angioblastic cords of the mesoderm. The aortic ends of the primitive heart tube become the aortic arches and dorsal aortae. The aortic arches develop into the great arteries of the neck and thorax, and the dorsal aortae develop branches, which supply the rest of the body. The paired dorsal aortae connect to the umbilical arteries, which carry blood to the placenta.

The umbilical veins carry oxygenated and nutrient-rich blood from the placenta to the foetus. The venous system (from the foetus, yolk sac and umbilical veins) drains into the sinus horns and subsequently into the venae cavae and right atrium.

The ductus venosus shunts a portion of blood from the umbilical vein directly into the inferior vena cava during gestation. This is vital, as it allows oxygenated blood to enter the right atrium and be pumped around the foetus.

The lungs are not functional during gestation, negating the need for a large pulmonary circulation. Pulmonary circulation is largely bypassed by two mechanisms:

- The foramen ovale enables most oxygenated blood in the right atrium to pass into the left atrium and systemic circulation.
- The ductus arteriosus develops from the sixth aortic arch and connects the pulmonary arteries to the aortic arch. This allows oxygenated blood not shunted through the foramen ovale to enter the systemic circulation. The duct is kept open during foetal life by prostaglandins, and this stimulation may be continued artificially early in the neonatal period.

Circulatory adaptations at birth

A series of changes convert the single system of blood flow around the foetus into dual systems at birth (Figs. 1.23 and 1.24). Blood flow in the umbilical vessels drastically declines in the first few minutes after birth because of:

- Compression of the cord.
- Vasoconstriction in response to cold, mechanical stimuli and circulating foetal catecholamines as a result of the stress of descending through the birth canal.

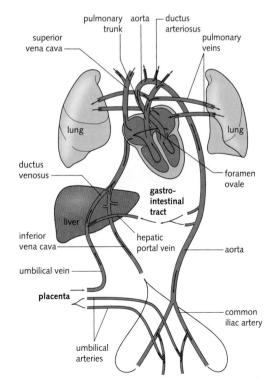

Fig. 1.23 Foetal circulation in utero.

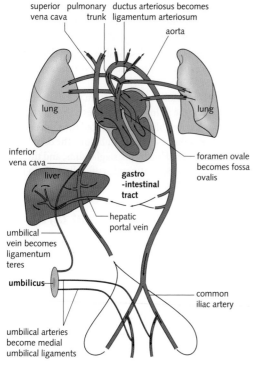

superior vena cava
pulmonary trunk
ductus arteriosus becomes ligamentum arteriosum
aorta
lung
lung
inferior vena cava
liver
gastro-intestinal tract
foramen ovale becomes fossa ovalis
hepatic portal vein
umbilical vein becomes ligamentum teres
umbilicus
common iliac artery
umbilical arteries become medial umbilical ligaments

Fig. 1.24 Neonatal circulation after birth. Note the closure of the foetal shunts (foramen ovale, ductus arteriosus and ductus venosus) and umbilical vessels.

At birth, pulmonary vascular resistance falls rapidly because:
- The thorax of the foetus is compressed, emptying amniotic fluid from the lungs.
- The mechanical effort of ventilation opens constricted alveolar vessels.

- Raising PO_2 and lowering PCO_2 causes vasodilatation of pulmonary vessels.

This produces increased pulmonary blood flow.

Sudden cessation of umbilical blood flow and opening of the pulmonary system cause a change in pressure balance of the atria, with a pressure drop in the right atrium and a pressure rise in the left atrium (caused by increased pulmonary venous return to the left atrium). This changes the pressure gradient across the atrial septum and forces the flexible septum primum against the rigid septum secundum, closing the foramen ovale. These septa fuse after about 3 months.

The ductus arteriosus closes 1 to 8 days after birth. It is thought that as pulmonary vascular resistance falls, the pressure drop in the pulmonary trunk causes blood to flow from the aorta into the pulmonary trunk through the ductus arteriosus. This blood is oxygenated and the increase in PO_2 causes the smooth muscle in the wall of the ductus to constrict due to decreased prostaglandin production, obstructing the flow in the ductus arteriosus. Eventually, the intima of the ductus arteriosus thickens – complete obliteration of the ductus results in the formation of the ligamentum arteriosum, which attaches the pulmonary trunk to the aorta.

The ductus venosus closes soon after birth and becomes a remnant known as the ligamentum venosum. The mechanism is unclear but is thought to involve prostaglandin inhibition.

Chapter Summary

- The cardiovascular system is vital to the survival of all other body tissues.
- The right ventricle pumps blood to the pulmonary circulation, and the left ventricle pumps blood to the rest of the body.
- Knowledge of coronary arterial anatomy is important when considering which region of the myocardium is affected in ischaemic heart disease and allows prediction of clinical sequelae.
- Appreciation of the development of foetal circulation and its changes after birth is essential to understanding congenital heart abnormalities and their effects.

CARDIAC ELECTROPHYSIOLOGY

Unlike skeletal muscle, the heart possesses intrinsic electrical activity and does not require nervous input to contract. This activity originates at the sinoatrial (SA) node, a cluster of specialized myocytes that depolarize spontaneously, sometimes referred to as the heart's pacemaker. Cardiomyocytes can be broadly divided into two categories in terms of electrophysiological behaviour, function and appearance of their action potentials:

- Fast depolarizing cells – atrial and ventricular myocardial cells, and cells of the His–Purkinje system.
- Slow depolarizing cells, such as those forming the SA node and atrioventricular (AV) node ('pacemaker/nodal cells').

The conduction system

For the heart to function effectively, the action potential generated by the SA node must propagate through the heart in a coordinated manner. This is facilitated by a specialized conduction system (Fig. 2.1) and the presence of low resistance gap junctions, which allow the direct spread of depolarization between cells. The SA node is located in the posterior wall of the right atrium at the junction with the superior vena cava. From the SA node, the impulse passes through the atrial myocardium to the AV node, where conduction is delayed by approximately 100 ms

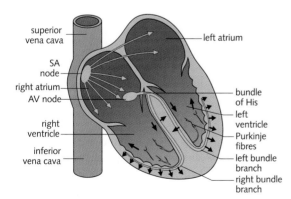

Fig. 2.1 Cardiac conduction pathway. The action potential is initiated in the sinoatrial (SA) node and spreads through the atria. It travels through the atrioventricular (AV) node and then to the bundle of His. From here, it travels down left and right bundle branches and into Purkinje fibres; then it spreads through the ventricles.

to allow completion of atrial contraction before ventricular depolarization.

The AV node, located at the top of the interventricular septum, is the only point where current can pass through the fibrous skeleton from the atria to the ventricles (in a healthy heart). The AV node is also able to act as a backup pacemaker in situations when the SA node ceases to function or communication between the SA and AV nodes is interrupted. The impulse then enters the bundle of His, which splits into right and left bundle branches. The left bundle branch is subdivided into anterior and posterior hemifascicles. These bundles give off fine fibres composed of specialized cardiomyocytes (called Purkinje fibres) that enter the ventricular myocardium.

HINTS AND TIPS

Remember that the cells comprising the conduction systems are specialized muscle cells, NOT nerves.

Resting membrane potential

The electrical potential across a plasma membrane is determined by two main factors:

- Distribution of ions across the membrane.
- Selective permeability of the cell membrane.

In cardiomyocytes, potassium (K^+) ions are the major determinant of resting membrane potential because large numbers of K^+ channels are open constitutively. These 'leak' K^+ channels mean permeability to K^+ is high and there is a constant efflux of K^+, referred to as the 'outward background current'. The resting membrane is only slightly permeable to sodium (Na^+), and because both the electrical and chemical gradients favour the inward movement of Na^+ ions, there is a very small inward Na^+ current, often referred to as the 'inward background current'. Intracellular and extracellular concentrations of these ions (Fig. 2.2) are maintained by the activity of the Na^+/K^+ ATPase on the cardiomyocyte cell membrane.

Cardiac action potential

An action potential is a transient depolarization of the cell membrane. Action potentials are initiated when the membrane is depolarized (i.e., becomes less negative) to a threshold potential. This can occur spontaneously (in nodal cells) but is usually

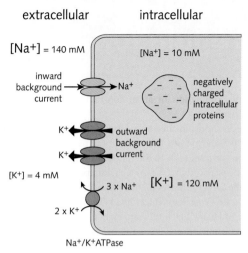

Fig. 2.2 Ion distribution and movement across the resting plasma membrane. Intracellular and extracellular concentrations of sodium [Na^+] and potassium [K^+] are shown. These concentrations are maintained by the action of the Na^+/K^+ ATPase.

stimulated by transmission from adjacent myocytes through gap junctions.

Fast cell action potential

Action potentials in fast depolarizing cells (Fig. 2.3) occur in five phases and are initiated by an action potential in an adjacent cell:

- Phase 0: rapid depolarization (upstroke). When the membrane is depolarized to its threshold potential, fast voltage-gated Na^+ channels open, allowing the rapid influx of Na^+ down its electrochemical gradient, causing further depolarization.
- Phase 1: initial repolarization. As the membrane potential approaches neutral, voltage-gated Na^+ channels become inactivated, terminating the rapid inward Na^+ current. The persistent outward background K^+ current causes slight repolarization. Phase 1 is most prominent in Purkinje fibres.
- Phase 2: plateau. This phase is mediated by the opening of L-type calcium (Ca^{2+}) channels. These are voltage-gated channels that are activated slowly. Slow inward Ca^{2+} current is balanced by K^+ efflux and thus membrane potential remains relatively steady. Towards the end of phase 2, Ca^{2+} channels close, and the steady potential is maintained by an inward current brought about by the action of the Na^+/Ca^{2+} exchanger. The plateau phase prolongs the cardiac action potential to 150 to 300 ms and is a key difference between the cardiac and neuronal action potentials. This prolongation is critical in allowing contraction to occur.
- Phase 3: repolarization. Additional K^+ channels open, increasing K^+ efflux. This brings about membrane

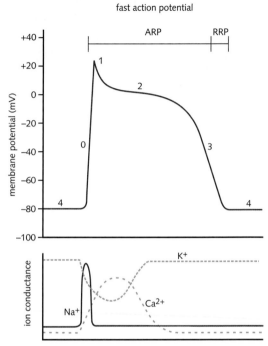

Fig. 2.3 Fast cell action potential. Phases of the action potential (0–4) and changes in membrane ion conductance are shown (*ARP*, absolute refractory period; *RRP*, relative refractory period).

repolarization to its resting potential. A delay or defect in the opening of K^+ channels caused by a genetic defect delays repolarization and manifests as a long QT syndrome.
- Phase 4: resting potential. When repolarization is complete, the membrane potential is restored to its resting value and the cycle repeats.

Slow cell action potential

Nodal cells do not have a stable resting membrane potential. There is a relatively lower density of constitutively open leak K^+ channels on these cells compared to fast depolarizing cells/work myocytes. This membrane potential decays (depolarizes) slowly until it reaches a threshold potential and an action potential is triggered spontaneously (Fig. 2.4). This decaying potential is a result of a gradual reduction in the K^+ permeability, reducing K^+ efflux, along with a gradual increase in Na^+ and Ca^{2+} influx through slow channels. This unstable pacemaker potential (phase 4) means that an action potential may occur spontaneously if the cell is not stimulated by adjacent cell depolarization.

Nodal cells do not express functional fast voltage-gated Na^+ channels and the upstroke of the action potential (phase 0) is produced by a slow inward Ca^{2+} current through L-type Ca^{2+} channels. As a result, the upstroke of the action potential is much

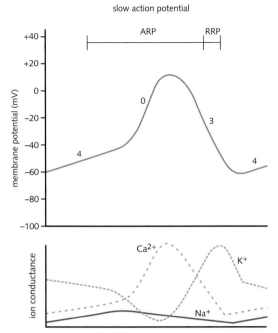

Fig. 2.4 Slow cell action potential. The phases of the action potential (0–4) and changes in membrane ion conductance are shown (*ARP*, absolute refractory period; *RRP*, relative refractory period).

slower than that of fast cells. After the upstroke, K$^+$ channels open and the outward K$^+$ current brings about repolarization (phase 3). There is no plateau phase in the nodal cell action potential.

The 'funny current'

The funny current (I$_f$ for short) is an electric current highly prevalent in spontaneously depolarizing areas of the heart (such as the nodal cells). It is so-named due to unusual features when compared to other ion channels in the heart (including mixed permeability to sodium and potassium ions, unusual kinetics and activation). The I$_f$ current is activated when the membrane potential is hyperpolarized (during diastole), supplying inward current and depolarization of the action potential. As a result, this current is important for bringing about the spontaneous activity of these nodal cells and, therefore, also the underlying heart rate. Ivabradine (an antianginal therapy) acts to inhibit this current, thereby preventing the I$_f$ current's contribution to depolarization of the nodal cells' action potentials and slowing the heart rate as a result.

Refractory period

During an action potential, cardiac cells are refractory to excitation, i.e., another action potential cannot be generated. There are two different refractory periods (Figs. 2.3 and 2.4):

- Absolute refractory period, during which another action potential cannot be elicited, no matter how great the stimulus.
- Relative refractory period, during which an action potential can be initiated by a strong stimulus.

The *absolute refractory period* begins at the onset of phase 0 and lasts until midway through phase 3. This refractory period prevents a new action potential from being initiated during the previous one, allowing adequate time for ventricular filling before the next contraction. The absolute refractory period in ventricular myocytes is approximately 250 ms in a healthy heart, thus the maximum rate the heart can beat in a coordinated manner is 240 beats per minute (bpm).

During phase 3, some fast voltage-gated Na$^+$ channels are reset and primed to be activated again; however, only a small number are primed so a large stimulus is required. This is the *relative refractory period*, which in fast depolarizing cells lasts until resting membrane potential is reached and can persist into phase 4 in nodal cells.

Control of heart rate

In nodal cells, the rate at which spontaneous depolarization occurs depends on the slope of the pacemaker potential. Both the SA and AV nodes are innervated by sympathetic and parasympathetic fibres, which exert opposing chronotropic stimuli (effects on heart rate) by altering the slope of the pacemaker potential. In a denervated heart, the SA node spontaneously depolarizes at a rate of approximately 100 bpm and the AV node at between 30 and 50 bpm. Under normal circumstances, the SA node is the dominant pacemaker and determines heart rate. If the SA node ceases to function or conduction from the SA node to the AV node is interrupted, the AV node becomes the dominant pacemaker.

Sympathetic fibres release norepinephrine, which acts on β_1 receptors, increasing the permeability of the nodal cell plasma membrane to Na$^+$ and Ca^{2+}, thereby increasing the slope of the pacemaker potential. This causes an increased firing rate of the SA node (increasing heart rate) and decreases the conduction delay at the AV node.

Parasympathetic fibres release acetylcholine, which acts on muscarinic M2 receptors, increasing the permeability to K$^+$ and decreasing the Na$^+$ and Ca^{2+} permeability. This decreases the slope of the pacemaker potential, decreasing heart rate. In addition, increased parasympathetic activity causes a slight hyperpolarization at the end of each action potential, further slowing heart rate.

Under resting conditions, the parasympathetic nervous system (PNS) exerts a constant influence on the SA node via the vagus nerve, resulting in a resting heart rate of approximately 70 bpm. If this parasympathetic influence is blocked (with atropine, for example), then the resting heart rate will increase. The effects of autonomic innervation on the action potential in the SA and AV nodes are shown in Fig. 2.5.

A

sympathetic → NA → β_1 receptor → ↑pNa⁺ + ↑pCa²⁺

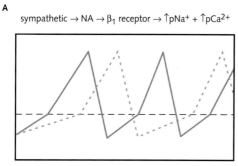

B

parasympathetic → Ach → M2 receptor → ↑pK⁺

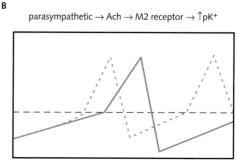

Fig. 2.5 Autonomic influences on the nodal action potential. (A) Sympathetic stimulation increases the slope of the pacemaker potential by acting on β_1 adrenoceptors and increasing Na⁺ and Ca²⁺ permeability. (B) Parasympathetic stimulation decreases the slope of the pacemaker potential and hyperpolarizes the plasma membrane by acting on M2 receptors and increasing K⁺ permeability. *Dotted lines* represent baseline trace; *solid lines* represent potential after given alteration in autonomic activity (*ACh*, acetylcholine; *NE*, norepinephrine).

HINTS AND TIPS

Pacemaker rate is also affected by temperature. This is why fever increases heart rate. It is estimated that heart rate increases by 10 bpm for every 1°C increase in temperature.

Excitation contraction coupling

Excitation contraction coupling (Fig. 2.6) is the process that couples an action potential with contraction in cardiac muscle, a process underpinned by an increase in cytosolic calcium concentration ([Ca²⁺]). During the plateau phase of the cardiac action potential (phase 2), calcium enters the cytosol through L-type Ca²⁺ channels. This stimulates further Ca²⁺ release from the sarcoplasmic reticulum (SR), a process termed 'Ca²⁺ induced Ca²⁺ release'. Once in the cytosol, Ca²⁺ ions bind troponin C, altering the position of tropomyosin and exposing the myosin heads to bind actin filaments, allowing contraction to occur. Greater increases in cytosolic [Ca²⁺] increase contraction strength. Therefore, the amount of Ca²⁺ entry determines myocyte contractility. Contractility is defined as the force generated by cardiac muscle for a given fibre length.

Following myocyte contraction, rapid reduction of cytosolic [Ca²⁺] is crucial to allow relaxation and ventricular filling during diastole (Fig. 2.7). The Ca²⁺ ATPase on the SR is activated by

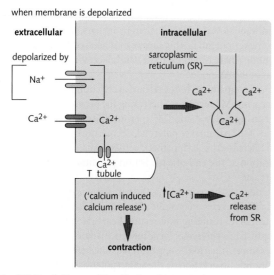

Fig. 2.6 Excitation and its effect on the myocyte.

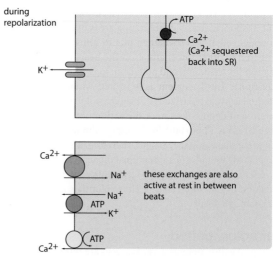

Fig. 2.7 Ion exchanges that take place during relaxation (*ATP*, adenosine triphosphate; *SR*, sarcoplasmic reticulum).

increased cytosolic [Ca^{2+}] and pumps approximately 80% to 90% of the Ca^{2+} back into the SR. The remainder is removed from the cell by the Na^+/Ca^{2+} exchanger on the plasma membrane, which utilizes the Na^+ gradient created by the activity of the Na^+/K^+ ATPase to remove Ca^{2+} from the cell.

THE CARDIAC CYCLE

The cardiac cycle is the sequence of pressure and volume changes that take place during cardiac activity (Fig. 2.8 and Table 2.1). At a resting heart rate of approximately 70 beats per minute (bpm), the cardiac cycle lasts 0.85 s. This is divided into diastole and systole, which last 0.6 s and 0.25 s, respectively. When considering the cardiac cycle, it is useful to remember:

- Blood flows down a pressure gradient.
- The position of a valve is dependent on the pressure gradient across it.

The ventricular cycle

The ventricular cycle consists of four phases. The duration and order of each of these are shown in Table 2.1.

1. Ventricular filling (diastole). The atria and ventricles are initially relaxed, with passive filling occurring due to central venous pressure (CVP) and pulmonary venous pressure. Filling distends the ventricle, raising pressure. Passive ventricular filling stops when ventricular pressure reaches central/pulmonary venous pressure. Atrial contraction further increases ventricular filling (the 'atrial kick'). This accounts for about 15% to 20% of ventricular filling at rest but is more important during exercise as the time for passive ventricular filling is reduced. The volume of blood in the ventricle at the end of diastole is termed end-diastolic volume (EDV).

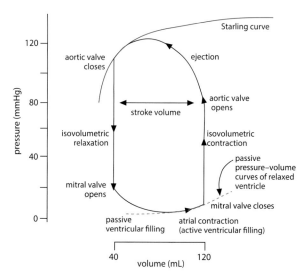

Fig. 2.8 Pressure–volume cycle of the left ventricle. The most significant pressure changes occur within the ventricles during the isovolumetric stages.

CLINICAL NOTES

The 'atrial kick' is absent in people with atrial fibrillation due to ineffective atrial contraction. This has little effect on cardiac output at rest.

2. Isovolumetric contraction (systole). Ventricular contraction increases ventricular pressure. As ventricular pressure rises above atrial pressure, the atrioventricular valves close early in systole. This creates a closed chamber as all valves are closed. Ventricular contraction continues, causing a rapid rise in ventricular pressure. No blood is ejected from the

Table 2.1 Summary table of the stages of the cardiac cycle

	Diastole	Systole		Diastole
Stage	Ventricular filling	Isovolumetric contraction	Ejection	Isovolumetric relaxation
Duration (s)	0.5	0.05	0.3	0.08
Atrioventricular (AV) valves	Open	Closed	Closed	Closed
Arterial valves	Closed	Closed	Open	Closed
Ventricular pressure	Falls then slowly rises	Rapid rise	Rises then slowly falls	Rapid fall
Ventricular volume	Increases	Constant	Decreases	Constant

Note: changes at fixed volume are referred to as isovolumetric and precede the later contraction or dilation of the ventricles.

ventricles because aortic/pulmonary pressure is greater than that in the ventricles, keeping the aortic and pulmonary valves closed.

3. Ejection (systole). As contraction continues, ventricular pressure rises, opening the aortic and pulmonary valves. This causes ejection of blood from the ventricles and a rapid rise in arterial pressure. The momentum of blood prevents immediate valve closure, even when ventricular pressure falls below arterial pressure. Eventually the arterial valves close, creating a brief fluctuation in arterial pressure called the dicrotic notch. The ventricle does not empty completely, with an end-systolic volume (ESV) of about 40% to 50%, which can be used to increase stroke volume (SV) when necessary. The ejection fraction (proportion of blood ejected during systole) is usually 50% to 60%.

4. Isovolumetric relaxation (diastole). Both sets of valves are closed as the ventricles relax. When ventricular pressure falls below atrial pressure, the atrioventricular valves open and the cycle repeats.

HINTS AND TIPS

Venous return = Right heart input/output = Pulmonary blood flow = Left heart input/output = Systemic blood flow. All of these are in series. This idea that 'what goes in must come out' is called the Fick principle.

The atrial cycle

The cardiac cycle pressure changes in the atria are different from those in the ventricles. The right atrium directly communicates with the internal jugular veins (IJVs) and the absence of valves between the two means that changes in right atrial pressure are reflected by changes in the jugular venous pressure (JVP). The JVP waveform is assessed when examining the cardiovascular system and is shown in Fig. 2.9. The JVP waveform has five components:

- The A wave – atrial contraction.
- The C wave – closure of the tricuspid valve.
- X descent – atrial relaxation.
- V wave – atrial filling during systole.
- Y descent – passive ventricular filling during diastole.

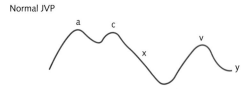

Fig. 2.9 The normal jugular venous pressure (JVP) waveform (a, a wave; c, c wave; v, v wave; x, x descent; y, y descent).

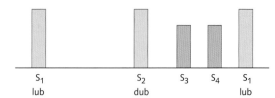

Fig. 2.10 Normal heart sounds (S_1, first heart sound; S_2, second heart sound) and the added third and fourth heart sounds (S_3, third heart sound; S_4, fourth heart sound).

Heart sounds

Normal heart sounds (see Fig. 2.10):

- First (S_1): produced by closure of the mitral and tricuspid valves.
- Second (S_2): produced by closure of the aortic and pulmonary valves.

Added heart sounds (see Fig. 2.10):

- Third (S_3): may be heard in early diastole and is due to rapid ventricular filling. A third heart sound is common in young people and athletes but also may be seen with heart failure.
- Fourth (S_4): occurs just before the first heart sound and is due to forceful atrial contraction against a stiff ventricle. This is always abnormal and can occur in ventricular hypertrophy.

HINTS AND TIPS

To get an idea of the timing of the S_3 and S_4, consider the cadence of the words Kentucky (mirrors S_3) and Tennessee (mirrors S_4).

During inspiration, physiological splitting of the second heart sound can occur (Fig. 2.11). Inspiration decreases intrathoracic pressure, increasing venous return (VR) and right ventricular preload. Simultaneously, the lungs expand, decreasing return to the left atrium and left ventricular preload. As a result, right ventricular systole lasts longer than left ventricular systole and the pulmonary valve closes after the aortic valve, causing a 'split' S_2.

Fig. 2.12 brings together the atrial/ventricular cycles and heart sounds, showing their relations to each other.

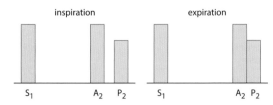

Fig. 2.11 Splitting of the second heart sound. S_2 may show physiological splitting into A_2 and P_2, which is usually more pronounced on inspiration (A_2, aortic component; P_2, pulmonary component).

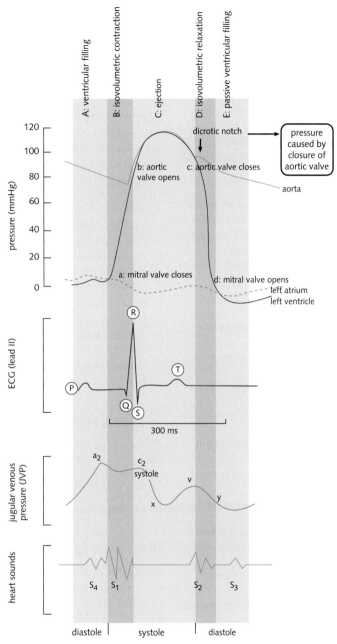

Fig. 2.12 Displayed at the top of the diagram are the pressures in the left atrium, left ventricle and aorta during the cardiac cycle. (A) Pressure in the left ventricle increases slightly as blood enters during left atrial contraction. (B) The most rapid increase in pressure occurs during isovolumetric contraction. The increase in pressure caused by ventricular contraction closes the mitral valve (a). (C) When left ventricular pressure just exceeds aortic pressure, the aortic valve opens (b), leading to ejection. Pressure rises to a peak and then falls, leading to aortic valve closure (c). (D) Isovolumetric relaxation then occurs and eventually left ventricular pressure is just below left atrial pressure, leading to opening of the mitral valve (d). (E) This allows passive ventricular filling. Below this, the normal electrocardiogram is displayed as it relates to the cardiac cycle. The jugular venous pressure (JVP) (shown below) reflects right atrial pressure due to the proximity of the central veins to the right atrium. Finally, the heart sounds are displayed (S_1, closure of the mitral and tricuspid valves 'lub'; S_2, closure of the aortic and pulmonary valves 'dub').

Murmurs

Murmurs (see Chapter 10) result from turbulent blood flow. They are most often due to valvular disease, although a benign 'flow' murmur may be present in young people or in high cardiac output (CO) states, e.g., pregnancy, anaemia. Murmurs may also be present in certain congenital heart defects.

CONTROL OF CARDIAC OUTPUT

Definitions and concepts

Cardiac output (CO) is the amount of blood ejected from the heart per minute. CO = heart rate (HR) × stroke volume (SV). In a normal adult, it ranges from 4 to 7 L/min at rest but is increased during exercise (up to 20 L/min) and decreased during sleep. Before considering how CO is regulated, it is important to understand several definitions:

- Stroke volume (SV): the volume of blood ejected in one ventricular contraction.
- End-diastolic volume (EDV): the volume of blood in the ventricle just before contraction.
- End-diastolic pressure (EDP): the pressure of blood in the ventricle just before contraction.
- End-systolic volume (ESV): the volume of blood left in the ventricle after contraction.
- Central venous pressure (CVP): the pressure of blood in the great veins as they enter the right atrium.
- Venous return (VR): the volume of blood returning to the right heart in 1 minute. In a healthy heart, VR = CO.
- Mean arterial pressure (MAP): the average blood pressure during a single cardiac cycle.
- Total peripheral resistance (TPR): the resistance to the flow of blood in the whole system (MAP/CO).
- Systemic vascular resistance (SVR): the resistance to blood flow offered by the systemic (not pulmonary) vasculature (MAP – CVP)/CO.
- Ejection fraction: the proportion of EDV that is ejected during systole.
  SV and therefore CO, are influenced by preload, afterload and contractility.

Preload

Preload is the degree of ventricular myocyte stretch at the end of diastole and is determined by EDV. The greater the EDV, the greater the preload. EDV is influenced by:

- Venous return.
- Heart rate.
- Atrial contraction (reduced if ineffectual, as in atrial fibrillation).

Afterload

Afterload is defined as the force or stress on myocytes during systole. It is determined by resistance to ventricular outflow. Aortic pressure and pulmonary artery pressure are the main determinates for the left ventricle and right ventricle, respectively.

Contractility

Contractility is the force of contraction for a given fibre length and is determined by the degree of calcium influx during the plateau phase (phase 2) of the cardiac action potential. Factors that influence contractility are termed inotropic factors and can have a positive or negative effect.

Positive inotropes include:

- Catecholamine (e.g., norepinephrine).
- β-Agonists (e.g., dobutamine).
- Phosphodiesterase inhibitors (e.g., milrinone).
- Ca^{2+} sensitizers (e.g., levosimendan).
- Cardiac glycosides (e.g., digoxin).

Negative inotropes include:

- β-Blockers (e.g., propranolol): inhibit catecholamine action on $β_1$ receptors.
- Ca^{2+} channel blockers (e.g., verapamil): block the L-type Ca^{2+} channels on ventricular myocytes, reducing Ca^{2+} influx.
- Hypoxia.

COMMON PITFALLS

Although sympathetic stimulation causes an increase in contractility, parasympathetic stimulation does NOT decrease contractility because parasympathetic innervation to the ventricular myocardium is sparse.

Starling's law of the heart

Starling's law of the heart (also called the Frank-Starling law) states that the energy released during contraction depends upon the initial fibre length, within physiological limits (Fig. 2.13). The greater the heart is stretched by filling (preload), then the greater the energy released by contraction. This is due to the stretch-dependent sensitivity of myocardial contractile proteins to calcium ions, which influences the numbers of actin-myosin cross-bridges formed. It is important to distinguish this from contractility.

Although initial stretch of the ventricular myocardium is produced by the EDV, EDP is easier to measure, and the relationship between the two is almost linear (if normal myocardial compliance). In the right ventricle, EDP is closely related to the CVP. EDP plotted against SV produces the Starling curve (Fig. 2.14). Excessively high filling pressures cause excessive myocyte stretch

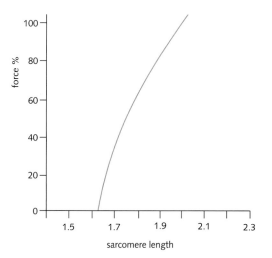

Fig. 2.13 Sarcomere length compared with tension. Increasing the initial sarcomere length increases tension up to the maximum stretch possible for an individual myocyte.

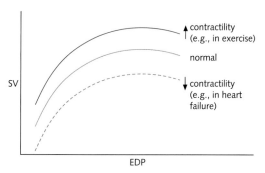

Fig. 2.14 Stroke volume (SV) compared with end-diastolic pressure (EDP). This produces the Starling curve, which shows that an increase in EDP (and therefore end-diastolic volume (EDV), as they have an almost linear relationship) causes an increased SV. There is, however, a limit at which the curve turns downwards and the relationship is no longer valid. The mechanism for this downturn is complex, and it mainly reflects excessive stretching of the ventricular myocytes. Changes in contractility are characterized by upward (positively inotropic) and downward (negatively inotropic) displacement of the Starling curve.

and the relationship is no longer valid, such that when a certain EDP is exceeded, any further increase will decrease SV.

Starling's law is the principle that matches right and left ventricular SVs and understanding it is central to understanding CO control.

Change in preload

Increased preload will increase CO. Within a few beats, increased right ventricular stretch and right ventricular SV will increase

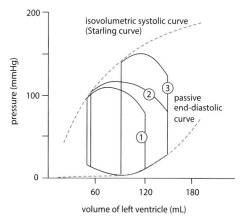

Fig. 2.15 Pressure–volume loops (1, normal state; 2, increased end-diastolic volume (EDV) leads to increased stroke volume (SV) if arterial pressure is constant; 3, increased EDV and increased mean arterial pressure (MAP) result in a decreased SV). The end-systolic points of the loops produce the Starling curve so long as contractility remains constant. The total loop area is equivalent to the mechanical work.

pulmonary pressures and thus left ventricular filling. This increases left ventricular SV. A decrease in preload will, in the same way, decrease CO.

Change in afterload

An increase in afterload will reduce left ventricle SV, therefore increasing ESV. This will result in a greater EDV during the next cycle. The increased preload increases the force of the next contraction to restore SV despite increased afterload. Fig. 2.15 shows the pressure-volume loop for the left ventricle and how this is affected by changes in EDV and contractility.

These pressure-volume loops are important in understanding the importance of:

- Adequate, but not excessive, filling of the ventricles (e.g., in heart failure, high EDV may be pathological).
- Keeping peripheral resistance as low as possible to maximize CO (reducing afterload).
- Maintaining a sufficient level of contractility.

These factors are particularly important when considering heart failure treatments.

HINTS AND TIPS

Remember that cardiac output is limited by venous return – without integrated regulation of the cardiovascular system, increased heart rate will be compensated for by reduced stroke volume.

HAEMODYNAMICS AND VASCULAR FUNCTION

Blood flow and velocity

In normal arteries and veins, blood flow is described as laminar (Fig. 2.16), flowing in several parallel planes, with those in the centre flowing faster than those towards the vessel wall. This occurs due to increased shear forces between the outermost layers of blood and the vessel wall, resulting in slower flow. Disruption of laminar flow can occur at areas of stenosis or branching. This promotes atherosclerosis.

HINTS AND TIPS

Alteration in normal blood flow (such as turbulence, stasis, etc.) is one of the three main contributing factors for thrombus formation, as described by Virchow's triad. The other two factors are endothelial injury/dysfunction and hypercoagulability.

The velocity of blood flow within the vessels is inversely related to the total cross-sectional area (Fig. 2.17). The branching nature of the circulatory system means that the total cross-sectional area of the capillaries is much greater than that of the large arteries or veins. 'Single-file' flow occurs in capillaries where the vessel diameter is the same or often less than that of the blood cells. This reduces flow rate in the capillaries, allowing time for diffusion.

Vascular resistance

The total vascular resistance (Fig. 2.18) is greatest in the arterioles, through a combination of their length and reduced radius without a significant change in total cross-sectional area. Total resistance is dependent upon the arteriolar radius, which is tightly controlled.

Capillary resistance is less than arteriolar resistance because capillaries are shorter (0.5 mm), large numbers of capillaries occur in parallel and they have single-file flow rather than laminar flow. Remember, however, that due to its smaller radius, a given length of capillary will have greater resistance than the same length of arteriole.

Blood viscosity

Viscosity is a measure of internal friction within a moving fluid. According to Poiseuille's law, resistance is proportional to viscosity, so blood viscosity therefore plays a role in determining flow. The main determinant of viscosity is the haematocrit (the percentage of red cells in the blood volume).

A normal haematocrit (generally 40%–50%) is the optimal level for oxygen delivery. An elevated haematocrit (polycythaemia) increases carriage of oxygen but increases viscosity, impeding flow and increasing cardiac work. Polycythaemia may occur with:

- Chronic hypoxia (e.g., severe respiratory disease).
- High altitude living – as a physiological adaptation.
- Myeloproliferative disease (e.g., polycythaemia rubra vera).
- Severe dehydration – haemoconcentration due to reduction in circulating volume without loss of red blood cells.
- Right to left shunting (e.g., Eisenmenger syndrome or cyanotic congenital heart disease).

Plasma viscosity is also determined by the level of plasma proteins (mainly albumins and globulins) and is increased in conditions such as myeloma, in which there is increased production of immunoglobulin. In addition to increasing plasma viscosity, this increase in plasma proteins promotes the aggregation of red blood cells, further increasing viscosity. Vessel diameter and the rate of flow also influence red blood cell aggregation and as a result, the viscosity of blood is different throughout the vascular system.

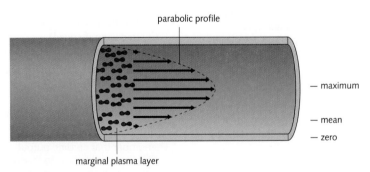

Fig. 2.16 Laminar flow. The dashed line indicates the parabolic profile of the different speeds across the vessel. Cells tend to accumulate in the centre of the flow, leaving a marginal plasma layer with fewer red cells at the periphery.

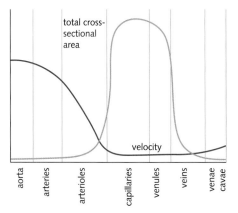

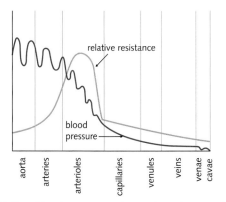

Fig. 2.17 Total cross-sectional area and mean velocity within the different anatomical classifications of vessels. Velocity on the arterial side varies during the cardiac cycle – the mean velocity is shown.

Fig. 2.18 How blood pressure and vascular resistance change across the vascular system. Pressure in the arterial side and in the great veins varies with the cardiac cycle.

Arteries

The pulse waveform

The waveform of arterial pressure during the cardiac cycle is shown in Fig. 2.19.

- During early systole, the rate of blood flowing into the aorta is greater than that into the peripheral circulation. This increases the volume and pressure of blood in the aorta. The peak pressure reached is the systolic blood pressure (SBP).
- As ejection declines and during diastole, flow from the aorta into the peripheral vessels is greater than flow into the aorta and the pressure drops. The minimum pressure (at the end of diastole) is the diastolic blood pressure (DBP).

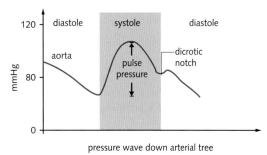

Fig. 2.19 Pulse waveform. The dicrotic notch is caused by the closure of the aortic valve.

- Closure of the aortic valve causes a small backflow of blood into the ventricles and a visible dip in pressure readings, referred to as the 'dicrotic notch'.

During systole, when aortic pressure increases, the elastic wall arteries are stretched and store some of the energy generated by ventricular contraction. They recoil during diastole to maintain pressure and convert the intermittent flow from the left ventricle into the aorta into more continuous flow into the peripheral vasculature, maintaining perfusion pressure.

Factors that alter the rate of ventricular ejection or outflow from the aorta to the peripheral circulation will alter the shape of the pulse waveform. Aortic stenosis decreases the rate of ejection and causes a 'slow rising' pulse, whereas aortic regurgitation, in which blood flows back into the heart through the aortic valve, causes a 'collapsing' pulse. These are shown in Fig. 2.20.

Arterial blood pressure

Arterial blood pressure is determined in the arteries and in the presence of steady venous pressures, it determines perfusion pressure of the body's tissues. Arterial blood pressure is expressed as SBP/DBP.

Normal blood pressure

Normal blood pressure for a healthy adult male at rest is 120/80 mmHg. However, this value can vary due to many factors:

- Ageing increases SBP due to decreased arterial compliance.
- During sleep, blood pressure falls because of decreased metabolic demands.
- Anger, sexual excitement and stress increase blood pressure as a result of sympathetically mediated responses.
- In the young, MAP falls by a small amount during inspiration because of a transient fall in SV.
- In pregnancy, blood pressure falls gradually in the first trimester, reaching a minimum in the second trimester and rising to normal in the third trimester.

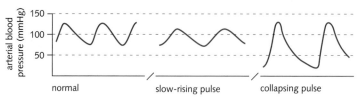

Fig. 2.20 Normal, slow-rising and collapsing pulse waveforms.

Mean arterial pressure

This is the average blood pressure over a single cardiac cycle and not the average of the systolic (SBP) and diastolic pressures (DBP). Mean arterial blood pressure is equal to CO multiplied by TPR. It can be estimated from DBP + 1/3 (SBP – DBP).

Pulse pressure

This is the difference between SBP and DBP. Pulse pressure can be altered by:

- Age: the aortic wall becomes less elastic with age. This causes greater increases in pressure during ventricular ejection, resulting in a higher SBP. DBP, on the other hand, is reduced due to lack of elastic recoil, meaning that pressure drops at a greater rate during diastole. This increases pulse pressure.
- Haemorrhage: when blood volume is reduced, SV is reduced due to decreased preload, decreasing SBP. To maintain MAP (and perfusion pressure), TPR is increased, raising DBP and decreasing pulse pressure.
- Aortic valve disease (see Fig. 2.20). Pulse pressure is decreased in aortic stenosis and increased in aortic regurgitation.

Arterioles

Arterioles are the site of greatest resistance to blood flow in the circulatory system. The abundant smooth muscle in the wall of these vessels allows tight control of lumen diameter. Control over arteriolar diameter has several important functions:

- Coordinated constriction or dilatation of a large proportion of arterioles will alter the TPR and thus arterial blood pressure.
- Constriction or dilatation of arterioles in single organs allows the distribution of the CO to different organs to be regulated.
- Constriction or dilatation of arterioles influences the hydrostatic forces in the capillaries and, as a result, affects fluid filtration. Constriction of arterioles increases resistance and causes a greater pressure drop, reducing the pressure in the distal vessels.

Control of vascular smooth muscle tone

Mechanisms to control arteriolar vascular smooth muscle tone can be broadly divided into local and systemic influences.

Vasoconstriction is an active process brought about by the contraction of vascular smooth muscle. Vasodilatation occurs when vascular smooth muscle relaxes.

Local factors are numerous and include:

- Intrinsic vascular smooth muscle tone – higher internal pressures cause increased myogenic constriction.
- Endothelium-derived dilator factors (e.g., nitric oxide).
- Endothelium-derived constrictor factors (e.g., endothelin 1, thromboxane A_2).
- Metabolic factors – locally produced products of metabolism relax smooth muscle, causing vasodilatation and increasing blood flow to tissues with high metabolic requirements.
- Various other factors – such as histamine, bradykinin and leukotrienes.

Local influences serve only the needs of the local tissues without taking into account the requirements of the whole body, including maintenance of blood pressure. Consider a situation in which all the tissues had increased requirements and local factors brought about vasodilatation in all the tissues simultaneously. This would cause a massive drop in blood pressure. To maintain blood pressure, there are several systemic influences on vascular tone that are superimposed on local factors:

- Sympathetic nervous system (SNS) activity – a basal level of sympathetic vasoconstriction is partly responsible for vessel tone at rest. Increased activation of these nerves causes contraction of smooth muscle and vasoconstriction. Conversely, vasodilatation can be brought about by a decrease in sympathetic nerve activity. Catecholamines (epinephrine and norepinephrine) are released from the adrenal medulla secondary to exercise, hypotension or 'fight-or-flight' situations. Catecholamines bind to β_1 receptors in the myocardium, increasing heart rate and contractility, and bind to α_1 receptors on vascular smooth muscle, causing vasoconstriction. Epinephrine has a high affinity for β_2 receptors in skeletal muscle and increases blood flow for 'fight-or-flight' responses.
- Parasympathetic nervous system (PNS) activity – parasympathetic vasodilator nerves innervate blood vessels in the genitalia, skin, salivary glands, pancreas and gastrointestinal mucosa. Their effect on blood pressure is small, but they are important for initiating an erection and in 'rest and digest' responses.

- Antidiuretic hormone (ADH) – released from the posterior pituitary following a rise in plasma osmolarity (or to a lesser extent with hypotension). ADH promotes water retention in renal tubules and vasoconstriction in most tissues (but vasodilatation in coronary and cerebral vessels).
- Natriuretic peptides – in response to increased cardiac filling pressures, specialized myocytes in the atria and ventricles secrete atrial natriuretic peptide (ANP) and brain natriuretic peptide (BNP), respectively. These peptides increase excretion of salt and water in renal tubules and have a mild vasodilatory effect.
- Renin-angiotensin system – described in detail hereafter.

The renin-angiotensin system

Renin is an enzyme produced by juxtaglomerular cells in the kidney. It converts circulating angiotensinogen to angiotensin I (Fig. 2.21). Renin production is increased by:

- A fall in blood pressure in glomerular afferent arterioles.
- Increased sympathetic activity to the renal arterioles by binding of epinephrine to β_1 receptors in the kidney.
- Decreased sodium in the macula densa of the adjacent distal tubule.

Angiotensin-converting enzyme (ACE) converts angiotensin I to the peptide angiotensin II, predominantly on the endothelium of the pulmonary vascular bed. Angiotensin II is the active component of the renin-angiotensin-aldosterone system (RAAS) and acts to:

- Increase aldosterone secretion from the adrenal cortex, leading to salt and water reabsorption in the distal renal tubules.
- Cause vasoconstriction by acting on vascular smooth muscle, augmenting release of norepinephrine and increasing SNS action.
- Stimulate the release of ADH from the posterior pituitary.

Capillaries

In most tissues, vascular smooth muscle tone in the supplying arteriole determines the perfusion of the supplied capillaries.

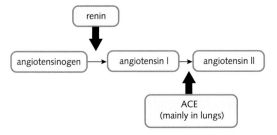

Fig. 2.21 Formation of angiotensin II. Angiotensinogen is secreted by the liver, acted on by renin (secreted by the kidney), and finally converted to the active angiotensin II by angiotensin-converting enzyme (ACE).

Vascular smooth muscle in capillaries has sparse innervation and tone is predominantly controlled by local factors. Changes in terminal arteriolar diameter and capillary perfusion pressure impact fluid filtration.

Capillary diameter is often smaller than red blood cell diameter (3–6 µm compared with 8–10 µm), but because the red blood cells can deform, they are still able to pass through the microvasculature.

HINTS AND TIPS

Raynaud's phenomenon is a condition where exposure of the extremities (fingers, toes, nose) causes excessive cutaneous vasoconstriction, impairing perfusion and causing ischaemia.

Veins and venules

Venules and veins are thin-walled, distensible vessels that return blood from capillaries to the right atrium.

Veins have valves that prevent backflow of blood and without them, VR would be limited. Valve failure can result in varicosities. Venous vessels have other important functions and influences:

- Venous pressure is a determinant of fluid filtration by altering capillary hydrostatic pressure.
- Due to their high compliance, venous vessels can function as a reservoir for blood.
- The venous vessels determine filling pressures of the heart and thus the EDV and SV according to Starling's law.

Skeletal muscle pump

Rhythmic exercise, especially of the leg muscles, produces a pumping effect, increasing the movement of venous blood and maintaining venous return. Pumping blood out of the active muscle lowers venous pressure in that muscle, increasing perfusion pressure and blood flow through active muscles. Incompetent valves make the skeletal muscle pump ineffective.

INTEGRATED CONTROL OF THE CARDIOVASCULAR SYSTEM AND CARDIOVASCULAR REFLEXES

Arterial baroreceptors and the baroreflex

The baroreceptor reflex is vital for minute-to-minute control of arterial blood pressure. Arterial baroreceptors are stretch receptors in the wall of the carotid sinuses and the aortic arch. They continuously generate impulses, with frequency dependent on the degree of vessel wall stretch. Increased stretch (due to increased pressure), also known as increased baroreceptor loading, increases firing rate. The impulses generated by the baroreceptors are carried to the nucleus tractus solitarius (NTS) in the medulla by the glossopharyngeal and vagus nerves (from the carotid sinus and aortic arch, respectively). In the NTS, these afferent impulses interact with other central pathways, regulating autonomic nervous system activity.

When blood pressure decreases, the baroreceptors are unloaded (stretch is reduced) and the firing rate to the medulla decreases. The effect is to decrease parasympathetic (PNS) and increase sympathetic (SNS) drive. This causes the following effects (Fig. 2.22):

- Increased heart rate and contractility, increasing CO (SNS and PNS).
- Peripheral vasoconstriction, increasing TPR (SNS).
- Venoconstriction, decreasing venous pooling and increasing VR and preload (SNS).
- Catecholamine secretion (SNS).
- Increased renin secretion and activation of the renin-angiotensin system, causing vasoconstriction and increasing circulating volume (SNS).

These actions increase CO and TPR, restoring blood pressure to normal. The baroreflex is rapid and very important in acute hypotension or haemorrhage. Increased loading of the baroreceptors has the opposite effect, decreasing CO and TPR.

Baroreceptor-mediated vasoconstriction primarily affects vascular beds in skeletal muscle and the gastrointestinal tract. Cutaneous circulation is important if the temperature is neutral. Cerebral and coronary circulations are largely unaffected by these changes in sympathetic activity.

The level of blood pressure that the baroreceptors take as 'normal' (the set point) can be reset by central or peripheral processes:

- Central resetting: in exercise or during fight-or-flight situations, the rise in blood pressure that occurs does not cause bradycardia because central influences reset the baroreflex set point and allow the blood pressure to increase.
- Peripheral resetting: chronic hyper- or hypotension leads to the set point being reset to this new pressure, allowing the baroreflex to operate in its optimal range. Because of this, the baroreflex is of little use for long-term control of blood pressure.

Arterial baroreceptors' sensitivity to changes in blood pressure is decreased by reduced compliance of arterial walls – this occurs with ageing and chronic hypertension.

Central pathways

The cardiovascular system is influenced by complex interactions between the medulla, hypothalamus and cortex.

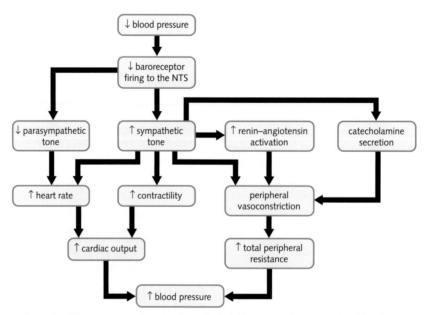

Fig. 2.22 The baroreceptor reflex. The responses to unloading of arterial baroreceptors to restore blood pressure to the set point (*NTS*, nucleus tractus solitarius).

Medulla

It is thought that there are complex signals between the hypothalamus, cortex and cerebellum, as well as signals within the vasomotor centre of the medulla:

- The rostral ventrolateral medulla is responsible for sympathetic outflow.
- The nucleus ambiguus is responsible for parasympathetic (vagal) outflow.

Together, these two areas mediate neural control of vascular tone and heart rate. Information from baroreceptors and other cardiovascular receptors is received at the NTS in the medulla. The afferent inputs are integrated and relayed to other areas in the brain.

Hypothalamus

The hypothalamus contains four areas of interest:

- Depressor area – receives input from the NTS and can produce the baroreflex.
- Defence area – responsible for the alerting (fight-or-flight) response.
- Temperature-regulating area – controls cutaneous vascular tone and sweating.
- ADH-secreting area – produces antidiuretic hormone (vasopressin).

Cardiorespiratory interactions

During inspiration, reduced intrathoracic pressure increases venous return. This increases SV by Starling's law. In addition to this mechanical interaction, there are also neurally mediated cardiorespiratory interactions.

Sinus arrhythmia

Sinus arrhythmia describes the physiological phenomenon of increased heart rate during inspiration and is more profound in young people. The mechanisms that underlie sinus arrhythmia are detailed in Fig. 2.23.

This also explains the increase in heart rate that occurs in any situation where the respiratory rate is increased. Examples include systemic hypoxia, exercise and stress.

Arterial chemoreceptors

Peripheral chemoreceptors are located in the carotid and aortic bodies. They are involved in the regulation of pH and oxygen/carbon dioxide levels in arterial blood. Their fibres travel with afferent baroreceptor fibres in the glossopharyngeal and vagus nerves. Their activity is increased by increased carbon dioxide, decreased oxygen and reduced pH in arterial blood.

Increased stimulation of these chemoreceptors results in increased parasympathetic drive to the heart, decreasing the

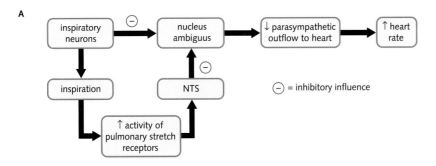

A

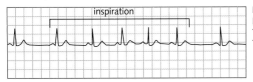

B

Sinus arrhythmia (change of heart rate due to inspiration and expiration)

Every QRS complex has a preceding P wave. There is a normal PR interval, but the heart rate increases during inspiration. This is seen by the decreased R–R interval. This is normal, especially in children and healthy adults.

Fig. 2.23 Sinus arrhythmia. (A) Neural pathways underpinning sinus arrhythmia and the increase in heart rate in response to an increased respiratory rate or increased tidal volume. (B) ECG trace of sinus arrhythmia (*NTS*, nucleus tractus solitarius).

heart rate and increasing sympathetic drive to the arterioles, causing vasoconstriction. This reflex is in place to reduce oxygen requirements; however, it is only apparent if the respiratory rate is not able to increase, for example, during artificial ventilation or in a foetus in the womb.

Under normal circumstances, when the respiratory rate can increase, increased stimulation of the chemoreceptors increases outflow from the inspiratory centre, increasing respiratory rate and tidal volume. This increases heart rate, and the greater degree of pulmonary stretch receptor stimulation that accompanies increased tidal volume further augments this response. Under normal circumstances, hypoxaemia will cause tachycardia. Remember that hypoxaemia will also cause vasodilatation in certain vascular beds, such as skeletal muscle and the brain, via local effects of reduced partial pressure of oxygen in the blood.

Other cardiopulmonary receptors

There are many cardiopulmonary receptors in the heart, great veins and pulmonary arteries with afferents to the NTS including:

- Atrial stretch receptors – these are located where the great veins join the atria and are stimulated by atrial stretch, which increases when blood volume increases. Stimulation produces a reflex tachycardia (the Bainbridge reflex) by increasing sympathetic drive to the SA node. It also reduces ADH secretion to reduce circulating volume.
- Unmyelinated mechanoreceptor fibres – these are present in the atria and left ventricle. Large degrees of distension in these chambers stimulate the receptors, causing reflex bradycardia and peripheral vasodilatation.
- Chemosensitive fibres – these are stimulated by bradykinin and other substances released by ischaemic myocardium. It is thought that the pain of angina and myocardial infarction is mediated by these fibres. Stimulation increases respiratory rate, reduces heart rate and peripherally vasodilates.

Coordinated cardiovascular responses

Orthostasis

Orthostasis means maintenance of an upright posture. When moving from a supine position to standing, gravity causes venous pooling in vessels below the heart, thereby increasing venous

pressures and distending veins. This reduces apparent circulation volume and venous return. Cardiac filling is reduced, and SV and CO fall. Arterial blood pressure drops, but only transiently, as the baroreceptor reflex corrects it almost immediately.

Valsalva manoeuvre

The Valsalva manoeuvre is a forced expiration against a closed glottis. This commonly occurs when coughing, defecating or lifting heavy weights. It causes increased intrathoracic pressure, which brings about the following response (Fig. 2.24):

1. Increased intrathoracic pressure increases blood flow from the pulmonary circulation into the left atrium. This increases left ventricular EDV and SV. Compression of the aorta increases blood pressure.
2. High intrathoracic pressure impedes venous return, decreasing SV and therefore blood pressure. During this period, there is a baroreceptor-mediated increase in heart rate.

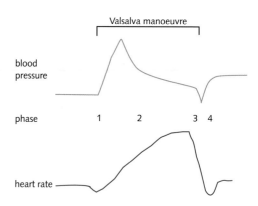

phase 1 BP↑: compression of thoracic aorta
2 BP↓: high intrathoracic pressure impedes venous return, filling pressure and stroke volume
3 BP↓: suddenly compression of aorta is stopped
4 BP↑: ↑venous return, ↑stroke volume, reflex bradycardia

Fig. 2.24 Response to the Valsalva manoeuvre (*BP*, blood pressure).

3. When the manoeuvre is released, compression on the aorta is stopped and left ventricular filling pressures are reduced temporarily as the pulmonary vessels re-expand. This causes a drop in blood pressure.
4. VR is restored, increasing cardiac filling pressures and SV. This increases BP, resulting in a baroreceptor reflex-mediated bradycardia and subsequent fall in BP to normal levels.

This manoeuvre is a useful test of baroreceptor competence. If the pressure fall in phase 2 continues and there is no bradycardia in phase 4, then the baroreflex is interrupted, and the person will be at risk of postural hypotension.

Diving reflex

The diving reflex occurs when cold water stimulates the sensory receptors of the trigeminal nerve and receptors in the nasopharynx and oropharynx. The body is expecting a period of submersion and responds to conserve the limited oxygen supply available and to preferentially divert it to the heart and brain. The reflex results in three changes:

- Apnoea – while apnoeic, changing concentrations of oxygen and carbon dioxide in the blood stimulate chemoreceptors, increasing vagal drive and decreasing heart rate.
- Bradycardia – intense vagal inhibition decreases the slope of the pacemaker action potential and decreases oxygen consumption.
- Peripheral vasoconstriction in the splanchnic, renal and skeletal muscle vascular beds – strong sympathetically mediated vasoconstriction increases TPR, allowing blood pressure to be maintained despite profound bradycardia.

HINTS AND TIPS

The diving reflex can be exploited clinically as one method to terminate supraventricular arrhythmias. Placing an icepack on the face or submersing the face in cold water elicits this response and slows the heart rate.

The alerting/defence response

This response (also known as the fight-or-flight response) is the body's response to a stressful stimulus and involves:

- Increased sympathetic outflow (increased epinephrine binding to myocardial β_1 receptors) and decreased parasympathetic outflow to the heart. This increases heart rate and contractility, increasing CO.
- Increased sympathetic outflow to the gastrointestinal tract, kidneys and skin causes vasoconstriction (due to increased epinephrine acting on α_1 receptors).

- Increased sympathetic outflow to skeletal muscle reduces arteriolar tone causing vasodilatation (due to increased epinephrine acting on β_2 receptors).

The net result is increased heart rate and blood pressure, and increased skeletal muscle blood flow. During this response, the baroreceptor reflex is inhibited so hypertension is not corrected. Changes in autonomic activity cause pupillary dilatation and piloerection. The intensity of the stimulus affects intensity of the response and the responses of two different people to the same stimulus may be very different.

Syncope (fainting)

Syncope is a sudden, transient loss of consciousness as a result of cerebral hypoperfusion. It may be initiated by standing, hypovolaemia, arrhythmia or psychological stress. There is often a presyncope period of tachycardia, cutaneous vasoconstriction, hyperventilation and sweating (due to the alerting response). Hyperventilation causes a reduction in the concentration of carbon dioxide in the blood and can cause paraesthesia in the fingers and around the mouth.

A vasovagal episode proceeds as follows:

1. A sudden large increase in vagal outflow causes bradycardia.
2. Profound peripheral vasodilatation occurs due to decreased sympathetic drive.
3. This causes a fall in blood pressure, reducing cerebral blood flow.
4. If it occurs at all, loss of consciousness results within seconds.

HINTS AND TIPS

Fits, faints and funny turns are common presentations of cardiovascular disease but it is important to remember there may also be nervous, respiratory and psychological causes of these episodes.

A person who has fainted falls to the floor. This raises intrathoracic blood volume and cardiac filling pressures. Coupled with the baroreflex, this increases CO and arterial pressure, restoring cerebral perfusion and consciousness. Raising the person's legs will cause a further increase in VR and thus CO.

HINTS AND TIPS

You should never hold a person who has fainted upright, as this prevents the beneficial effects of increasing intrathoracic blood volume and may maintain cerebral hypoperfusion.

Shock and haemorrhage

Haemorrhage

Haemorrhage describes the loss of blood from the vascular compartment. The body has several responses in place to initially compensate for the reduction in circulating volume and eventually to replace that volume. Acute haemorrhage can be classified according to either the amount of blood loss or the percentage of total blood volume lost. Table 2.2 shows this classification and the changes in physiological parameters that occur at each stage.

In the absence of compensatory cardiovascular changes, haemorrhage will reduce circulating volume and blood pressure. Reduction in blood pressure would be dependent on the amount of blood lost, as that would determine the degree to which ventricular filling (preload) was reduced. In reality, however, compensatory changes do take place and can be divided into three sets based on the timeframe in which they occur (Fig. 2.25).

The primary aims in the treatment of haemorrhage are first to stop the bleeding and then to replace circulating volume with intravenous fluids as appropriate. The key is to restore circulating volume to ensure CO is sufficient to maintain organ perfusion; in major haemorrhage, early transfusion of blood products is advised.

Shock

Shock is an acute failure of the cardiovascular system to adequately perfuse the tissues, which may result in cellular injury and organ dysfunction. There are four broad categories:

- Hypovolaemic shock – due to a fall in circulating volume. This may be caused by internal or external losses, e.g., vomiting, diarrhoea, haemorrhage.
- Distributive shock – the result of abnormal distribution of blood flow, e.g., septic shock, anaphylaxis, neurogenic shock.
- Cardiogenic shock – when the heart is unable to maintain CO. This usually has an acute precipitant, e.g., myocardial infarction, arrhythmia.

- Obstructive shock – when there is physical obstruction to blood entering or leaving the great vessels, e.g., tamponade, massive pulmonary embolism.

Most types of shock (apart from septic shock) cause a characteristic clinical picture as the result of compensatory changes that occur in response to a decrease in CO and blood pressure, including:

1. Pale, cold, clammy skin caused by cutaneous vasoconstriction in an effort to maintain adequate blood flow to vital organs.
2. Sweating caused by sympathetic stimulation.
3. Rapid, weak pulse caused by compensatory tachycardia and decreased SV.
4. Reduced pulse pressure due to reduced SV (reduced SBP) and increased TPR (increased DBP).
5. Rapid, shallow breathing as a result of chemoreceptor stimulation from metabolic acidosis caused by anaerobic cellular respiration (in the presence of inadequate oxygen delivery).
6. Reduced urine output due to renal hypoperfusion and reduced glomerular filtration.

Septic shock is the most common type of circulatory shock. Sepsis is caused by toxins (e.g., endotoxin) released from certain bacteria. This initiates a profound systemic inflammatory response, with the production of cytokines and inflammatory mediators. Widespread vasodilatation and increased capillary permeability reduce TPR. Fluid moves from the vascular compartment into the interstitium. Reduced circulating volume in combination with the decrease in TPR significantly decreases blood pressure. Although the baroreceptor reflex causes tachycardia and increases myocardial contractility, increasing CO, the peripheral vasoconstriction is ineffective. The patient will have a tachycardia but warm skin and low blood pressure due to widespread vasodilatation. Treatment is with fluid replacement, antibiotics and, if severe, cardiovascular support with norepinephrine may be required.

Table 2.2 Changes in vital signs in response to acute haemorrhage

Parameter	Severity of circulatory shock			
	Class I	Class II	Class III	Class IV
Blood loss (%)	0–15	15–30	30–40	>40
Blood loss (mL)	0–750	750–1500	1500–2000	>2000
Pulse rate	↔	↑	↑	↑↑
Respiratory rate	↔	↑	↑↑	↑↑
Capillary refill time	↔	↔	↑	↑↑
Blood pressure	↔	↔ and narrow pulse pressure	↔/↓ and narrow pulse pressure	↓

Note that higher classes of shock indicate increased severity.

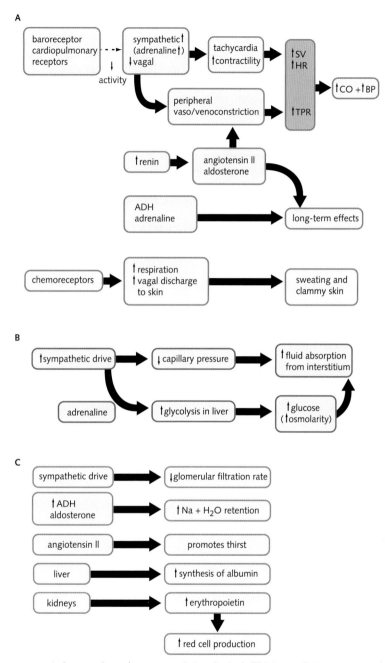

Fig. 2.25 (A) Immediate response to haemorrhage (over seconds to minutes). (B) Intermediate response to haemorrhage (over minutes to hours). (C) Long-term response to haemorrhage (over hours to days) (*ADH*, antidiuretic hormone; *BP*, blood pressure; *CO*, cardiac output; *HR*, heart rate; *SV*, stroke volume; *TPR*, total peripheral resistance).

● Chapter Summary

- Electrical activity in the heart originates in the SA node and propagates through the atria and to the ventricles via the AV node. The AV node can function as a backup pacemaker.
- Nodal cells spontaneously depolarize and initiate action potentials without outside stimulus. The other cardiomyocytes are stimulated by adjacent cells depolarizing.
- CO is a product of SV and heart rate, and is determined by preload, afterload and cardiac contractility.
- Complex changes in cardiac volumes and pressures occur throughout the cardiac cycle.
- Blood flows in a laminar fashion in the blood vessels; disruption of this can result in atherosclerosis.
- There are several important local and systemic influences that provide closely regulated control of blood pressure, vascular resistance and organ perfusion.
- The body has several mechanisms in place to ensure homeostasis when the requirements placed upon the cardiovascular system are altered (e.g., hypotension, haemorrhage, exercise, etc.).

UKMLA Conditions
Vasovagal syncope

UKMLA Presentations
Blackouts and faints
Heart murmurs

THE ELECTROCARDIOGRAM

The electrocardiogram (ECG) is a recording of the heart's electrical activity obtained by measuring changes in electrical potential difference across the body surface. It is usually the first investigation used to diagnose arrhythmias and the underlying cause of chest pain.

As a wave of depolarization spreads through the myocardium, there will be, at any one moment, areas of myocardium that have been excited and areas that have not yet been excited. As a result, there is a difference in potential between them: one area is negatively charged (excited) and the other is positively charged (not excited) with respect to the charge in the extracellular space. These areas can be thought of as two electrical poles that comprise the cardiac dipole. This dipole depends on both the size of the charge (which depends on the amount of muscle excited) and the direction the wave of depolarization is travelling in. In the absence of electrical activity in the heart and skeletal muscle, the electrical potential across the surface of the body is uniformly positive. The cardiac dipole (electrical activity in the heart) alters the electrical potential across the body, and by placing electrodes in certain positions, the cardiac dipole and other changes in potential can be measured in different directions. This provides the basis for electrocardiography.

Fig. 3.1 depicts how a wave of depolarization affects the potential difference between two electrodes, and thus how this is translated onto an ECG trace. Remember that as the dipole has both charge (amplitude) and direction, the shape of the ECG varies depending on the position of the recording electrode. As current travels towards the positive electrode, there is an upward deflection of the ECG waveform. As the current travels towards the negative electrode (or away from the positive one), there is a downward deflection of the ECG waveform. If the current is moving perpendicular to the recording pair of electrodes, there is a biphasic waveform.

The 12-lead ECG

Conventionally, the ECG is recorded using 12 'leads' (Fig. 3.2). Note that the term 'lead' is used to denote the direction in which the potential is measured and not a physical electrode – only 10 electrodes are used to produce 12 leads that allow us to view the direction and magnitude of electrical activity in both the frontal and transverse planes.

A 'unipolar lead' measures potential difference towards the lead from an estimate of zero potential, whereas a 'bipolar lead' measures potential difference between two leads.

Limb leads

The limb leads view the heart in the frontal plane. To produce these leads, one electrode is placed on each arm and leg. The right leg electrode is important in reducing noise/artefact – it is not a direct contributor to produce the lead traces. It can be placed anywhere on the body but is usually right leg by convention.

Unipolar limb leads (also called the 'augmented limb leads') measure positive potential difference directed towards a limb electrode from an estimate of zero potential and include aVL, aVR and aVF. The zero potential for these leads is estimated by averaging the potential of electrodes on the other two limbs (e.g., $aVR = RA - 1/2(LA+LL)$).

The bipolar leads make up Einthoven's triangle around the heart (see Fig. 3.2). They record the differences in potential between pairs of limb leads:

- Lead I: right arm to left arm; left arm positive.
- Lead II: right arm to left leg; left leg positive.
- Lead III: left arm to left leg; left leg positive.

ECG traces from each of the limb leads are shown in Fig. 3.3.

Chest leads

The chest leads (V1–V6) are unipolar leads that measure potential difference in the transverse plane between positive electrodes arranged around the left side of the chest (as in Fig. 3.2) and a negative central point derived from average of the three limb electrodes.

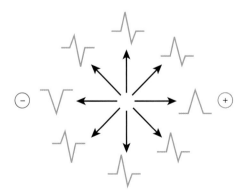

Fig. 3.1 The influence of the direction of depolarization on the ECG trace. Repolarization produces a deflection in the opposite direction.

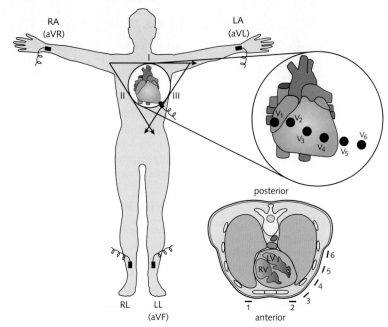

Fig. 3.2 Placement of ECG electrodes. The electrodes on the right arm *(RA)*, left arm *(LA)* and left leg *(LL)* give the electrocardiogram trace for the limb leads (i.e., I, II, III, aVL, aVR and aVF). The right leg *(RL)* lead doesn't contribute to the ECG trace directly. Einthoven's triangle around the heart is shown. Anterior chest lead placement is shown in the frontal and transverse planes. V1 is placed in the fourth intercostal space on the right sternal edge and V2 on the left sternal edge. V4 is placed in the fifth intercostal space in the mid-clavicular line, V5 in the anterior axillary line and V6 in the mid-axillary line. V3 is placed between V2 and V4 *(LV, left ventricle; RV, right ventricle)*.

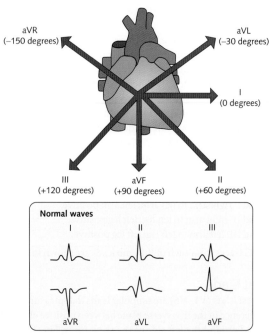

Fig. 3.3 Lead directions in the anterior plane. (Redrawn with permission from Epstein, O., et al., 1997. *Clinical examination*, second ed. Mosby International, New York.)

HINTS AND TIPS

Rarely, electrodes may be placed on the posterior chest wall (usually to confirm posterior myocardial infarction). Posterior leads V7 to V9 are placed in the same horizontal plane as V6. V7 is placed in the left posterior axillary line, V8 at the tip of the left scapula and V9 in the left paraspinal region.

The ECG trace

The components that make up an ECG tracing (Fig. 3.4) are:

- P wave – due to atrial depolarization.
- PR interval – from onset of the P wave to the onset of the QRS complex (approximately 120–200 ms). This represents the time taken for depolarization to propagate through the atria and the impulse to conduct through the atrioventricular node to the bundle of His.
- QRS complex – due to ventricular depolarization and is usually less than 100 ms in duration; greater than 120 ms is considered to be prolonged. The definitions of each wave within the QRS complex are depicted in Fig. 3.5.

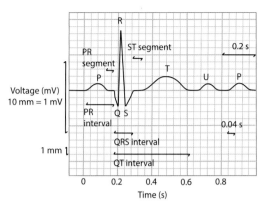

Fig. 3.4 Components of the ECG trace.

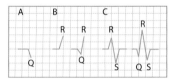

Fig. 3.5 Definitions of the ECG waves. (A) If the wave following the P wave is negative, it is a Q wave. (B) If a positive deflection follows the P wave, it is called an R wave, whether it is preceded by a Q wave or not. (C) Any following negative deflection is known as an S wave, whether there has been a preceding Q wave or not.

- ST segment – coincides with the plateau phase of the ventricular action potential and ventricular contraction. It is usually isoelectric (flat) as the ventricles are depolarized throughout. Abnormalities of the ST segment can indicate ischaemia or infarction.
- T wave – due to ventricular repolarization.

- QT interval – from the onset of the Q wave to the end of the T wave (approximately 400 ms). This represents electrical depolarization and repolarization of the ventricles.
- U wave – sometimes seen as a small deflection following the T wave (and usually in the same direction). The source of the U wave is unclear – they are seen most classically in hypokalaemia but are also seen in a number of other conditions (including hypocalcaemia, hypomagnesaemia and hypothermia). It is thought they may represent delayed repolarization of Purkinje fibres.

Q waves

Small, nonsignificant Q waves are often seen in the left-sided leads due to the depolarization of the septum from left to right. Significant (pathological) Q waves:

- Are more than 0.04 s (one small square) in duration and more than 25% of the following R wave in depth.
- Occur after transmural myocardial infarction (MI) where the myocardium on one side of the heart dies. This myocardium has no electrical activity and therefore the leads facing it are able to pick up the electrical activity from the opposite side of the heart (effectively like looking through an electrical hole in the heart). The myocardium depolarizes from the inside out; therefore, the opposite side of the heart depolarizes away from these leads, resulting in a negative deflection or Q wave.
- May also occur in patients with hypertrophic cardiomyopathy due to depolarization of the thickened septum. This may lead to an erroneous diagnosis of previous MI.

R wave progression

The wave of depolarization in the ventricles starts in the septum and then spreads into the left and right ventricles (Fig. 3.6). Because the left ventricle is usually larger than the right, the

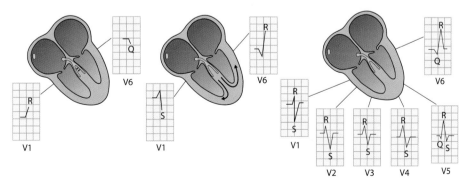

Fig. 3.6 The different anterior chest leads show different QRS traces due to the changing directions of the electrical activity. Lead V4 is usually over the interventricular septum and therefore usually shows equal R and S waves. Note the changing relative heights of Q, R and S waves between leads. The changing height of the R wave from V1 to V6 is known as 'R wave progression'.

average depolarization heads towards the left ventricle. This means that V1 and V2 will have a predominant S wave (i.e., negative deflection) and a small R wave, whereas V5 and V6 will have a predominant R wave (i.e., positive deflection) and a small S wave. The interventricular septum lies where there are equal positive and negative deflections (i.e., R and S waves) and is usually at V3 or V4. This steady increase in the size of the R wave is sometimes termed R wave progression. If this is normal, then there is said to be 'good' R wave progression.

ECG abnormalities in noncardiac disease

Noncardiac diseases may have a number of impacts on the ECG trace, for example:

- Hypokalaemia – prolonged QT interval, small T, U wave.
- Hyperkalaemia: tall 'tented' T, wide QRS, absent P.
- Hypercalcaemia: short QT interval.
- Hypocalcaemia: long QT interval.
- Hypothermia: bradycardia, J waves/Osborn waves (positive deflections at the junction between QRS complex and ST segment), baseline artefact due to shivering, risk of arrhythmia as the patient is warmed up.
- Digoxin – downsloping ST segment ('reverse tick' shape), T wave inversion.
- Digoxin toxicity – atrioventricular block, atrial tachycardia, ventricular arrhythmias.

    Some of these abnormalities are seen in Fig 3.7.

Assessment of cardiac axis

The average direction of the wave of depolarization is the electrical axis of the heart, usually referred to as the cardiac axis

(Fig. 3.8). This usually lies closest to lead II but is within normal limits if between − 30 and + 90 degrees. Any deviation from this range is referred to as right or left axis deviation. Right axis deviation can be caused by right ventricular hypertrophy and left axis deviation by left ventricular hypertrophy. When interpreting an ECG, it must be established whether the axis is normal or not.

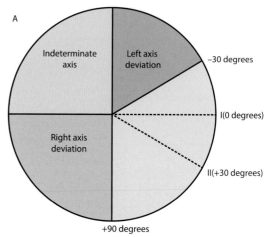

B	Causes of left axis deviation	Left bundle branch block, left anterior hemiblock, left ventricular hypertrophy, ostium primum atrial septal defect
	Causes of right axis deviation	Right bundle branch block, cor pulmonale, right ventricular hypertrophy, ostium secundum atrial septal defect

Fig. 3.8 (A) Cardiac axis. (B) Causes of left and right axis deviation.

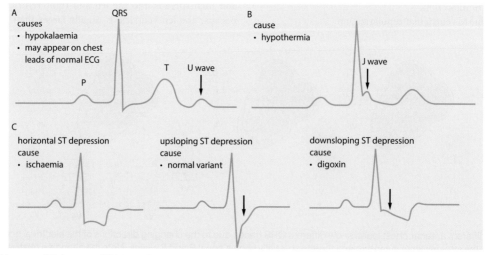

Fig. 3.7 (A) U waves. (B) J waves. (C) Not all ST depression is due to ischaemia.

When the depolarization wave in the ventricles is moving towards a lead, then the R wave will be larger than the S wave in that lead. When the ventricular depolarization wave is moving away from a lead, then the S wave will be larger than the R wave in that lead. If the S wave and R wave are equal, then the depolarization is moving (on average) at right angles to that lead. The simplest way to assess the cardiac axis is to look at leads I and II. If the overall deflection in leads I and II is positive (both pointing upwards), then the axis is normal. If lead I is positive and II is negative (pointing away from each other), it is left axis deviation. If lead I is negative and II is positive (pointing towards each other), then it is right axis deviation. If both are negative (both pointing downwards), check that you have the leads on correctly!

HINTS AND TIPS

Do not get confused between the orientation of the heart and the cardiac axis. The cardiac axis is an electrical entity and is the angle at which the maximum amplitude R wave is generated.

The vector method for calculating the cardiac axis

The cardiac axis can be calculated more accurately by considering the net deflection (in terms of numbers of small squares) from the isoelectric line in leads I and aVF. The net deflection values can then be plotted as vectors (Fig. 3.9) to calculate the cardiac axis.

Note that positive displacement in aVF is plotted down the y-axis. If the net deflection in a lead is negative, it should be

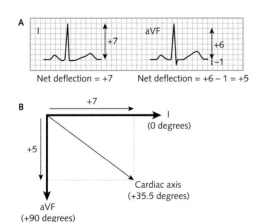

Fig. 3.9 Calculation of the cardiac axis. The net positive displacement of the QRS in leads I and aVF is (A) measured and (B) plotted on a graph. The angle subtended by a line between this point and 0 degrees is equal to the mean QRS axis.

plotted in the opposite direction to that lead (i.e., 180 degrees for a negative displacement in lead I and 270 degrees for a negative displacement in aVF).

Assessment of rate and rhythm

The standard paper speed is 25 mm/s, which means that in 1 second, the paper has moved by five large squares (i.e., 0.2 s per large square and 0.04 s per small square). The rate can be measured in a variety of ways:

- Divide 300 by the number of large squares between QRS complexes. That will give you the rate in beats per minute (bpm).
- Count the number of beats in the rhythm strip, which represents 10 seconds of electrical activity on a standard trace, and multiply this number by 6.

Assessing rhythm is usually achieved by looking at lead II (often used to form the rhythm strip), but looking at V1 is also helpful, as P waves cannot always be seen in lead II. Note whether the distance between the R wave peaks is consistent. If it is not, try and establish whether it is regularly irregular or irregularly irregular. See Chapter 14 for more detail.

COMMON PITFALLS

ECG machines will often attempt to interpret the ECG trace. Do not accept this without question, as it is often wrong!

Ambulatory ECG monitoring

A standard 12-lead ECG, gives a 10-second snapshot of the heart's rhythm. In some cases, a longer recording may be beneficial. Ambulatory ECG monitoring allows continuous monitoring of cardiac electrical activity, normally over a period of 24 hours or longer. The patient wears an ambulatory ECG device (sometimes called a Holter monitor) for the monitoring period. See Chapters 8 and 14 for more details.

PRESENTING AN ECG

When reading or presenting an ECG, it is helpful to have a systematic approach to ensure no abnormalities are missed. The following is an example of such an approach, but with experience, you may develop your own system:

- Name, age and sex of the patient.
- Date and time the ECG was taken.
- Rate.

- Rhythm.
- Axis.

Next, note any abnormalities and in which lead they occur:

- P waves – width and height.
- PR interval.
- QRS complex – width and height.
- QT interval.
- ST segment – any elevation or depression
- T waves – negative/positive and height.

If there are abnormalities, look to see whether they are global or territorial. Remember the territories:

- Anterior – V3 to V4.
- Septal – V1 to V2.
- Inferior – II, III and aVF.
- Lateral – I, aVL, V5 to V6.
- Posterior – V7 to V9 (may see reciprocal changes in V1–V2).

CLINICAL NOTES

Abnormalities may be present across more than one territory. For example, an anterolateral ST elevation myocardial infarction may be seen as ST elevation in leads V3 to V6, I and aVL.

● Chapter Summary

- A standard 12-lead ECG has 6 limb leads and 6 chest leads. There are, however, only 10 physical electrodes.
- P waves represent atrial depolarization. QRS complexes represent ventricular depolarization. T waves represent ventricular repolarization.
- Not all ECG abnormalities are the result of cardiac disease.
- When reading an ECG, ensure a methodical approach is used to avoid missing abnormalities.

UKMLA Conditions
Acute coronary syndromes
Arrhythmias

UKMLA Presentations
Chest pain
Palpitations

Other cardiac investigations 4

COMMON CARDIAC BLOOD TESTS

The main blood tests that it is important to know about are:

- Troponin – a complex of three proteins (troponin C, troponin I and troponin T) that plays an important role in the contraction of cardiac and skeletal muscle, being one of the key components of thin filaments (along with tropomyosin and actin). The subtype of these proteins varies between cardiac and skeletal muscle. If heart muscle cells are damaged (e.g., in myocardial infarction (MI), myocarditis, etc.), then the cardiac subtype of troponin is released into the bloodstream and can be detected via a blood test. Certain other noncardiac conditions (e.g., acute kidney injury) can also raise troponin levels. See Chapter 12.
- Brain natriuretic peptide (also known as B-type natriuretic peptide, BNP) is a hormone released by the ventricles in response to increased wall stretch. High levels of BNP usually signify heart failure. See Chapter 13.

EXERCISE ECG

Indications for exercise testing

Current National Institute for Health and Care Excellence (NICE) guidelines recommend that exercise ECG testing should not be used routinely to diagnose or to exclude stable angina in people without known coronary artery disease.

NICE states that exercise ECG can be used as an alternative to functional imaging in patients who have confirmed coronary artery disease when there is uncertainty as to whether their symptoms are caused by myocardial ischaemia. It can be helpful to aid diagnosis in some cases and can provide prognostic information.

Other indications include:

1. To detect exercise-induced arrhythmias – increased catecholamine levels and metabolic acidosis caused by exercise may potentiate arrhythmias in patients vulnerable to this. This gives an indication of prognosis and whether treatment is required or not.
2. Driver and Vehicle Licensing Agency (DVLA) requirements, e.g., for holders of a Group II or Heavy Goods Vehicle (HGV) licence.
3. Risk assessment in hypertrophic cardiomyopathy.

4. Cautiously may be used in patients with aortic stenosis and unclear symptoms.
5. Preoperative noncardiac surgery assessment.

Methods of exercise

The aim of the exercise test is to stress the cardiovascular system; hence, it is referred to as an exercise stress test (EST) or exercise tolerance test (ETT). All exercise protocols have a warm-up period, a period of exercise with increasing grades of intensity and a cool-down period.

The best method is treadmill exercise. Other methods, such as bicycle testing, are often less effective because many patients are not used to the cycling action, and leg fatigue may set in before cardiovascular fatigue, resulting in early test termination. However, bicycle testing has the advantage that the workload can be controlled and recorded in watts.

The Bruce protocol is often used in conjunction with treadmill testing. This involves 3-minute stages starting with a speed of 1.7 mph and a slope of 10 degrees. Subsequent stages are at incrementally higher speeds and steeper gradients. The final stage (stage 6) is at a rate of 5.5 mph and a gradient of 20 degrees.

The modified Bruce protocol is sometimes used for patients likely to have poor exercise tolerance. An additional two stages are added to the beginning of the standard Bruce protocol. Again, they are 3 minutes in duration and at a speed of 1.7 mph, but the gradient starts at 0 degrees and increases to 5 degrees in the first and second stages, respectively.

Preparation

All patients should have a detailed history and examination to ensure no contraindications to testing (see later). The test, its indications and risks should have been fully explained to the patient. Certain patients may be advised to stop medication before the test. The operator should be aware if patients are still taking their medication (especially drugs affecting the heart rate, such as β-blockers) because these affect the response to exercise. Other medicines, such as digoxin, can give rise to ST segment abnormalities and false positive results.

Variables measured

The following variables are measured before, during and after exercise. Measurements are stopped once all variables have returned to preexercise levels.

- 12-lead electrocardiogram – using standard ECG equipment. Poor electrode contact is avoided by shaving hair if necessary.
- Blood pressure (BP) – this should normally increase following exercise. Inadequate response or a fall in BP may indicate coronary artery disease (most commonly), cardiomyopathy, left ventricular outflow tract obstruction (e.g., aortic stenosis), or use of antihypertensive medications.
- Heart rate – should normally increase following exercise. Inadequate response may indicate ischaemic heart disease or sinoatrial node disease (or use of medications including β-blockers and calcium channel antagonists). Excessive increase in heart rate indicates reduced cardiac reserve secondary to left-ventricular failure (LVF) or anaemia.

Test end-points

The following denote successful test completion:

1. Attainment of maximal heart rate (maximal heart rate is 220 minus age in years; however, attainment of 85% of maximal heart rate is satisfactory).
2. Completion of all stages of the test with no untoward symptoms.

Appropriate premature termination of the exercise test is indicated if any of the following occur:

1. The patient requests to stop due to excessive dyspnoea or fatigue – the most common cause.
2. Chest pain.
3. Dizziness or faintness.
4. Any arrhythmia.
5. Failure of blood pressure to increase with exercise (or a fall in blood pressure).

6. An excessive increase in blood pressure (e.g., systolic 220 mmHg).
7. Failure of heart rate to increase.
8. ST segment depression or elevation greater than 1 mm.

Positive exercise test

The following are indications of a positive exercise test:

1. ST segment depression (horizontal or downsloping) of more than 1 mm in two or more contiguous leads. (Upsloping ST segments are normal with exercise) (Fig. 4.1).
2. ST segment elevation.
3. Characteristic angina.
4. Ventricular arrhythmias.
5. Exertional hypotension.

Causes of ST segment depression are listed in Table 4.1.

COMMON PITFALLS

Exercise testing has variable sensitivity (40%–60%) and specificity (80%–90%) for detecting coronary artery disease, with both values lower in women. It cannot be used to definitively rule in or rule out coronary artery disease. This is most problematic in low-risk populations where positive results are more likely to be a false-positive. Problems arise when clinicians do not fully understand how to use or interpret the test. Beware of a negative exercise test with good history of angina; other investigations will be more helpful.

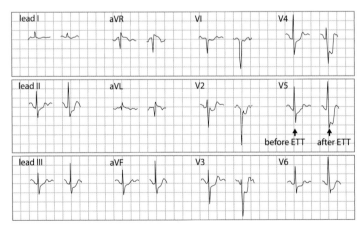

Fig 4.1 Computer-averaged exercise ECG report showing ST depression after exercise *(right-hand trace)* compared with resting ECG *(left-hand trace)* in each of the ECG leads. The ST depression is in the lateral leads V3–V6 and the inferior leads II, III and aVF. *ETT*, Exercise tolerance test.

Table 4.1 Causes of ST-segment depression

Source	Pathology
Cardiac	Ischaemia, aortic stenosis, left ventricular hypertrophy, intraventricular conduction defect (e.g., left bundle branch block)
Noncardiac	Hypokalaemia, digoxin, hypertension

Contraindications to exercise testing

This list includes conditions in which additional stress on the heart may be hazardous:

1. Severe aortic stenosis with a gradient >40 mmHg and normal left-ventricular function.
2. Severe hypertrophic cardiomyopathy – except in specific cases to assess for surgical treatment.
3. Uncontrolled cardiac failure.
4. Unstable angina or acute MI.
5. Myocarditis or pericarditis.
6. Second- or third-degree atrioventricular block.
7. History of sustained ventricular arrhythmias.
8. Severe uncontrolled hypertension.

Despite adhering to these rules, exercise testing does have a mortality rate of approximately 0.5–1/10,000. In all cases, there should be trained staff and full cardiopulmonary resuscitation facilities available.

COMMUNICATION

You need to have a working knowledge of the common cardiac investigations so that you can explain to patients what is involved and how findings may guide management.

ECHOCARDIOGRAPHY

Echocardiography (echo) is the use of ultrasound to investigate the structure and function of the heart. The frequency of the ultrasound waves used is between 1 and 10 MHz. This is above the upper limit of audible sound (20 kHz).

The ultrasound waves are generated by a piezoelectric element within the transducer. Certain structures (e.g., blood) transmit waves much more than others (e.g., muscle or bone), and wave reflection varies with different tissue interfaces. The transducer picks up the reflected waves and, by knowing the time taken for the sound to return and the speed of the waves through the medium, the distance of the reflecting object from the transducer can be calculated.

By rapidly generating waves and detecting reflected waves, a picture of the heart can be built up.

Although this is a noninvasive, harmless and well-tolerated investigation, this approach has certain inadequacies:

1. Ultrasound does not transmit well through air or bone; therefore, the presence of lung between the heart and chest wall impedes ultrasound travel, and only windows that avoid the lungs, ribs and sternum are useful.
2. The posterior part of the heart is furthest from the transducer and may not be viewed adequately, particularly when searching for thrombi and vegetations; therefore, transoesophageal echocardiography (TOE) may be required.
3. Operator dependent – requires a user skilled in the production and interpretation of images.
4. Patient dependent – limited in overweight/obese patients.

M mode echocardiography

The transducer is stationary and records only a single line through the heart, producing an image on a moving page. The activity along the beam is seen changing with time. This mode of echocardiography allows rapid motion to be visualized and accurate timing of cardiac events. It is useful for:

1. Visualizing the movement of the mitral and aortic valve leaflets.
2. Assessing left-ventricular dimensions and function.
3. Assessing aortic root size.
4. Assessing left atrial size.

Two-dimensional echocardiography

The ultrasound generator moves from side to side so a sector of the heart is visualized, and the series of scan lines are brought together to form a two-dimensional (2D) image. This is the mainstay of echocardiography and provides anatomical reference for other imaging modalities.

Standard views of the heart are taken in transthoracic echocardiography (Fig. 4.2) to provide information on:

1. Valve structure and function.
2. Ventricular contractility.
3. Size of the chambers.
4. Congenital malformations.
5. Pericardial disease.

Doppler echocardiography

This records blood flow within the heart and great vessels by using the Doppler shift phenomenon, where the change in frequency of ultrasound reflected off moving objects (e.g., blood cells) varies according to their speed and direction of movement. Colour Doppler echocardiography assigns colours to different directions of blood flow to enable the operator to assess both the speed and the direction of blood flow.

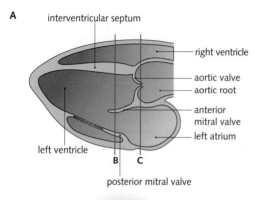

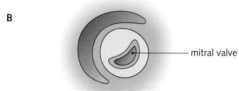

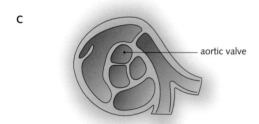

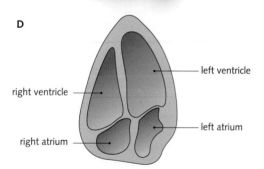

Doppler echocardiography is used for assessment of:

1. Valve stenosis and regurgitation.
2. Atrial and ventricular septal defects, patent ductus arteriosus and other congenital anomalies.
3. Pulmonary hypertension.

Tissue Doppler imaging uses the same principles to assess the motion of the myocardium, rather than of the blood. This can give enhanced information about left-ventricular systolic function and, in particular, diastolic relaxation of the heart.

3D echocardiography

Three-dimensional (3D) echo can produce detailed anatomical images of cardiac valves and chambers, which can be used to accurately calculate chamber volumes as well as plan interventions. Real-time 3D echo can also be used to guide interventions and procedures (e.g., transcatheter aortic valve implantation (TAVI)). Miniaturized echo probes can be deployed through catheters to produce intracardiac echo images. These modalities may become more common in the future.

Transoesophageal echocardiography

TOE uses a flexible probe with a 2D transducer incorporated into the tip. Images are obtained by introducing the transducer into the distal oesophagus (Fig. 4.3). The advantage of TOE is that images are much clearer because the transducer is in close apposition to the heart. This is why TOE is the investigation of choice for assessment of:

1. Intracardiac thrombus – transthoracic echocardiography (TTE) is unreliable.
2. Prosthetic valve function – the planes used in TTE result in a great deal of artefact generated by the prosthesis.

Fig. 4.2 Two-dimensional echocardiography. (A) Long axis view of the heart taken from the left parasternal position with the transducer at the left sternal edge. Rotating the probe 90 degrees gives the parasternal short axis view. (B) Shows the mitral valve (MV), looking like the mouth of a fish. (C) Tilting the probe upwards from this point shows the three-pointed star of the aortic valve and downwards shows the apex of the left ventricle. (D) Placing the probe over the apex of the heart gives the apical four-chamber view. Tilting the probe anteriorly to include the left-ventricular outflow tract and aortic valve gives a five-chamber view.

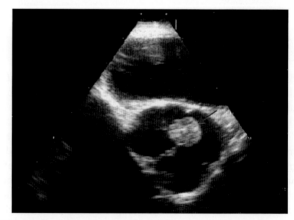

Fig. 4.3 Transoesophageal echocardiography showing a fibroelastoma on the aortic valve.

3. Valve vegetations – usually cannot be excluded without TOE.
4. Congenital heart lesions (e.g., atrial and ventricular septal defects).

TOE imaging can be performed in multiple planes, whereas TTE is restricted to a few planes. TOE can be used during cardiac surgery to provide information on valve function and left-ventricular function.

Stress echocardiography

This can be used to look for the presence of myocardial ischaemia. When myocardium is ischaemic, it contracts less strongly and efficiently. Stress echo aims to demonstrate transient reduced function in a region of myocardium supplied by a narrowed coronary artery.

The patient's heart is stressed with a drug such as dobutamine, which increases the rate and force of contraction and causes peripheral vasodilatation, thus mimicking exercise. With a skilled operator, echocardiography images are obtained before, during and after dobutamine. Areas of ischaemia are seen as areas of regional wall motion abnormality that recover with rest.

COMPUTED TOMOGRAPHY CORONARY ANGIOGRAPHY

To obtain clear, detailed images of a moving structure such as the heart is inherently challenging. The advent of rapid acquisition of images has allowed heart motion artefact to be overcome and led to the use of computed tomography (CT) as a noninvasive alternative for imaging the coronary arteries (Fig. 4.4). Injection of intravenous contrast and ECG monitoring (or 'gating') is used to guide image acquisition – the scan is carried out when cardiac motion is at a minimum (usually towards the end of diastole). Modern scanners give ever-higher spatial and temporal resolution at a lower dose of radiation and can image the whole heart within one heartbeat.

CT coronary angiography (CTCA) has recently become the first-line investigation in patients with new chest pain due to suspected coronary artery disease and is now arguably the gold standard investigation in the majority of cases. Coronary artery lesions and their degree of obstruction can be assessed accurately. CTCA also has the benefit of giving additional information that may not be demonstrated on conventional angiography via cardiac catheterization, including:

- Assessment of atherosclerotic plaques that do not narrow the lumen (these may be missed/occult on cardiac catheterization).
- Additional structural information regarding the heart (including chamber size, valve thickening/calcification and pericardial appearance).

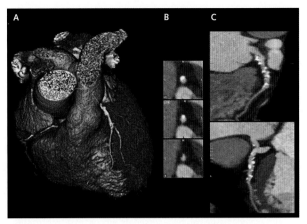

Fig. 4.4 CT coronary angiography. (A) A 3D CT rendering of the heart with automated detection of the coronary arteries (depicted with green line). (B) CT allows cross-sectional assessment of the vessel lumen. (C) Curved planar reformatted images allow curved structures such as vessels to be displayed in a single plane to make visual assessment easier.

- Assessment of any other potential cause for patient symptoms (the central pulmonary arteries and some of the lungs will be imaged during CTCA – pathologies relating to these may account for chest pain or breathlessness).

HINTS AND TIPS

CTCA does not carry the risks of an invasive procedure but clearly does not allow the option to intervene, and some cases may benefit from further invasive angiography for angioplasty. CTCA requires the patient to have a heart rate of around 60 beats per minute to ensure images are not degraded by motion – this can be difficult to achieve in some patients, especially in patients who cannot tolerate β-blockers. This examination may also not be possible if the patient cannot tolerate IV contrast (e.g., poor renal function or contrast allergy).

CT calcium scoring also uses ECG gating but does not use intravenous contrast. Calcium scoring gives information about the volume and density of coronary artery calcification to calculate a risk score for future MI and cardiac death. It can also be used to assess valvular calcification, which can be helpful in grading the severity of disease in cases where echocardiography is equivocal. However, it cannot assess for noncalcified plaque, does not provide as much anatomical information as CTCA and doesn't provide any functional information.

CARDIAC MAGNETIC RESONANCE

Cardiac magnetic resonance (CMR) is increasingly common. It has a number of advantages:

1. It is noninvasive.
2. It does not expose the patient to ionizing radiation.
3. It can be gated by an ECG trace, so as to produce detailed still images from each stage of the cardiac cycle. These images can be used to produce video sequences of the heart in motion.

Depending on which imaging sequences are used, MRI has a number of uses in the assessment of:

1. Ischaemic heart disease. Myocardial perfusion and scar (infarcted) tissue can be assessed using contrast techniques. Myocardial function before and after pharmacological stress can be assessed.
2. Cardiomyopathy. Particularly useful in the assessment of the degree of myocardial fibrosis and occasionally in rare diseases associated with deposition of proteins or lipids into the myocardium (e.g., amyloidosis or Fabry disease).
3. Congenital heart disease.
4. Valvular heart disease.
5. Myocarditis.
6. Aortic disease.

Possible contraindications include:

1. Permanent pacemaker or implantable cardioverter defibrillator (ICD), or temporary pacing wires – modern pacemakers are usually 'MRI conditional'. This means patients can undergo MRI if certain specific conditions are met (usually this requires a technician to download diagnostic information from the pacemaker or ICD before and after the scan and for the device mode to be adjusted for the scan itself).
2. Intracerebral clips.
3. Metallic foreign bodies – may be an absolute or relative contraindication depending on nature, location of the foreign body and how long it has been present. Orthopaedic metalwork is generally not a contraindication.
4. Severe claustrophobia.

CARDIAC CATHETERIZATION

Although CTCA is now the most frequently performed procedure for the assessment of coronary artery disease, this invasive investigation is the gold standard for luminal assessment of the coronary arteries and assessment of obstructive disease. Invasive angiography has better temporal and spatial resolution than CTCA at present.

Technique

Access to the left side of the heart is gained by a peripheral artery (e.g., right radial or femoral artery).

Access to the right side of the heart (right heart catheterization) is gained by a large vein (e.g., right antecubital fossa, femoral or internal jugular vein).

The vessel is punctured using a large hollow (Seldinger) needle and a wire is passed through the needle. The needle is then removed, and a sheath is passed over the wire. Using a long radio-opaque guide-wire, hollow catheters can then be passed through the sheath to the heart and inserted into the desired chamber or vessel, where a number of investigations may be carried out:

- The pressure in the chamber or vessel can be recorded.
- Oxygen saturation of the blood can be measured at different locations.
- Radiopaque contrast can be injected via the catheter to provide information, depending on the location of the catheter. For example, if in the aortic root (aortography), the size and tortuosity of the aortic root can be seen by the outline of contrast within it, and aortic regurgitation can be detected.

Left heart catheterization and coronary angiography

Indications

This can be indicated for patients who have:

- Confirmed or suspected coronary heart disease, e.g., positive exercise test or myocardial perfusion scan, a good history of and multiple risk factors for ischaemic heart disease.
- Valvular heart disease.
- Previous cardiac arrest.
- Heart failure.
- Occupational reasons – for patients who have chest pain, even if noninvasive tests are negative (e.g., airline pilots).

Note that the list of indications is more complicated, but you only need to have a general idea of the common indications.

Patient preparation

The following must be completed prior to the procedure:

- A detailed history to ensure that the indications are appropriate and that the patient has no other serious diseases that may affect the decision to proceed. Any history of allergy to iodine must be noted.
- Examination to ensure that the patient is well enough.
- The procedure and its risks must be carefully explained to the patient.
- Informed consent is obtained.

- Peripheral pulses must all be felt for and their absence or presence noted. If the femoral approach is to be used, the groin area will need to be shaved just before the procedure.

Left ventriculography

This assesses left-ventricular cavity size and function and mitral regurgitation. Contrast is injected rapidly to fill the left ventricle. X-ray images are obtained to visualize left-ventricular contractility and the direction in which contrast is ejected from the left ventricle.

Coronary angiography

The left and right coronary ostia are located in turn and contrast is gently injected into the arteries. Several images are obtained of each artery from different angles so a detailed picture of the anatomy and patency of the arteries can be obtained. Images are recorded using fluoroscopy (X-ray video recording). See Figs. 12.1 and 12.2 for images of normal coronary arteries and a coronary stenosis, respectively.

Complications of coronary angiography

The average mortality or serious complication rate of coronary angiography is 1/1000 cases. The following complications may occur:

- Haemorrhage from the arterial puncture site – more common from a femoral approach compared to a radial approach. Firm pressure should be applied to the site of bleeding; rarely, operative repair is necessary. Patients should all have a clotting screen performed preprocedure to reduce risk of this.
- Formation of a pseudoaneurysm – this results from weakening of the femoral artery wall and may require surgical repair.
- Infection of the puncture site or (rarely) septicaemia. Blood cultures and intravenous antibiotics may be required.
- Thrombosis of the artery used – this results in a cold white or blue foot or hand if there is no collateral supply. This necessitates urgent peripheral angiography and referral to the vascular surgeons.
- Contrast reaction – ranging from mild urticaria and pyrexia to anaphylactic shock.
- Arrhythmias – these may occur during the angiography due to coronary spasm, dissection or occlusion by the catheter. Any arrhythmia may occur but ventricular arrhythmias are more common.
- Pericardial tamponade – rare and occurs as a result of coronary artery tear or left-ventricular tear. The patient becomes acutely cyanosed and hypotensive. Pericardial aspiration is required urgently.
- Displacement of atherosclerotic fragments, which embolize distally, may result in myocardial infarction, stroke, ischaemic toes, etc.
- Death.

HINTS AND TIPS

Coronary angiography is mandatory before a patient can undergo a coronary artery bypass graft (CABG) operation. It provides detailed information on the severity and location of coronary disease, without which surgery cannot be undertaken. Older patients undergoing valve replacement surgery also have coronary angiography before surgery to exclude coexistent coronary artery disease. If this is found, CABG may be undertaken at the same time as valve replacement.

Right heart catheterization

A catheter can be passed to measure pressures in the right atrium, right ventricle and pulmonary arteries. A balloon tip on the end can be 'wedged' into the pulmonary artery to obtain the 'wedge' pulmonary artery pressure, an approximation of left atrial filling pressure, useful in some critically ill patients. Cardiac shunts can be identified by measuring the oxygen saturations in different parts of the heart, and thermodilution techniques (where cold fluid is injected and the rate of change of temperature with time can be used to calculate blood flow) can measure cardiac output.

RADIONUCLIDE IMAGING

Myocardial perfusion imaging

This investigation uses radiolabelled agents (e.g., technetium-99m or thallium-201), which are taken up by the myocardium proportional to local myocardial blood flow. If the image early after stress demonstrates areas of reduced uptake and the later image demonstrates normal uptake in the same areas, this suggests the presence of reversible ischaemia. It is more sensitive and specific than exercise testing alone but much more resource-intensive.

Methods of stressing the heart

Wherever possible, exercise should be used to create actual physiological stress.

For patients who are unable to exercise due to poor mobility, peripheral vascular disease or respiratory disease, pharmacological agents may be used to mimic physiological stress. (Patients who have severe aortic stenosis or cardiac failure should, in general, not have stress testing.)

The commonly used agents for pharmacological stress are:

- Dipyridamole – this blocks the reabsorption of adenosine into the cells, increasing intravascular adenosine concentrations. Adenosine is a powerful vasodilator and vasodilates normal coronary arteries but not diseased coronary arteries. It therefore redistributes blood flow away from diseased vessels. This relative hypoperfusion of diseased areas is picked up by radionuclide myocardial imaging.

- Adenosine – a direct infusion of adenosine may be used.
- Dobutamine – mimics exercise by increasing heart rate and myocardial contractility.

Note that both dipyridamole and adenosine are contraindicated in patients who have bronchospasm.

Multigated acquisition scanning

Multigated acquisition (MUGA) scanning is a radionuclide technique for evaluating cardiac function. Technetium-99m label is applied to the patient's red blood cells. The amount of radioactivity detected within the left ventricle is proportional to its volume, and its degree of contraction will affect this. The imaging of the cardiac blood pool is synchronized to the ECG trace. Images throughout hundreds of cardiac cycles are recorded and an overall assessment of the left-ventricular ejection fraction can be made using the averaged values for end-systolic and end-diastolic volume. This is used less often than in the past, but it remains superior to echocardiography for the accurate assessment of ejection fraction.

Positron emission tomography

Positron emission tomography uses radionuclides, such as 18F-fluorodeoxyglucose, rubidium-82 and nitrogen-13 ammonia, to provide images of the metabolic processes or perfusion of the myocardium. It is expensive, but 18F-fluorodeoxyglucose can be used to assess myocardial viability or endocarditis when conventional techniques have given equivocal results.

● Chapter Summary

- Exercise ECG has been superseded by CT coronary angiography as a first-line test to provide evidence for suspected angina. However, when used judiciously, it can still provide useful information with regard to risk.
- Echocardiography is commonly used for the diagnosis and assessment of valvular disease and to diagnose and assess severity of heart failure. Stress echocardiography also has a role in assessing coronary artery disease.
- Cardiac catheterization is the gold standard for assessing coronary artery disease and allows for percutaneous intervention at the same time, if suitable. However, there are low rates of significant risks involved with this procedure.
- MRI does not expose the patient to ionizing radiation and can provide detailed cross-sectional images of the heart and great vessels to evaluate congenital anomalies, problems with the great vessels and inflammatory/infiltrative diseases of the myocardium. Contrast also allows the assessment of myocardial perfusion and infarction.
- Radionuclide imaging is decreasing in use due to improvements in other cross-sectional imaging techniques and due to its cost and radiation exposure, although it can still be useful in selected cases.
- A detailed understanding of these investigations is important to select the most likely investigation to be useful, to prepare the patient for what the test involves, and to allow timely treatment and judicious use of resources.

Section 2

PRESENTING COMPLAINTS

History and examination of the cardiovascular system

5

This chapter will cover some basic principles of history and examination. These will be elaborated on in subsequent chapters.

HISTORY

Presenting complaint

As with any history, you should let the patient tell you the natural history of the complaint, but symptoms you should specifically ask about that are relevant to the cardiovascular system include:

- Chest pain.
- Shortness of breath, orthopnoea and paroxysmal nocturnal dyspnoea.
- Oedema/leg swelling.
- Palpitation.
- Syncope (fainting) or dizziness.

Past medical history

Important past medical conditions to note include:

- Ischaemic heart disease (e.g., myocardial infarction and angina) and any previous interventions, including angioplasty, coronary artery bypass graft (CABG), etc.
- Hypertension.
- Dyslipidaemia/high cholesterol.
- Diabetes mellitus.
- Any pacemakers or other implantable devices.
- Other vascular diseases (e.g., stroke/transient ischaemic attack, peripheral vascular disease).
- Rheumatic fever.
- Renal disease.

Social history

It is particularly important to ask regarding smoking history (as an atherosclerotic risk factor) and regarding alcohol intake (alcohol has a toxic effect on the myocardium). Recreational drug use may also be relevant (cocaine may cause vasospasm or myocardial infarction, injecting drug users are at risk of infective endocarditis).

Family history

Ask whether there is any incidence of the following diseases in close relatives:

- Myocardial infarction – a positive family history for myocardial infarction is regarded as <55 years for a male first-degree relative and <65 years for a female first-degree relative.
- Stroke.
- Angina.
- Cardiomyopathy or sudden cardiac death.

CLINICAL NOTES

If the history is consistent with any form of cardiovascular disease, it is useful to make a list of risk factors for atherosclerosis that the patient does and does not have. This can help to formulate a management plan tailored specifically to that individual patient.

Review of systems

Remember to review the other systems:

- Respiratory system – cough, sputum or haemoptysis may occur in a patient with pulmonary oedema. A dry cough is a side effect of angiotensin-converting enzyme (ACE) inhibitors.
- Gastrointestinal system – abdominal (particularly epigastric) pain or retrosternal 'heart burn' might be caused by a myocardial infarction/ischaemia. Ascites, nausea and abdominal discomfort may be the result of heart failure.
- Genitourinary system – diabetes mellitus and diuretic therapy may cause urinary frequency. Nocturia is common in heart failure.

CLINICAL EXAMINATION

Before beginning your examination, it is important to introduce yourself to the patient, gain consent and ensure they are adequately exposed. The patient should be seated at 45 degrees, if possible, and the whole upper body exposed.

General appearance

Note from the end of the bed the general appearance of the patient. Think about whether they look comfortable or are in pain. The patient may be obviously short of breath, pale or cyanosed (blue tinge to the skin). Make a note of any oxygen masks or intravenous infusions that the patient is receiving. You may also hear the clicking sound of a mechanical heart valve replacement.

Hands and arms

Both hands should be inspected on the anterior and posterior aspects. Signs that may be present in the hands are shown in Table 5.1.

CLINICAL NOTES

Fingernail clubbing is an important sign of disease and should always be checked for. It progresses as follows:

1. Increased fluctuation of the nail bed only.
2. Loss of the normal angle at the base of the nail.
3. Increased convexity of the nail fold.
4. Clubbed or 'drumstick' appearance of the fingertip.

Radial pulse

Palpate the radial pulse with the tips of the fingers and gently compress the radial artery against the distal radius. The radial pulse is used to assess heart rate and rhythm. The pulse character and volume, however, are best assessed at the carotid artery. The rate should be counted for about 30 seconds and then doubled to give a rate per minute. A normal pulse is between 60 and 100 beats per minute (bpm). Anything outside this range is termed bradycardia (<60 bpm) or tachycardia (>100 bpm). The rhythm may be:

- Regular: normal rhythm; remember sinus arrhythmia is normal (an increased rate during inspiration).
- Regularly irregular: commonly caused by ectopic systolic beats or second-degree heart block.
- Irregularly irregular: usually caused by atrial fibrillation, but an ECG is required to confirm this.

Radioradial delay is delay of one radial pulse compared with the other. Radiofemoral delay is delay of the femoral pulse compared with the radial. These findings are usually caused by coarctation of the aorta but may be seen in other conditions (e.g., subclavian artery stenosis, aortic dissection).

Checking for a collapsing pulse (see later) is also often performed at the wrist. The flats of the examiner's fingers should be placed over the radial artery and the arm raised above the patient's head. A positive result is a bounding pulse, which rapidly falls – a so-called 'water hammer' pulse. It is worthwhile

---

Table 5.1 Examination of the hands

Area	Sign observed	Diagnostic inference
Nails	Clubbing (loss of the angle at the base of the nail). normal / gap present / clubbed / loss of angle	Cardiac causes include subacute bacterial endocarditis and cyanotic congenital heart disease. Numerous other noncardiac causes including bronchial carcinoma, bronchial empyema/abscess, bronchiectasis, fibrosing alveolitis, mesothelioma, inflammatory bowel disease, and cirrhosis. May be idiopathic.
	Splinter haemorrhages (small, splinter-like, linear haemorrhages under the nail).	Infective endocarditis; commonly found after trauma to the nail, especially in manual workers.
Fingers	Tobacco stains.	Smoking.
	Osler nodes (red, painful, transient swellings on pulp of fingers and toes).	Infective endocarditis. Occur due to immune complex deposition.
Palms	Janeway lesions (small, erythematous macules on the thenar and hypothenar eminences that blanch under pressure).	Infective endocarditis. Occur due to septic emboli, forming microabscesses.
Dorsum	Tendon xanthomas (yellow nodules over the extensor tendons).	Familial hypercholesterolaemia.

checking with the patient before carrying out this manoeuvre, as some patients may find this uncomfortable, for example, if they have osteoarthritis of the shoulder.

Brachial pulse

Palpate just above the medial aspect of the antecubital fossa and compress the brachial artery against the humerus. If you have trouble, palpate the tendon of biceps and move your fingers medial to it. People will usually assess the brachial pulse OR the carotid pulse for the pulse volume and character.

Blood pressure

A measurement of blood pressure should be taken in all patients. As well as observing whether the blood pressure is high or low, think about whether the pulse pressure is normal, increased or decreased.

Face and neck

Signs that may be found in the face are shown in Table 5.2.

Carotid pulse

The carotid pulse should be palpated by pressing backwards at the medial border of the sternocleidomastoid and lateral to the thyroid cartilage. The two pulses should never be palpated at the same time or you will risk restricting the cerebral blood supply. The carotid pulse should be used to assess the character of the pulse (Fig. 5.1). This may be difficult, and it is important to note that there are variations of normal pulse character. The important pulses to note are:

- Slow rising pulse – the pulse rises slowly to a peak and then falls slowly. It is of small volume. This suggests aortic stenosis.
- Collapsing (water hammer) pulse – a rapid rise to the pulse and then a rapid fall. It is usually found in aortic regurgitation but may also be found in patent ductus arteriosus.
- Bisferiens pulse – two pressure peaks are seen (both in systole). This is indicative of aortic stenosis and regurgitation (mixed aortic valve disease).
- Pulsus alternans – alternating strong and weak pulses, indicative of severe left ventricular dysfunction.

Table 5.2 Examination of the face

Area	Sign observed	Diagnostic inference
Eyes	Corneal arcus (crescenteric opacity in the periphery of the cornea).	Common in old people; hypercholesterolaemia.
	Xanthelasma (lipid deposits above or below the eye).	Hypercholesterolaemia.
	Conjunctival pallor.	Anaemia.
	Exophthalmos (protrusion of the eyeballs from their sockets).	Thyrotoxicosis.
Retina	Microaneurysm (small vascular leaks caused by capillary occlusion).	Diabetes mellitus.
	Cotton-wool spots (white exudate around the macula).	Hypertension; arterial occlusion; retinal ischaemia.
	Flame-shaped haemorrhages (haemorrhage around optic disc spreading outwards).	Hypertension.
	Papilloedema (swelling of the optic nerve head caused by raised intracranial pressure).	Malignant hypertension; chronic meningitis; brain tumour or abscess; subdural haematoma.
	Roth spots.	Infective endocarditis.
Skin	Malar flush (peripheral cyanosis on cheeks).	Mitral stenosis.
Lips and tongue	Central cyanosis.	Pulmonary–systemic shunting; lung disease; haemoglobinopathy.
Palate	High arched.	Marfan syndrome.
Oral cavity	Poor dentition and oral hygiene.	May be more prone to infective endocarditis.

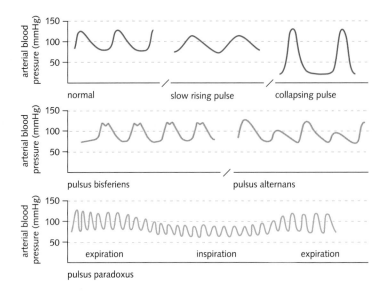

Fig. 5.1 Characters of pulses. The various pulse waveforms that can result are shown here.

- Pulsus paradoxus – a pulse that is weaker or even disappears on inspiration. Although blood pressure can decrease slightly during inspiration in a normal individual, if it drops by more than 10 mmHg, it is defined as pulsus paradoxus and is abnormal. It can occur in cardiac tamponade, constrictive pericarditis, status asthmaticus or a tension pneumothorax.

Pulse volume should also be assessed. Low volume implies a decreased stroke volume. High volume (sometimes described as bounding) may be caused by high cardiac output (e.g., anaemia, thyrotoxicosis, sepsis, etc.).

Jugular venous pressure

The internal jugular venous pressure (JVP) reflects right atrial pressure. The reasons behind this and the components of the normal waveform are described in Chapter 2. You should observe the maximum height of the internal jugular venous pulsation and the character of the pulsation as follows (Fig. 5.2):

1. Place the patient at a 45-degree angle with the neck supported to relax the neck muscles. You may need to turn the patient's head away from you slightly.
2. Observe the junction of the sternocleidomastoid with the clavicle and then look up along the route of the jugular veins to see if you can see visible pulsation.
3. Try palpating the pulse. If you can feel it, then the pulse is probably from the carotid artery. The venous pulse is also usually complex, with two impulses and a dominant inward

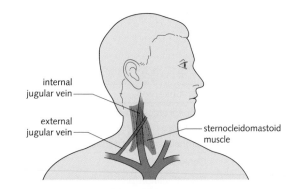

Fig. 5.2 The course of the internal and external jugular veins.

wave, whereas the arterial pulse is usually a simple dominant outward wave. The JVP decreases with inspiration under normal circumstances.

4. Measure the vertical height of the pulse from the manubriosternal angle (angle of Louis). This measurement is the JVP (in cmH$_2$O), which can be used to calculate right atrial pressure (by adding 5 cmH$_2$O to the JVP measurement).

The external jugular vein is often easier to see, as it is lateral to the sternocleidomastoid and more superficial. However, it is an unreliable indicator of central venous pressure. It contains valves and moves through many fascial planes, and so it is affected by

Table 5.3 Common abnormalities in JVP

Abnormality	Diagnostic inference
Dominant a wave	Pulmonary stenosis, pulmonary hypertension, tricuspid stenosis.
Cannon a wave	Complete beat block, paroxysmal nodal tachycardia, ventricular tachycardia.
Dominant v wave	Tricuspid regurgitation.
Absent x descent	Atrial fibrillation.
Exaggerated x descent	Cardiac tamponade, constrictive pericarditis.
Sharp y descent	Constrictive pericarditis, tricuspid regurgitation.
Slow y descent	Right atrial myxoma.

Normal JVP for reference.

compression from structures in the neck. Some common abnormalities of the JVP waveform are described in Table 5.3.

A raised JVP (pulsation >4 cm above the manubriosternal angle with the patient positioned at 45 degrees) is usually indicative of:

- Right heart failure.
- Superior vena cava obstruction (this also abolishes any pulsations).
- Intravascular volume overload (e.g., acute nephritis, excess fluid therapy).

If the JVP rises (rather than falls) on inspiration (Kussmaul sign), then consider:

- Constrictive pericarditis.
- Cardiac tamponade.
- Tension pneumothorax.

HINTS AND TIPS

Observing the JVP is a difficult clinical skill to master. Distinguishing the JVP from carotid pulsation is important. The JVP falls on inspiration, has a complicated waveform, fills from the top when occluded, is nonpalpable and is exaggerated by the hepatojugular reflex and the Valsalva manoeuvre.

If the JVP is not visible, you may attempt to elicit the hepatojugular reflex. This involves applying pressure over the liver, which should increase venous return, raise central venous pressure and cause the JVP to rise and become visible. If the internal jugular venous pulsation was originally so high that it was not visible in the neck (i.e., the venous pulse was above the level of the jaw), then this manoeuvre will not elicit any change.

Central venous pressure (and therefore right atrial pressure) can be measured more accurately by the placement of a central line in the internal jugular vein. Normal central venous pressure is 0 to 10 cmH$_2$O.

Thorax

Inspection

Thorough inspection of the thorax should include asking the patient to lift their arms. Look for scars (Fig. 5.3), chest wall deformities, abnormal pulsations and a pacemaker/implantable cardioverter-defibrillator (usually just below the clavicle on the left). Important scars to be aware of include a median sternotomy, lateral thoracotomy and mitral valvotomy scar (may be hidden under the breast in a female patient).

Palpation

The apex beat should be palpated first. The apex beat is defined as the most inferior-lateral point at which the cardiac impulse can

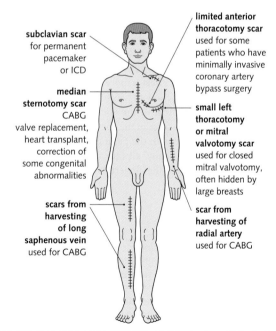

Fig. 5.3 Common scars related to cardiac surgery. Note that a larger left lateral thoracotomy is used for correction of coarctation and patent ductus arteriosus. *CABG,* coronary artery bypass grafting; *ICD,* implantable cardioverter defibrillator.

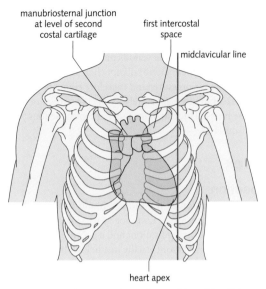

Fig. 5.4 Position of the apex beat. As a guide to identifying intercostal spaces, the second rib lies lateral to the manubriosternal angle; the second intercostal space is below this rib. The lateral position can also be described relative to the anterior axillary line and the mid-axillary line.

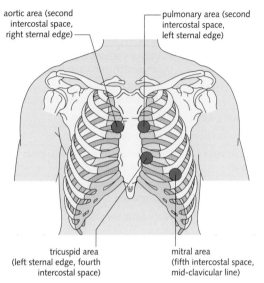

Fig. 5.5 Auscultatory areas. This shows where the valve sounds are best heard. These areas are not the surface markings of where the valves actually are.

be felt and is normally located in the left fifth intercostal space in the mid-clavicular line (Fig. 5.4). If the apex beat is displaced (usually inferolaterally), it generally indicates cardiac dilatation. In left ventricular hypertrophy, due to hypertension or aortic stenosis for example, the apex beat is more forceful. It is important to remember the distinction between ventricular dilatation (which causes displacement of the apex beat) and hypertrophy (which increases the force of the apex beat). The left sternal edge should be palpated with the palm of the hand for a right ventricular heave, and finally, all four valve areas (see later) should be palpated with the fingertips for thrills (palpable murmurs).

HINTS AND TIPS

The apex beat may be difficult to palpate in obese patients and in patients with emphysema or pleural/pericardial effusion. If the apex beat is completely absent on the left side of the precordium, consider checking the other side: the patient may have dextrocardia! This is something that may come up in medical student exams from time to time.

Auscultation

The stethoscope has two ends, the diaphragm (which has a flat membrane across it like a drum) and the bell. The diaphragm is better for listening to higher-pitched sounds; therefore it is best for hearing:

- First and second heart sounds.
- Third and fourth heart sounds.
- Systolic murmurs.
- Aortic diastolic murmurs (aortic incompetence).

The bell of the stethoscope is best for low-pitched sounds and is best for hearing the rumbling diastolic murmur of mitral stenosis. The bell should not be placed too tightly to the skin, as it will then function as a diaphragm.

There are certain areas where auscultation should be performed (Fig. 5.5); these are the areas where murmurs from heart valves are best heard.

Heart sounds

Auscultate the heart sounds while palpating the carotid pulse; this will allow you to determine where sounds are localized within the cardiac cycle. The heart sounds (both normal and abnormal) are discussed in Chapter 2.

Patients may also have prosthetic heart valve sounds if they have previously undergone valve replacement; this is discussed in Chapter 15 (Valvular Disease).

CLINICAL NOTES

S_3 occurs during ventricular filling and is a normal finding in some patients (e.g., young patients, athletes) but is often related to ventricular dilatation in adults (e.g., in cardiac failure). S_4 is almost always pathological and relates to a stiff, noncompliant ventricle.

Murmurs

Murmurs are additional sounds caused by turbulent blood flow at a valve or an abnormal communication within the heart. The presence of a murmur does not always indicate disease, and the intensity does not correlate with the severity of the lesion. The common murmurs that you are likely to encounter (and how to examine for them) are discussed in Chapter 10.

Lung bases

Use the stethoscope diaphragm to auscultate the bases of the lungs to check for signs of pulmonary oedema (i.e., fine crackles) or pleural effusion (absent breath sounds).

Abdomen

If there are any signs of heart failure, it may be useful to palpate the liver. An enlarged liver can occur due to venous congestion in heart failure affecting the right ventricle. In tricuspid regurgitation, the liver may be pulsatile.

Legs

Inspect for scars that may indicate previous vein harvesting for use in coronary artery bypass grafting.

It is important to always check the ankles for pitting oedema, which is a sign of heart failure. Gently press for at least 10 seconds on the skin over a bony landmark, such as the medial malleolus, and if pitting oedema is present, an imprint of your finger will be left after you remove it. You should comment on whether it is unilateral or bilateral and how far it extends up the legs. In patients who are in bed, sacral oedema may develop, so it is often useful to check while the patient is leaning forward for you to auscultate to their lung bases.

CARDIOVASCULAR EXAMINATION SUMMARY

Examination is best practised on real patients; for a template of examination and some of the signs you might find, see Table 5.4.

Table 5.4 Template for examination of the cardiovascular system

Wash your hands, introduce yourself to the patient, obtain consent and expose the patient. Position ideally supine at 45 degrees.	
General inspection	General appearance, oxygen, fluids, medications, etc.
Hands	Peripheral cyanosis, fingernail inspection (clubbing, splinter haemorrhages), tar staining, tendon xanthomata, Osler nodes and Janeway lesions. Feel temperature and check capillary refill time.
Radial pulse	Rate, rhythm, volume. Examine for radioradial and radiofemoral delay and for collapsing pulse.
Blood pressure	Note pulse pressure. Consider erect and supine measurements.
Face	Central cyanosis, conjunctival pallor, corneal arcus, xanthelasma, malar flush. Consider retinal examination for Roth spots (rarely carried out).
Neck	JVP (height and waveform), carotid pulse (character and volume).
Inspection of precordium	Scars, deformity, visible pulsation/heave.
Palpation of precordium	Apex beat position and character, left parasternal heave, thrills (palpable murmurs).
Auscultation of precordium	• Mitral area, tricuspid area, pulmonary area, aortic area. • Areas of murmur radiation – axilla (e.g., mitral regurgitation), carotids (e.g., aortic stenosis). • Manoeuvres to amplify diastolic murmurs.
Back	Auscultate lung bases for crepitations. Palpate for sacral oedema.
Abdomen	Palpate liver (for hepatomegaly and/or pulsation).
Legs	Peripheral pulses and ankle oedema.
Concluding remarks: Review of observation chart (if not done initially), appropriate investigations if present.	

● Chapter Summary

- As with any system, a comprehensive history is vital for diagnosis and to understand the patient's concerns.
- The main presenting complaints for cardiovascular disease include chest pain, breathlessness, peripheral oedema, palpitations, dizziness and syncope.
- Cardiovascular disease can present with a wide range of clinical signs. It is important to be methodical to avoid missing these.
- Certain elements of the cardiovascular examination can be very difficult (e.g., JVP inspection, auscultation of murmurs); repeated practice is necessary to become competent.

Chest pain is one of the most common presenting complaints, not just in cardiology but in medicine as a whole. There are many causes of chest pain. Some are life-threatening and require prompt diagnosis and treatment, while other causes are more benign.

DIFFERENTIAL DIAGNOSIS

The differential diagnosis of chest pain is diverse, as shown in Table 6.1. History taking is important to focus examination and investigation.

HINTS AND TIPS

In shingles (herpes zoster reactivation), chest pain can often present prior to the rash. It is useful to bear in mind if the patient describes unilateral burning/tingling pain from the back to the chest confined within a dermatome. Postherpetic neuralgia is also common.

Table 6.1 Differential diagnosis of chest pain (Red denotes potentially immediately life-threatening)

System	Pathology
Cardiac	Angina pectoris (myocardial ischaemia) Myocardial infarction Pericarditis/myocarditis Arrhythmia Prolapse of the mitral valve
Vascular	Aortic dissection Aortic aneurysm
Respiratory (most can be associated with pleuritic pain)	Pulmonary embolus/infarct Pneumothorax Pneumonia Pulmonary neoplasm
Gastrointestinal	Oesophagitis/oesophageal spasm Oesophageal tear/rupture Peptic ulcer Biliary disease Pancreatitis
Musculoskeletal	Musculoskeletal strain Rib fracture Costochondritis (Tietze syndrome)
Neurological	Herpes zoster (shingles) Nerve root compression by disc prolapse

HISTORY

If there is severe ongoing chest pain, signs of poor perfusion or haemodynamic instability, urgent action is required. History and examination will be more focused to allow timely investigation and management.

Nature of presenting complaint

In most cases, a detailed history of the patient's pain is vital. The mnemonic SOCRATES outlined in Table 6.2 is helpful initially. Time of onset and duration are important for ischaemic chest pain algorithms. Missing important points, such as onset, duration and exacerbating factors, does not only lose points in exams but can also miss the diagnosis, causing possible harm to the patient or unnecessary investigations.

In clinical practice, you will find your own way of taking a history smoothly. There is no need to stick to rigid structures, such as SOCRATES, once you are fluent. For example, radiation follows naturally from site of pain. Adapt your history to the patient and what they tell you about first. As with any system, starting with open questions identifies the patient's main concerns before narrowing the differential with closed questions.

Characteristics to help distinguish selected diagnoses are in Table 6.3.

COMMON PITFALLS

Do not use response to glyceryl trinitrate (GTN) to diagnose ischaemic chest pain, as this has been shown to be unreliable. Interestingly, oesophageal spasm, or indeed any muscular spasm, can be relieved by GTN, and ongoing chest pain not relieved by GTN can signify a myocardial infarction.

For an idea of symptom severity, previous and current 'exercise tolerance' clarifies the degree of deterioration. How far can they walk on the flat? On stairs/hills? Pain at a reproducible distance or effort is typical of angina.

Past medical history

This can provide clues including:

- History of ischaemic heart disease – increases risk of further ischaemic events. Even if the presentation is

Table 6.2 Evaluating the nature of chest pain (SOCRATES)

Site	Where is the pain (e.g., retrosternal, epigastric, interscapular, left or right)? Is it diffuse or localized?
Onset	When did the pain start? What was the patient doing at the time? Did it start gradually or suddenly?
Character	What is the quality of the pain (e.g., crushing/heavy, tight, sharp/stabbing, burning)?
Radiation	Does the pain go anywhere else? Neck/jaw/shoulders/arms? Back – from the chest to the back or vice versa?
Associated features	Associated symptoms (e.g., breathlessness, palpitations, nausea, sweating, change in colour).
Timing	Was the pain constant or intermittent? How long did it last?
Exacerbating and relieving factors	Did anything improve or worsen the pain (e.g., exertion, inspiration, food, posture, localized movement, emotion)?
Severity	Usually a numerical score (e.g., out of 10, 10 being the most severe pain ever experienced/imaginable).

Table 6.3 Classical characteristics of different types of chest pain

Characteristic	Myocardial ischaemia/ infarction	Pericarditis	Pleuritic pain	Oesophagitis/ reflux	Musculoskeletal	Aortic dissection
Quality	Crushing, heavy, dull ache, tight, bandlike	Sharp (may be dull or crushing)	Sharp	Specific to cause (e.g., burning, gnawing)	Usually sharp, although can be dull	Tearing, sharp, stabbing
Site	Central anterior chest, diffuse	Central anterior, left-sided	Anywhere in the chest, usually localized	Epigastric or retrosternal	Related to muscle involved	Retrosternal, interscapular
Radiation	Neck, jaw, arms left > right	Usually none, occasionally shoulder	Usually none	Specific to cause, occasionally throat	Related to muscle involved	Usually along the course of dissection
Exacerbating factors	Exertion, cold weather, anxiety	Recumbent position, deep inspiration	Deep inspiration, coughing, moving	Recumbent position, food, NSAIDs	Palpation of chest wall, movement by patient	Nil particular
Relieving factors	Rest (not in infarction), glyceryl trinitrate	Sitting forward, NSAIDs	Shallow breathing	Antacids	Resting affected muscles/joints	Nil particular
Associated features	Breathlessness; if infarction, can be associated with nausea, sweating and shock or syncope	Fever, recent viral illness (e.g., rash, arthralgia)	Cough, haemoptysis, breathlessness, fever with pneumonia/PE, shock with large volume PE	Can be associated with nausea and sweating	Other affected joints; the patient will usually look very well	Unequal radial and femoral pulse/BP; aortic regurgitation murmur may occur, end-organ symptoms (e.g., neuro deficit)

unrelated (e.g., sepsis or severe anaemia), the presence of chest pain in the context of preexisting coronary artery disease may signify an inability to compensate and resultant myocardial ischaemia (e.g., type 2 myocardial infarction (MI)).

- Risk factors for ischaemic heart disease (e.g., diabetes mellitus, hypertension, dyslipidaemia, other vascular disease).
- Previous arrhythmia may indicate a propensity to arrhythmia, which may cause decompensation and myocardial ischaemia.
- Hypertension is also an important risk factor for aortic dissection.
- Pericarditis might be preceded by a prodromal viral illness.
- Recent cardiothoracic surgery can cause many complications, including pericarditis, mediastinitis, arrhythmia, myocardial ischaemia, pulmonary embolus and pneumonia.
- Pulmonary embolus risk is increased in patients with previous venous thromboembolism, active malignancy, a recent operation or illness, or other causes of prolonged inactivity.
- Other preexisting diseases may provide the diagnosis. Previous reflux with typical symptoms of reflux would be reassuring of the same process.
- Protracted recent vomiting could increase the risk of oesophageal tear or rupture.

Medication history, family history and social history

Other risk factors for ischaemic heart disease include a positive family history and smoking. Heavy alcohol intake and nonsteroidal antiinflammatory drug (NSAID) ingestion may predispose to gastritis and peptic ulcer disease.

CLINICAL NOTES

A positive family history of early ischaemic heart disease is present if there is ischaemic heart disease in first-degree male relatives <55 years old or first-degree female relatives <65 years old.

EXAMINATION

The aim of examination is to identify the severity of the condition immediately, find signs to support the underlying diagnosis and refute other differentials or place them in a sensible order, and to identify complications. Points to note are detailed in Fig. 6.1.

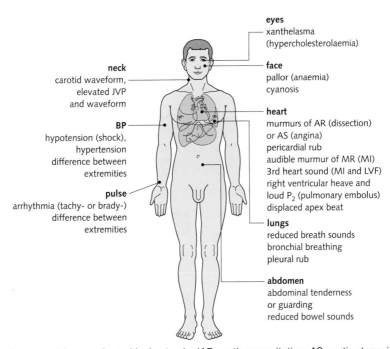

eyes
xanthelasma
(hypercholesterolaemia)

face
pallor (anaemia)
cyanosis

neck
carotid waveform,
elevated JVP
and waveform

heart
murmurs of AR (dissection)
or AS (angina)
pericardial rub
audible murmur of MR (MI)
3rd heart sound (MI and LVF)
right ventricular heave and
loud P_2 (pulmonary embolus)
displaced apex beat

BP
hypotension (shock),
hypertension
difference between
extremities

pulse
arrhythmia (tachy- or brady-)
difference between
extremities

lungs
reduced breath sounds
bronchial breathing
pleural rub

abdomen
abdominal tenderness
or guarding
reduced bowel sounds

Fig. 6.1 Points to note when examining a patient with chest pain. (*AR,* aortic regurgitation; *AS,* aortic stenosis; *BP,* blood pressure; *LVF,* left ventricular failure; *MI,* myocardial infarction; *MR,* mitral regurgitation.)

Observations, including heart rate, blood pressure, respiratory rate, oxygen saturations and temperature, are important to risk-stratify patients and inform the differential diagnosis.

The following points are specific to this chapter and omit differentials of examination findings that would not cause chest pain.

Inspection

- Shock (e.g., pallor, sweating, poor perfusion) – points more towards the life-threatening causes outlined in red earlier.
- Cyanosis, tachypnoea or increased work of breathing – may indicate MI leading to left ventricular failure or a respiratory cause.
- Vomiting – suggests MI or a gastrointestinal cause.
- Coughing – suggests a respiratory cause or, less commonly, left ventricular failure.

Cardiovascular system

- Perfusion of tissues is the best indicator of how well the cardiovascular system is functioning. This is in the form of end-organ perfusion, e.g., skin (capillary refill time, peripheral colour and warmth), brain (confusion/reduced consciousness), etc.
- Pulse and blood pressure – is there an abnormal rhythm, rate or character? A slow rising pulse may be due to severe aortic stenosis causing angina. A collapsing pulse due to aortic regurgitation is a classic but rare complication of aortic dissection. Is there hypotension/hypertension? Uncommonly, inequalities of the pulses or blood pressure between extremities will be found and may indicate aortic dissection.
- Conjunctival pallor could suggest anaemia, which may exacerbate angina.
- Oral mucous membranes can demonstrate central cyanosis due to hypoxia or can be dry due to tachypnoea or intravascular volume depletion.
- Raised jugular venous pressure – right heart failure as a result of MI or pulmonary embolus (PE).
- Carotid pulse – useful to palpate to check if a murmur is systolic or diastolic. If there is such significant hypotension that only large central pulses are palpable, urgent action is required!
- Displaced apex beat in the context of chest pain may be a result of dilatation/aneurysm from previous MI. A nondisplaced heaving apex beat may suggest preexisting hypertensive heart disease. A parasternal right ventricular heave may suggest a PE.
- Auscultation – pericardial rub suggests pericarditis; a pansystolic murmur may be heard in mitral regurgitation as a result of MI; a third heart sound may be found as a result of

left ventricular failure; angina caused by aortic stenosis would reveal an ejection systolic murmur; an early diastolic murmur may be heard in aortic regurgitation complicating dissection.
- Bilateral crepitations may suggest left ventricular failure, and sacral oedema/peripheral pitting oedema may be due to right ventricular or biventricular failure.
- Leg pulses may be delayed and diminished or absent in aortic dissection, and lower limb perfusion may be compromised.

CLINICAL NOTES

Interestingly, there is often no significant finding on examination of patients with angina. There may be signs of risk factors for angina (e.g., xanthomata/xanthelasma, tar staining/smell of tobacco, the heave of hypertensive heart disease and fingertip marks from BM testing or upper arm glucose monitors in diabetes).

Respiratory system

- Unequal hemithorax expansion – may be present in pneumonia and pneumothorax.
- Abnormal percussion note – dullness may be present in pneumonia and hyperresonance in pneumothorax.
- Bronchial breathing and unilateral crepitations – suggestive of pneumonia.
- Pleural rub – pleural irritation (e.g., pneumonia, pulmonary infarction secondary to PE).

Gastrointestinal system

- Abdominal tenderness or guarding – looking for causes of high abdominal/lower chest pain.
- Scanty/absent bowel sounds – abdominal pathology (e.g., peritonitis due to perforated peptic ulcer is a rare cause of lower chest pain).

INVESTIGATIONS

See Table 6.4 for urgent investigations; those lower in the table would only be considered if there was clinical concern.

Blood tests

- Cardiac biomarkers – Serial high-sensitivity troponins are used to diagnose or rule out MI. However, troponin may be elevated in other conditions, such as severe sepsis, major pulmonary embolism or acute kidney injury, and may reflect myocardial injury rather than infarction.

Table 6.4 First-line tests to exclude a chest pain emergency

Tests	Diagnosis
ECG	Demonstrates ST elevation in an anatomical territory in STEMI. ST depression or T wave inversion in an anatomical territory may signify NSTEMI if troponin is raised or ischaemia if it is not raised. Widespread concave ST elevation in pericarditis. May show signs of PE including right heart strain if large clot load.
Biochemical markers	Significant elevation usually suggests MI. Often protocols require repeat testing at 3 or 6 hours if initially mildly elevated.
CXR	Signs of LVF, pneumothorax or consolidation. Widened mediastinum can be seen with aortic dissection.
Arterial blood gases	In unwell patients, this will quantify hypoxaemia and severity of hypoperfusion (metabolic acidosis) rather than provide direct evidence for PE, LVF or pneumonia.
CT scan	Urgently required if aortic dissection or PE is suspected.

LVF, left ventricular failure; *NSTEMI,* non-ST elevation myocardial infarction; *PE,* pulmonary embolus; *STEMI,* ST elevation myocardial infarction.

- Arterial blood gases – useful for quick results in unwell patients. Hypoxia can be seen in pulmonary oedema, PE and other respiratory causes. Hypocapnoea can be seen with tachypnoea when lung gas exchange is preserved. Lactic acidosis is concerning for tissue hypoperfusion. Other electrolyte disturbances may contribute to arrhythmia and can cause myocardial ischaemia.
- Full blood count – anaemia may exacerbate angina; raised white cell count may suggest inflammation or infection.
- Renal function and electrolytes – may be abnormal due to cardiogenic shock and hypoperfusion, vomiting, diuretic therapy, etc. and will be important in decisions regarding further therapy.
- Liver function tests and amylase may be deranged in certain gastrointestinal pathologies.
- Thyroid function tests may provide an exacerbating (increased output or arrhythmic) cause of angina.
- Although lipids and glucose are less immediately important, if this is ischaemic chest pain, these will be important risk factors to tackle in ongoing management.

Electrocardiography

Relevant findings may include:

- ST elevation in contiguous leads in the same anatomical territory may indicate acute ST-elevation myocardial infarction (STEMI). Very rarely it can be due to Prinzmetal angina (MI secondary to coronary vasospasm).
- New bundle branch block (BBB) in the presence of typical chest pain may indicate MI; however, this is often difficult to diagnose unless recent ECGs without BBB are instantly accessible. The results of cardiac markers may help to make the diagnosis.
- ST depression or T wave inversion in an anatomical distribution in the presence of typical chest pain suggests non-STEMI or myocardial ischaemia. (Remember ST depression may be reciprocal change in STEMI.)

- Fully developed Q waves in an anatomical territory – indicates an old MI or late presentation of STEMI.
- Nonterritorial widespread 'saddle-shaped' ST elevation is typical of pericarditis.
- Arrhythmia causing myocardial ischaemia or as a result of cardiac or pulmonary disease.
- Rarely, acute aortic dissection can cause STEMI if it leads to coronary artery dissection (usually of the right coronary artery).

It is worth bearing in mind that there are other causes of ST elevation, including left ventricular aneurysm (deep Q waves and ST elevation in an anatomical distribution) and rarer causes, such as Brugada syndrome (ST elevation and partial right BBB in V1–2 with a 'coved' morphology) and ventricular pacing (similar to left BBB morphology with pacing spikes).

There are other causes of ST depression less pertinent to chest pain. Digoxin can cause 'reverse tick' ST depression. Hypokalaemia can cause widespread ST depression with T wave flattening/inversion and other changes. Other causes include right ventricular hypertrophy and right BBB morphology.

COMMON PITFALLS

Posterior ST elevation MIs can be easily missed if it is not appreciated that they cause anterior horizontal ST depression, along with dominant R waves (equivalent of Q waves) and prominent upright T waves.

The classic changes in PE are:

- Sinus tachycardia (most commonly seen).
- Anterior T wave inversion (common).
- Atrial fibrillation.
- Tall P waves in lead II (right atrial dilatation).
- Right axis deviation and right BBB.
- S wave in lead I, Q wave in lead III and inverted T wave in lead III (the classic but relatively uncommon, S1Q3T3 pattern).

An exercise 12-lead ECG or computed tomography (CT) coronary angiogram may be performed in intermittent stable exertional chest pain to risk stratify suspected angina if there are no contraindications. For this and other investigations in stable chest pain, see Chapter 12.

Chest X-ray

Signs include:

- Signs of heart failure – cardiomegaly, pulmonary oedema, effusions, upper venous diversion, septal lines.
- Pulmonary abnormalities corresponding to respiratory causes.
- Oligaemic lung fields in PE – this is rarely seen and unreliable; CT pulmonary angiography (CTPA) is required if PE is suspected.
- Pericardial effusion – better assessed with echocardiography.
- Mediastinal widening in aortic dissection.

Echocardiography

This may reveal:

- Regional myocardial dysfunction – a feature of infarction or ischaemia, although less useful in the acute setting.
- Pericardial effusion – suggests pericarditis or dissection.
- Aortic dissection with false lumen.
- Valve or septal abnormalities.
- Evidence of right heart strain in an unwell patient with suspected PE.

Computed tomography

A CT aortogram may be acutely required to diagnose aortic dissection. CTPA is a sensitive and specific test for PE. These are rapid tests and can also identify other causes of pain (e.g., a pulmonary cause). Increasingly, CT coronary angiography is being used to diagnose or exclude coronary artery disease.

Ventilation/perfusion scan

This is only sensitive for PE in selected patients (e.g., anaphylaxis to IV contrast) and is rarely performed now.

Angiography, myocardial perfusion imaging or stress echocardiography

For further information about both acute and stable chest pain, see Chapter 12.

NEW ONSET CENTRAL CHEST PAIN AT REST IN AN ILL PATIENT

This is clearly a medical emergency requiring rapid diagnosis and treatment. It is necessary to rapidly distinguish between:

- MI (high risk of hypoperfusion, arrhythmia and arrest).
- Crescendo angina (high risk of MI).
- Arrhythmia.
- Pericarditis.
- Dissection of the thoracic aorta.
- Mediastinitis secondary to oesophageal rupture.
- PE.

CLINICAL NOTES

Mediastinitis is uncommon but should be considered where there is a possibility of oesophageal leak, most likely after endoscopy or oesophageal surgery. Occasional oesophageal rupture occurs following protracted vomiting and is known as Boerhaave syndrome.

These are described in detail in the relevant chapters later in the book.

Therefore, urgent actions include:

- Rapid clinical assessment.
- Intravenous access with blood tests including troponin.
- ECG.
- Chest X-ray.
- Further imaging if required.

Myocardial infarction/ischaemia

RED FLAG

ST elevation MI usually indicates proximal occlusion of a major coronary artery. If untreated, myocardial necrosis begins within 30 minutes. Urgent restoration of coronary blood flow (reperfusion) prevents further myocardial damage and improves prognosis. Immediate treatment is detailed below. Primary percutaneous coronary intervention (PCI) is the preferred reperfusion option; thrombolysis is still used within 12 hours of pain onset if PCI is not available within 120 minutes of when thrombolysis could be given. This is discussed further in Chapter 12.

Immediate treatment for STEMI and non-STEMI includes (follow local acute coronary syndrome protocols):

- Targeted O_2 therapy if SaO_2 <90%; aim for 94% to 98%.
- Cardiac rhythm monitoring.
- Glyceryl trinitrate.
- Intravenous opiate analgesia titrated to pain and intravenous antiemetic.
- Aspirin 300 mg orally.
- Second antiplatelet by local protocol (clopidogrel, ticagrelor, prasugrel).
- Transfer to specialist cardiac unit.
- If not transferring direct to primary percutaneous coronary intervention (PCI) or considering thrombolysis,

antithrombotic by local protocol (fondaparinux, low-molecular-weight heparin).

- Local protocols regarding further treatment.

RED FLAG

If chest pain is related to extreme tachyarrhythmia or bradyarrhythmia, this is an adverse sign signifying resultant ischaemia and urgent action is required as outlined in the Resuscitation Council algorithms in Chapter 14.

Chapter Summary

- In a patient presenting with chest pain, a clear history provides more information than examination to narrow the differential diagnosis and will ensure appropriate investigations are chosen. This is achieved through careful consideration of the differential diagnoses and their features.
- Examination will indicate how unwell a patient is and may provide additional important clues.
- Information gathered directs immediate investigation. Potentially life-threatening causes to look for (or rule out) include acute coronary syndrome, arrhythmia-related myocardial ischaemia, PE, pneumothorax, aortic dissection and oesophageal rupture.
- Urgent treatment of life-threatening causes reduces risk of death and serious complications.
- Treatment of STEMI not only involves some universal principles but also involves carefully planned protocols suited to the setting (e.g., proximity to cardiology intervention units); therefore, familiarize yourself with local protocols.

UKMLA Conditions

Acute coronary syndromes
Aortic dissection
Arrhythmias
Ischaemic heart disease
Myocardial infarction
Pericardial disease
Pulmonary embolism
Unstable angina

UKMLA Presentations

Chest pain
Cough

Breathlessness and peripheral oedema

Shortness of breath, also known as dyspnoea, is an uncomfortable awareness of one's own breathing. It is a normal sensation on heavy exertion and considered abnormal only when it occurs at a level of physical activity not normally expected to cause a problem. This is a common presenting complaint with a number of possible underlying causes – the majority are cardiovascular or respiratory in nature.

Peripheral oedema is caused by an increase in extracellular fluid. This fluid follows gravity and therefore tends to affect the ankles initially. Ankle swelling is indicative of oedema if there is no local acute or chronic traumatic cause. Oedema may be a feature of generalized fluid retention or obstruction of fluid drainage.

DIFFERENTIAL DIAGNOSIS

There is a wide range of differential diagnoses for patients presenting with dyspnoea or breathlessness (Table 7.1).

Similarly, peripheral oedema may be the result of a number of different pathologies (Table 7.2).

In the patient presenting with dyspnoea and ankle swelling, the main diagnosis of concern is heart failure (see Chapter 13). There are many causes of cardiac failure, including:

- Ischaemic heart disease.
- Hypertension.
- Valvular disease.
- Cardiomyopathies.
- Chronic lung disease (cor pulmonale).
- Pulmonary embolism (PE).
- Primary pulmonary hypertension.

The multitude of underlying causes means that a detailed cardiovascular and respiratory history and examination is needed to identify possible causes of the patient's symptoms.

HISTORY

When taking a history from a patient presenting with dyspnoea, be sure to include:

- Timing – is the dyspnoea acute or chronic? Continuous or intermittent?
- Exacerbating and relieving factors – exertion, lying flat (orthopnoea), sleep (the patient may describe paroxysmal nocturnal dyspnoea – waking up gasping for breath).

Table 7.1 Differential diagnosis for patients presenting with dyspnoea

Diagnosis	Features of breathlessness
Pulmonary oedema	Acute or chronic; exacerbated by lying flat (orthopnoea) or patient may be woken at night by episodes of severe breathlessness (paroxysmal nocturnal dyspnoea); may have cough with pink frothy sputum.
Ischaemic heart disease	Acute; exacerbated by exertion and cold weather, relieved by rest and nitrates; associated with chest pain and sweating.
Chronic obstructive pulmonary disease (COPD)	Chronic; exacerbated by respiratory infections; may be associated with cough and sputum; almost always associated with smoking.
Interstitial lung disease	Chronic; no real exacerbating/relieving factors; may have history of exposure to occupational dusts or allergens.
Pulmonary embolus	Acute; associated pleuritic chest pain and/or haemoptysis.
Pneumothorax	Acute; pleuritic chest pain.
Pneumonia	Acute; may be systemic features of infection; may be associated with cough, sputum and pleuritic chest pain.
Lung malignancy	May be associated with history of weight loss, cough, haemoptysis and pleuritic chest pain.
Anaemia	History of blood loss, change in bowel habit, epigastric pain, peptic ulcers, recent operations, etc.
Anxiety	Associated with stress; may have associated perioral or peripheral paraesthesia.
Pregnancy	Gradual progression due to splinting of diaphragm (and sometimes anaemia).
Obesity	Gradual progression due to effort of moving and restriction of chest wall.
Trauma/musculoskeletal	Shortness of breath due to pain.

Table 7.2 Differential diagnosis for patients presenting with oedema

Diagnosis	Notes
Cardiac failure	Due to increased sodium retention secondary to activation of the renin-angiotensin-aldosterone system (RAAS).
Hypoalbuminaemia	Loss of fluid from the intravascular space due to low oncotic pressure within the capillaries.
Hepatic failure/ cirrhosis	Due to a number of mechanisms: hypoalbuminaemia, peripheral vasodilation and activation of RAAS with sodium retention.
Renal failure	Reduction in sodium excretion, resulting in water retention.
Other	Drugs (including corticosteroids, calcium channel blockers), venous disease, obesity, lymphoedema.

- If there is cough – ask for details of sputum production. Yellow-green sputum suggests pneumonia or exacerbation of chronic obstructive pulmonary disease (COPD); pink frothy sputum suggests left ventricular failure (LVF); haemoptysis can be a feature of PE or malignancy.
- If there is wheeze – this is suggestive of airways obstruction (i.e., asthma, COPD or, less commonly, neoplasm of the lung causing airway obstruction). Wheeze can also occur during LVF.
- If there is chest pain – ask for details of location, nature of pain, radiation, etc.
- If there are palpitations – ask about rate and rhythm; may suggest arrhythmia.

CLINICAL NOTES

Some patients may have breathlessness as their only symptom of ischaemic heart disease; this is sometimes called 'angina equivalent'.

If there is peripheral oedema, the patient's dyspnoea may be the result of cardiac failure and pulmonary oedema, but it is important when taking the history to remember other pathologies. A full systemic enquiry is important for this purpose, for example:

- Change in bowel habit, epigastric discomfort or dyspepsia may raise suspicion of anaemia.
- Diarrhoea, poor appetite or weight loss may raise suspicion of hypoalbuminaemia.

Past medical history

A detailed history of previous illnesses and operations will provide clues in patients with long-standing cardiac, respiratory, renal or liver disease.

Drug history

Important points include the following:

- Some drugs may be nephrotoxic (e.g., nonsteroidal antiinflammatory drugs, angiotensin-converting enzyme inhibitors).
- Some drugs may be hepatotoxic (e.g., methotrexate).
- Dihydropyridine calcium channel blockers (such as amlodipine) cause ankle oedema in approximately 8% of patients.

CLINICAL NOTES

Oedema commonly occurs in patients treated with dihydropyridine calcium channel blockers (e.g., nifedipine, amlodipine). This is due to disturbance of oncotic and hydrostatic pressures in the tissue, not due to general fluid retention. This type of oedema should not be treated with diuretics, which cause electrolyte depletion.

Social history

Important findings may include:

- Cigarette smoking – a risk factor for ischaemic heart disease and lung disease.
- Alcohol abuse – not only a risk factor for hepatic cirrhosis but also a common cause of cardiomyopathy.
- Intravenous drug abuse – a risk factor for PE, infective endocarditis (with associated valvular dysfunction), and hepatitis.
- Recent social stressors – may suggest a psychogenic cause for breathlessness (or rarely Takotsubo cardiomyopathy).

CLINICAL NOTES

Causes of localized oedema in either the arms or legs include:

- Local deep venous thrombosis, cellulitis or trauma.
- Lymphoedema secondary to impaired lymphatic drainage – either due to obstruction (e.g., secondary to malignancy) or as the result of previous lymph node clearance.

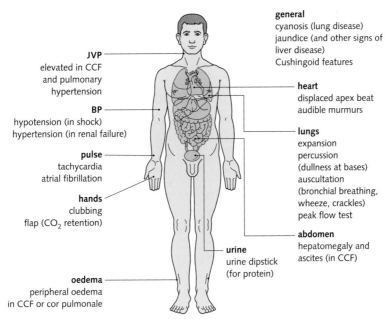

JVP
elevated in CCF
and pulmonary
hypertension

BP
hypotension (in shock)
hypertension (in renal failure)

pulse
tachycardia
atrial fibrillation

hands
clubbing
flap (CO_2 retention)

oedema
peripheral oedema
in CCF or cor pulmonale

general
cyanosis (lung disease)
jaundice (and other signs of
liver disease)
Cushingoid features

heart
displaced apex beat
audible murmurs

lungs
expansion
percussion
(dullness at bases)
auscultation
(bronchial breathing,
wheeze, crackles)
peak flow test

abdomen
hepatomegaly and
ascites (in CCF)

urine
urine dipstick
(for protein)

Fig. 7.1 Points to note when examining a patient presenting with dyspnoea or ankle swelling. *BP*, blood pressure; *CCF*, congestive cardiac failure; *JVP*, jugular venous pressure.

EXAMINATION

A thorough examination is needed due to the wide range of differential diagnoses; see Fig. 7.1 for a summary.

Inspection

Note the following:

- Signs of shock (e.g., pallor, sweating) – suggest acute LVF, pneumonia or PE.
- Signs of anaemia (e.g., conjunctival pallor).
- Appearance of hands and fingers – e.g., clubbing, flapping tremor (carbon dioxide retention or liver flap).
- Laboured or obstructed breathing, tachypnoea or cyanosis. One or more are usually seen with resting dyspnoea.
- Cough – may suggest acute LVF, pneumonia; note the appearance of the sputum (always ask to look in the sputum pot if it is present).
- Appearance of chest – a barrel-shaped chest (hyperexpansion) is a feature of emphysema; kyphoscoliosis may impede ventilation.
- Signs of chronic liver disease, such as jaundice, spider naevi, gynaecomastia, loss of body hair or testicular atrophy. Confusion may be indicative of encephalopathy.

- There might be evidence of ongoing dialysis, either of fistulae (usually in the forearms) or tubing attached to the abdomen in ambulatory peritoneal dialysis.
- Pyrexia – suggests infection (although note PE and myocardial infarction may be associated with a low-grade pyrexia).

Cardiovascular system

Check the following:

- Pulse and blood pressure – check for abnormal rhythm, tachycardia (often seen in cardiac failure), bradycardia, hypotension, and hypertension (common in both ischaemic heart disease and chronic renal disease).
- Mucous membranes – pallor suggests anaemia; cyanosis suggests hypoxaemia (e.g., LVF, COPD, PE, pneumonia and lung collapse).
- Carotid pulse waveform and jugular venous pressure (JVP) – JVP is elevated in fluid retention, cardiac failure and conditions causing pulmonary hypertension with associated right heart failure (e.g., PE, COPD). JVP assessment is one of the most important signs to elicit when looking for signs of heart failure. Assess it carefully.
- Palpation – lateral displacement of apex beat suggests cardiac enlargement, and a left parasternal heave

suggests right ventricular hypertrophy or pulmonary hypertension.

- Heart sounds – note any audible murmurs (valvular lesions may cause LVF) or added heart sounds (third and fourth heart sounds may be heard in LVF).
- Dip the urine – this is part of every examination of the cardiovascular system. Proteinuria is a feature of nephrotic syndrome and other causes of renal impairment. Haematuria is seen in some diseases causing renal impairment.
- Peripheral oedema.

Examination of oedema

Oedema of generalized fluid retention is pitting in nature. To demonstrate this, the area in question should be pressed firmly for at least 10 s – this will leave an indent. Be careful: ankle oedema may be tender. The severity of oedema can be gauged by the extent to which the oedema can be felt up the leg. Lymphoedema and chronic venous oedema do not 'pit'.

Respiratory system

Check the following:

- Expansion – unequal thorax expansion is a sign of pneumonia, pneumothorax or effusion.
- Vocal resonance/fremitus – when enhanced, suggests consolidation; is a sign of effusion or pneumothorax when reduced.
- Abnormal dullness over hemithorax with reduced expansion – suggests pneumonia.
- Stony dullness at one or both lung bases – suggests pleural effusion.
- Hyperresonance over hemithorax with unilaterally reduced expansion – suggests pneumothorax.
- Bilateral hyperresonance with loss of cardiac dullness – suggests emphysema.
- Bronchial breathing – suggests pneumonia.
- Crepitations – coarse crepitations are heard in bronchitis, emphysema and pneumonia. Bilateral basal fine inspiratory crepitations suggest LVF. Fine mid-inspiratory crepitations may suggest pulmonary fibrosis.
- Wheeze – asthma, COPD, cardiac asthma in LVF.
- Peak flow test – ask to perform this test as part of any respiratory examination. Explain the technique to the patient clearly, and then perform three attempts and take the best result out of the three. Peak flow will be reduced in active asthma and COPD.

Gastrointestinal system

Examine for hepatomegaly and ascites – seen in congestive cardiac failure, isolated right-sided failure and hepatic failure.

INVESTIGATION

A summary of immediate investigations for emergency causes of dyspnoea is shown in Table 7.3.

Blood tests

These include:

- Full blood count – might reveal anaemia or leucocytosis (in pneumonia).
- Urea and electrolytes – may be deranged due to diuretic treatment or possible syndrome of inappropriate antidiuretic hormone secretion in pneumonia. This will be abnormal in primary renal disease and commonly in liver disease.
- Cardiac biomarkers – elevated if dyspnoea is secondary to myocardial infarction or myocarditis. Modest elevations are also seen with ongoing heart failure.
- Liver function tests – this is abnormal in liver disease but note that hepatic congestion due to cardiac failure also causes abnormal liver function tests.

Table 7.3 Important immediate tests to investigate for dyspnoeic emergencies

Test	Diagnosis
Chest X-ray	Acute left ventricular failure – pulmonary oedema, cardiomegaly, effusions, Kerley B lines, upper lobe venous diversion.
	Acute asthma – clear overexpanded lungs.
	Pneumothorax – absence of lung markings between lung edge and chest wall, deviation of mediastinum if tension present.
	Pneumonia – consolidation (may be lobar or diffuse).
Electrocardiography	Look for evidence of myocardial infarction, ischaemia, pulmonary embolus.
Arterial blood gases	Hypoxia suggests left ventricular failure or significant lung disease (use the level of hypoxia to guide the need for oxygen therapy or artificial ventilation).
Peak flow	Reduced in airway obstruction (asthma, chronic obstructive pulmonary disease), but may also be reduced in sick patients because of weakness (it is an effort-dependent test).

Table 7.4 Examples of arterial blood gas results in dyspnoeic patients[a]

	Examples	PO_2 (kPa)	PCO_2 (kPa)	pH
Normal ranges		10.5–13.5	4.5–6.0	7.35–7.45
Type 1 respiratory failure (hypoxaemia without hypercapnoea)	Left ventricular failure, pulmonary embolus, acute severe asthma (without exhaustion)	↓ (<8.0)	↓	– / ↑
Type 2 respiratory failure (hypoxaemia with hypercapnoea)	Chronic obstructive pulmonary disease, life-threatening asthma	↓ (<8.0)	↑ (>6.0)	↓
Acute hyperventilation	Anxiety states	–	↓	↑

[a]The low pH in type 2 respiratory failure is secondary to acute retention of carbon dioxide. The high pH in acute hyperventilation results from a loss of carbon dioxide (respiratory alkalosis). The pH in type 1 respiratory failure may be increased (due to loss of carbon dioxide) or may be normal due to raised lactic acid levels/metabolic compensation.

- Plasma albumin concentration – hypoalbuminaemia predisposes to both peripheral and pulmonary oedema.
- Thyroid function tests – hyperthyroidism and hypothyroidism may precipitate cardiac failure. Hypothyroidism can cause non-pitting oedema: myxoedema.
- Arterial blood gases (Table 7.4).
- D-dimer – a fibrin degradation product (elevated in pulmonary embolus). High sensitivity but low specificity, generating a lot of false positive results. Sometimes useful as a 'rule-out' test.
- C-reactive protein – elevated in inflammatory processes, such as pneumonia.

- Severe asthma with acute CO_2 retention – the pH falls as the PCO_2 rises, as there has been insufficient time for metabolic compensation to occur.
- Metabolic acidosis can occur in liver and renal failure (with normal oxygen and normal or low carbon dioxide if compensating).

CLINICAL NOTES

Life-threatening carbon monoxide poisoning might not cause prominent dyspnoea but could present as coma.

Arterial blood gases

Arterial blood gases must be performed for all dyspnoeic patients at presentation. See Table 7.4 for examples of common findings.

Points to note:

- In acute conditions, such as acute LVF, pulmonary embolus, pneumothorax and early asthma – a respiratory alkalosis occurs (i.e., a low PCO_2 and a high pH). The kidneys have not yet compensated by excreting bicarbonate.
- Hypoxaemia – oxygen therapy causes the blood PO_2 to rise and the respiratory drive to fall, so ventilation is reduced and the blood PCO_2 rises. In asthma, exhaustion causes the ventilatory drive to fall off and the PCO_2 to rise; this precedes respiratory arrest and is an indication for artificial ventilation of the patient.
- COPD with chronic CO_2 retention – the pH is normal because metabolic compensation has occurred and bicarbonate levels rise as a result of renal retention of bicarbonate (this takes a few days to occur).

Electrocardiography

This might show:

- Ischaemic changes in patients with coronary artery disease.
- Sinus tachycardia with right axis deviation/anterior T wave inversion/right bundle branch block/S1Q3T3 pattern in patients who have a PE.
- Atrial fibrillation secondary to any lung pathology or ischaemia.

COMMON PITFALLS

Despite the S1Q3T3 pattern (deep S wave in lead I, Q wave and inverted T wave in lead III) being seen as a classic finding in pulmonary embolism, it is not a particularly sensitive or specific test for PE by itself. The commonest ECG changes in pulmonary embolism are sinus tachycardia and anterior T wave inversion.

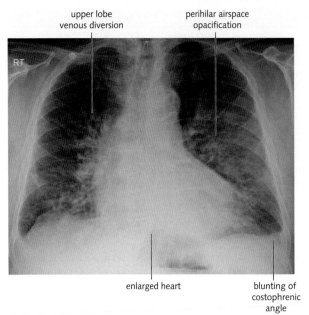

upper lobe venous diversion

perihilar airspace opacification

RT

enlarged heart

blunting of costophrenic angle

Fig. 7.2 Chest X-ray with features of pulmonary oedema.

Chest radiography

Note the following:

- Cardiomegaly in cardiac failure – increased cardiothoracic ratio.
- Signs of pulmonary oedema – bat's wing shadowing, upper lobe blood diversion, Kerley B lines (Fig. 7.2).
- Focal lung consolidation in pneumonia (opacification of an area of lung with air bronchograms).
- Pleural effusion – suggests infection, malignancy or cardiac failure.
- Hyperexpanded lung fields in emphysema (flattening of the diaphragm, ability to count more than six anterior ribs above the diaphragm at the level of the midclavicular line); bullae may be seen in emphysema.
- Presence of a pneumothorax – ask for erect radiograph in full inspiration if suspected.
- Occasionally wedge-shaped peripheral infarct or oligaemic portion of the lung(s) in PE (but usually appears normal).

Echocardiography

This may reveal:

- Left ventricular (LV) systolic dysfunction.
- Valve lesions.
- Ventricular hypertrophy and pulmonary hypertension.

Computed tomography

This is used to obtain detailed visualization of pulmonary fibrosis, tumours, lobar collapse, consolidation and pulmonary oedema. CT pulmonary angiography (CTPA) is used to analyze blood flow in the pulmonary system and is the gold standard for identifying pulmonary emboli.

Urine tests

If there is no evidence of cardiac disease and the plasma albumin is low, consider urine testing. Nephrotic syndrome causes loss of at least 3 g protein in 24 hours. The albumin:creatinine ratio may be used to estimate proteinuria, avoiding the need for 24-hour collections.

Pulmonary function tests

These tests are used to investigate:

- Lung volumes – increased in COPD, reduced in restrictive lung disease.
- Flow-volume loop – scalloped in COPD.
- Carbon monoxide transfer – reduced in many diseases including restrictive lung diseases (with normal airway function) and PE.

Ultrasound

Consider ultrasound of the pelvis in patients with no evidence of cardiac, renal or liver disease and bilateral ankle oedema to investigate for venous thrombosis or a mass lesion causing external compression.

RECENT ONSET DYSPNOEA AT REST IN AN ILL PATIENT

If a patient is unwell with dyspnoea, this is a cardiopulmonary emergency requiring rapid diagnosis and treatment. It is necessary to distinguish between the following life-threatening causes:

- Acute LVF.
- PE.
- Tension pneumothorax.
- Life-threatening asthma.
- Pneumonia.

Acute left ventricular failure

The detailed management of acute LVF is discussed in more detail in Chapter 13. Classic signs of LVF can be seen and include:

- Severe dyspnoea.
- Central cyanosis.

- Patient sits upright.
- Bilateral basal fine end-inspiratory crepitations (in severe LVF, the crepitations extend upwards to fill both lung fields).
- Hypotension secondary to poor LV output (common).
- Blood gases show hypoxia and often hypocapnoea due to hyperventilation. There is usually a metabolic acidosis as a result of poor tissue perfusion.

Treatment includes high-concentration inhaled oxygen via a mask and intravenous diuretic (furosemide). Current National Institute for Health and Care Excellence (NICE) guidance no longer advises routine use of opiates and nitrates in this situation.

Pulmonary embolism

This can present in a number of ways, for example:

- Severe dyspnoea.
- Collapse and syncope.
- Hypotension.
- Cardiorespiratory arrest (often with pulseless electrical activity).

If PE is suspected, anticoagulation should be commenced immediately with subcutaneous low-molecular-weight heparin (LMWH), direct-acting oral anticoagulant or an intravenous heparin infusion.

Haemodynamic instability may suggest massive PE – thrombolysis may be administered or emergency pulmonary angiography carried out in an attempt to disrupt the embolus.

Other respiratory causes of breathlessness

Refer to *Crash Course: Respiratory System*, 5th edition for more detail.

Pneumothorax

Pneumothorax may be an acute or chronic cause of dyspnoea. In pneumothorax, there is a connection between the pleural space and the atmosphere (via either the chest wall or the airways). This may be the result of trauma or rupture of bullae on the surface of the lung (may occur in emphysema, but also sometimes in young healthy patients).

Tension pneumothorax can occur if the air continues to accumulate in the pleural cavity, resulting in a progressive increase in pressure and displacement of the mediastinum away from the side of the pneumothorax. This is characterized by the following clinical signs:

- Severe and worsening dyspnoea.
- Displaced trachea and apex beat. Hyperresonance on the affected side with reduced breath sounds.
- Progressive hypotension due to reduced venous return and therefore reduced filling of the right ventricle.
- Eventual collapse and cardiac arrest.

Treatment should be immediate, with insertion of a large-bore needle into the second intercostal space in the mid-clavicular line on the affected side to allow gas to escape spontaneously from the pleural cavity. A chest drain should then be inserted.

Acute asthma

Patients may present with breathlessness and wheeze. Signs suggestive of a severe asthma attack include:

- The patient being unable to talk in full sentences due to dyspnoea.
- The patient sitting forwards and using accessory muscles of respiration.
- Tachycardia.
- Peak flow less than 50% of patient's best (or predicted).
- Pulsus paradoxus – drop in systolic blood pressure of >10 mmHg on inspiration.

Silent chest due to severe airflow limitation, peak flow less than 33% of predicted or cyanosis suggest life-threatening asthma. Hypercapnoea on blood gas analysis suggests exhaustion and respiratory arrest could be imminent – this may occur before severe hypoxia. The patient should be considered for intubation and artificial ventilation.

This is a medical emergency and appropriate treatment with oxygen therapy, bronchodilators and intravenous hydrocortisone should be commenced immediately.

Pneumonia

Patients may have a cough (either productive or non-productive). There may be pyrexia or even signs of septic shock (e.g., hypotension, renal failure). Blood gases may reveal hypoxia or increased lactate. The chest radiograph might show consolidation. Radiographic changes can be deceptively mild in certain atypical infections.

Blood and sputum cultures should be taken (if possible) and antibiotic therapy according to local guidelines should be started as soon as possible.

● Chapter Summary

- There is a wide differential diagnosis in patients presenting with dyspnoea, including cardiac (e.g., LVF, ischaemic heart disease), respiratory (e.g., asthma exacerbation, pneumothorax), and other pathologies (e.g., anaemia, anxiety).
- There is also a wide differential in patients presenting with ankle/leg oedema, including cardiac failure, hypoalbuminaemia, renal failure, hepatic failure and medication side effects, as well as a number of other causes.
- Cardiac failure is the main diagnosis of concern in the patient who presents with dyspnoea and peripheral oedema. Detailed history taking and examination is vital to establishing an accurate diagnosis.
- It is important to know how life-threatening causes of dyspnoea should be investigated and managed.

UKMLA Conditions
Cardiac failure
Pulmonary embolism

UKMLA Presentations
Breathlessness
Cough
Cyanosis
Peripheral oedema and ankle swelling
Wheeze

Palpitations are an abnormal awareness of the heartbeat. Palpitations may be rapid, slow or just particularly forceful beats occurring at a normal rate.

DIFFERENTIAL DIAGNOSIS

Palpitations may occur in a number of different disorders (Table 8.1). Any condition producing a change in cardiac rhythm, rate or stroke volume may cause palpitations.

Table 8.1 Differential diagnosis of palpitations

	Diagnosis
Arrhythmia	Bradycardia
	Sinus arrhythmia
	Sinus tachycardia
	Atrial fibrillation/flutter
	Atrial tachycardia
	Atrial/ventricular ectopic beats
	Supraventricular tachycardia
	Ventricular tachycardia
Nonarrhythmic cardiac causes	Septal defects
	Congestive heart failure
	Congenital heart disease
	Cardiomyopathy
	Valvular disease
Extra-cardiac causes	Anaemia
	Electrolyte abnormality
	Hypoglycaemia
	Fever
	Hyperthyroidism
	Hypovolaemia
	Pregnancy
	Phaeochromocytoma
Drugs and medications	Alcohol
	Caffeine and other stimulant drugs
	Sympathomimetic drugs (e.g., β-agonists, antimuscarinics, etc.)
	Nicotine
Psychiatric	Anxiety or depression
	Panic attacks

Arrhythmias of greater concern are highlighted in red.
Life-threatening features to watch out for are **shock, syncope, myocardial ischaemia or severe heart failure**. Many of the other causes of palpitations can potentially be severe or life-threatening, such as profound anaemia or fever secondary to severe sepsis.

Rapid palpitations

Rapid palpitations may be either regular or irregular in rhythm. Regular palpitations may be a sign of:

- Sinus tachycardia.
- Atrial flutter.
- Atrial tachycardia.
- Supraventricular tachycardia (SVT).
- Ventricular tachycardia.

    Irregular palpitations may indicate:

- Atrial fibrillation (i.e., with a fast ventricular response rate).
- Multiple atrial or ventricular ectopic beats.

CLINICAL NOTES

Remember, many patients presenting with palpitations do not have evidence of arrhythmia and many patients presenting with arrhythmia do not have palpitations!

Slow palpitations

Patients may describe these as missed beats or particularly forceful beats. After a brief pause in the heart rhythm, the following beat is often more forceful due to longer ventricular filling time and therefore higher end-diastolic volume and higher stroke volume. Causes of slow palpitation include:

- Ectopic beats with compensatory pauses.
- Atrioventricular (AV) block.
- Sick sinus syndrome.

Disorders causing increased stroke volume

An increase in stroke volume may be the result of:

- High-output states (e.g., anaemia, pregnancy, fever, thyrotoxicosis, etc.).
- Valvular lesions (e.g., mitral or aortic regurgitation).

HISTORY

When taking a history from a patient presenting with palpitations, aim to answer the following questions:

1. What is the nature of the palpitations?

2. What is the likely underlying cause?
3. Do they represent a severe or life-threatening process?

This will help to structure your approach and present your findings.

Nature of the palpitations

Often it is helpful to ask patients to describe the palpitation by tapping it out themselves. This gives an idea of rate and rhythm (i.e., fast or slow, regular or irregular). Do the episodes involve single particularly forceful beats or longer runs of palpitations? Are the episodes paroxysmal (i.e., intermittent) or continuous in nature? Is the onset sudden or gradual?

Likely underlying causes of palpitation

Certain features of the history may be suggestive of the recognized causes of arrhythmia shown in Table 8.2.

> **CLINICAL NOTES**
>
> Hyperthyroidism is well recognized to predispose to palpitations, tachycardia and sometimes atrial fibrillation. It is somewhat less well recognized that *hypo*thyroidism can predispose to ventricular arrhythmias.

Table 8.2 Features in the history that might suggest the cause of an arrhythmia

Cause of arrhythmia	Features in the history
Ischaemic heart disease	Exertional chest pain or breathlessness, history of myocardial infarction/coronary intervention or bypass grafting, risk factors for coronary disease
Thyroid disease	Tremor, excessive sweating, unexplained weight loss, lethargy, obesity
Valvular heart disease	History of rheumatic fever, previous valve surgery, intravenous drug use
Anaemia	Menorrhagia, peptic ulcer disease, recent operations
Proarrhythmic agents	Alcohol, caffeine, stimulant drugs, antiarrhythmic agents
Anxiety	Anxiety, paraesthesia in fingertips

Are the palpitations severe or life-threatening?

It is important to clarify whether palpitations are innocent or whether severe pathology is underlying (i.e., is the underlying rhythm life-threatening or are palpitations occurring in the context of heart failure, ischaemia or thromboembolic events?).

Are palpitations associated with:

- Breathlessness, dizziness or syncope? This suggests cardiac output is compromised.
- Angina? This suggests the palpitations are causing (or perhaps being caused by) myocardial ischaemia.
- History of transient ischaemic attack, stroke or limb ischaemia? Certain arrhythmias (atrial fibrillation in particular) are associated with thromboembolic complications.

EXAMINATION

Examination is aimed towards identifying both signs of the underlying cause and any complications of palpitations. This is summarized in Fig. 8.1.

General observation

Look for:

- Cyanosis – suggestive of cardiac failure or lung disease (remember pulmonary embolus is a well-recognized cause of tachyarrhythmia).
- Dyspnoea – suggestive of cardiac failure or lung disease.
- Pallor – suggestive of anaemia.
- Fever – pyrexia, sweating, etc. may be suggestive of underlying infection (may precipitate arrhythmias, such as atrial fibrillation).
- Thyrotoxic or myxoedematous facies.

> **COMMON PITFALLS**
>
> Cardiac disease can both cause and be caused by disease in other systems, so be sure to examine all systems thoroughly.

Cardiovascular system

Pulse

Palpate the pulses to assess for rate, rhythm, volume and character for at least 15 s.

- Rate. Bradycardia can be associated with higher stroke volume due to a longer period for ventricular filling between

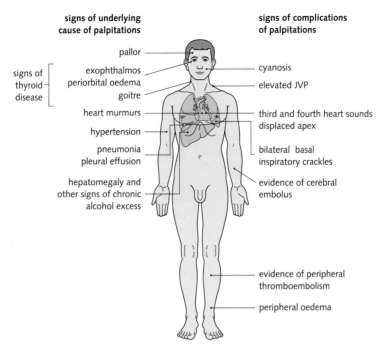

signs of underlying
cause of palpitations

signs of complications
of palpitations

pallor

exophthalmos
periorbital oedema
goitre

signs of
thyroid
disease

heart murmurs

hypertension

pneumonia
pleural effusion

hepatomegaly and
other signs of chronic
alcohol excess

cyanosis

elevated JVP

third and fourth heart sounds
displaced apex

bilateral basal
inspiratory crackles

evidence of cerebral
embolus

evidence of peripheral
thromboembolism

peripheral oedema

Fig. 8.1 Important points to note when examining a patient who has *palpitations*. *JVP*, jugular venous pressure.

beats. This may result in forceful beats. Tachycardia (of any cause) can predispose to awareness of palpitations.

- Rhythm. Is the rhythm regular? If not, is it regularly irregular (as in some bigeminal rhythms or heart blocks) or irregularly irregular (as in atrial fibrillation)?
- Volume. A high-volume pulse (due to high-output states and aortic or mitral regurgitation) is most easily felt at the radial pulse. Volume may vary from beat to beat in certain rhythms, such as atrial fibrillation, due to variation in ventricular filling time and therefore stroke volume. In these cases, low-volume ventricular contractions may not conduct a palpable pulse to peripheral arteries. This is called a 'pulse deficit'. Radial pulse assessment may give an inaccurate reflection of the true heart rate, particularly in tachycardia. Assessment of rate at the cardiac apex is more accurate.
- Character. Abnormal character may suggest underlying valvular heart disease (see Chapter 15).

CLINICAL NOTES

Sinus arrhythmia is a term for sinus rhythm with a beat-to-beat variation in the P–P interval (interval between subsequent P waves). This usually occurs due to changes in vagal tone due to different stages of the respiratory cycle and is a normal physiological phenomenon most commonly seen in the young.

Blood pressure

Hypertension is a well-recognized cause of atrial fibrillation (and ischaemic heart disease). Pulse pressure may give information as to valvular causes of palpitation, with a narrow pulse pressure suggesting aortic stenosis and a wide pulse pressure suggesting aortic regurgitation.

Jugular venous pressure

Jugular venous pressure may be elevated if the patient has congestive cardiac failure as a consequence of an uncontrolled tachycardia or has atrial flutter or fibrillation secondary to pulmonary embolism.

Apex beat

This may be displaced in the patient with left ventricular failure. The apex beat in hypertrophic cardiomyopathy is classically forceful in nature, with a double impulse if the left ventricular outflow tract is obstructed. Individuals with hypertrophic cardiomyopathy are more at risk of arrhythmia.

Heart sounds

A third or fourth heart sound may be heard. Mitral or aortic regurgitation are possible causes of high output state and may cause murmurs. A murmur of mitral stenosis may be heard, as this condition leads to atrial dilatation and therefore increases risk of atrial fibrillation.

Respiratory system

Bilateral basal inspiratory crepitations may be heard in patients with left ventricular failure. There may be signs of underlying chest infection, a common cause of palpitations.

Gastrointestinal system

Hepatomegaly and ascites may be signs of congestive cardiac failure or alcoholic liver disease. Alcohol is one of the commonest causes of tachyarrhythmias. Look for other signs of liver disease if this is suspected.

Limbs

Examine for:

- Peripheral oedema – may be a sign of congestive cardiac failure.
- Tremor – may be a sign of thyrotoxicosis or alcohol withdrawal.
- Brisk reflexes – seen in thyrotoxicosis.
- Abnormal neurology – may be a sign of previous cerebral embolus.

INVESTIGATIONS

Biochemical tests

The following tests may aid diagnosis:

- Serum electrolytes – deranged levels of potassium and calcium in particular can predispose to arrhythmia.
- Full blood count – look for anaemia or raised white cell count.
- Inflammatory markers – may be relevant if palpitations arise in context of sepsis.
- Thyroid function tests – palpitations may result from both hyperthyroid and hypothyroid states.
- Liver function tests – deranged in congestive cardiac failure or alcoholic liver disease.
- 24-hour urinary catecholamines – not routinely done but may be useful to exclude phaeochromocytoma in some cases.

Electrocardiography

12-lead electrocardiography

This may enable instant diagnosis if palpitations are present at time of testing. However, if palpitations are paroxysmal, the ECG may be normal.

There may be clues to the cause of the palpitations on the ECG, for example ischaemia, or presence of a delta wave or short PR interval (as seen in some congenital causes of paroxysmal tachyarrhythmias, such as Wolff-Parkinson-White syndrome).

Ambulatory electrocardiography

Ambulatory ECG monitoring (e.g., for 24 hours) may reveal paroxysmal arrhythmias. Patients press an alert button when they have symptoms, marking that period of the recording for review.

Longer-term monitors may be necessary to document infrequent episodes. This may involve external monitoring for an extended period or, in some cases, use of an implantable loop recorder. A loop recorder is a small subcutaneous ECG monitoring device that may be left in for 2 to 3 years.

Patients may also now own smart watches or other personal ECG monitoring devices (some of which can produce up to a 6-lead ECG). These are being increasingly used by patients and, in some circumstances, can be helpful to identify infrequent arrhythmias; this requires patients using them correctly and results are not always reliable. The automated assessment by these devices is, however, prone to both false negatives and false positives (something which is likely to improve over time as this technology develops).

COMMUNICATION

Ask about frequency of episodes; remember, a normal 24-hour recording does not exclude arrhythmia if the arrhythmia is paroxysmal and the patient has not had any symptoms when monitored.

Exercise electrocardiography

This test can be used to reveal exercise-induced arrhythmias. Examples of ECGs illustrating atrial fibrillation, atrial flutter and SVT are shown in Fig. 8.2.

Vagotonic manoeuvres

Such manoeuvres include:

- Valsalva manoeuvres – (e.g., blowing into a large syringe).
- Carotid sinus massage – there is a risk of stroke in patients with carotid artery disease (due to embolization of plaque) so avoid in patients with carotid bruits and be cautious in the elderly or those with prior transient ischaemic attack or stroke.
- Diving reflex – this involves submerging the face in water (or applying a cold wet towel to the face). This is particularly effective in infants in whom the diving reflex is better preserved.

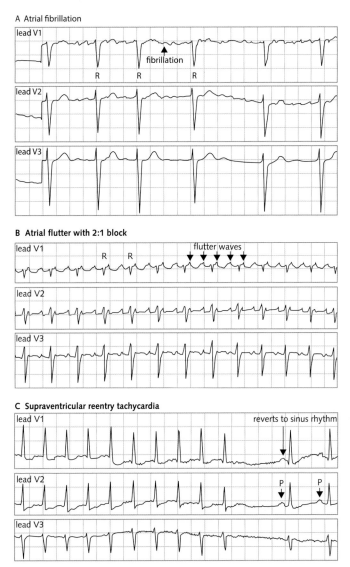

Fig. 8.2 Electrocardiograms illustrating atrial fibrillation, atrial flutter and supraventricular reentry tachycardia. (A) Note the irregularly irregular rhythm (variable R-R), underlying 'fibrillation' and absence of P waves preceding QRS complexes. (B) Note a regular rhythm at a rate divisible into 300 (150 beats/min in this case). Sometimes underlying flutter waves can be seen at a rate of 300 per min. (C) Note the fast, regular rhythm (usually 140–240 beats/min). P waves are present but not always easy to see; they may occur before or after the QRS (and are sometimes hidden by the QRS complex). Note normal P waves are visible when the rhythm reverts to sinus rhythm.

HINTS AND TIPS

A modified Valsalva manoeuvre has been shown to be much more effective for reverting supraventricular tachycardia to sinus rhythm than standard Valsalva manoeuvres. Position the patient semi-recumbent in the bed. Have him or her perform a Valsalva manoeuvre as normal, but immediately following the manoeuvre, the patient should be repositioned supine and legs passively raised. This increases venous return and accentuates vagal response.

Table 8.3 Characteristic features of atrial fibrillation, atrial flutter and supraventricular reentry tachycardia

	Atrial fibrillation	Atrial flutter	Supraventricular tachycardia
Rate	Any rate, pulse deficit may be present if fast	Atrial flutter rate is 300/min; the ventricular rate is usually divisible into this (e.g., 150 or 100 beats per minute) (due to 2:1 or 3:1 conduction)	140–260/min
Rhythm	Irregularly irregular	Regular	Regular
Response to adenosine/ Valsalva manoeuvre	Unnecessary – irregularly irregular rhythm should be recognizable; adenosine can be dangerous if accessory pathway present	Slowing of ventricular rate reveals 'saw-tooth' flutter waves	Blocking the atrioventricular node may 'break' the reentry circuit, terminating the tachycardia

These manoeuvres act to increase vagal tone, which in turn increases the refractory period of the AV node. This enables differentiation between three common tachyarrhythmias that are sometimes indistinguishable on ECG recording:

- Atrial flutter.
- Atrial fibrillation.
- SVT.

Characteristic features of these tachyarrhythmias are listed in Table 8.3.

Adenosine administration

Adenosine is a purine nucleoside that acts to block the AV node. When administered intravenously, it will achieve complete AV block. Its half-life is very short (only a few seconds), so this effect is very short-lived. Adenosine can be useful in both the diagnosis of arrhythmia (differentiation of tachyarrhythmias) and in terminating reentrant tachyarrhythmias involving the AV node (see Table 8.3).

Side effects of adenosine include bronchospasm, so avoid in asthmatics. In individuals with asthma, verapamil might be used as an alternative. Adenosine has a higher rate of minor adverse effects but verapamil is associated with higher risk of significant hypotension.

COMMUNICATION

It is important to mention before administering adenosine that the side effects can be quite unpleasant but should settle within seconds. Patients may experience nausea, flushing, light-headedness, a metallic taste and classically a 'sense of impending doom'.

Chest X-ray

Chest X-ray may reveal evidence of heart failure, either as a direct cause of palpitations or as a result of cardiac decompensation secondary to arrhythmia.

Echocardiography

This may reveal valvular pathology, evidence of congenital heart disease or cardiomyopathy. Echocardiography enables evaluation of chamber size and of ventricular function, which may both be deranged due to arrhythmia.

Electrophysiological study

This is useful in investigating patients suspected of having tachyarrhythmias due to abnormal reentry pathways. The technique enables localization of the reentry circuit, which may then be ablated using a radiofrequency thermal electrode placed inside the heart.

Other investigations

Various other investigations may be required to identify a suspected cause of palpitations, for example:

- Computed tomography pulmonary angiography – if a pulmonary embolus is likely.
- Coronary angiogram – if coronary artery disease is suspected.

PALPITATIONS IN THE UNWELL PATIENT

Many causes of palpitations can be severe or life-threatening. In the patient presenting acutely unwell and complaining of palpitations, investigation and treatment is comprised of supportive treatments and treatment of the underlying cause of the palpitations. This may involve for instance:

- Blood transfusion in severe anaemia.
- Antibiotic treatment in sepsis.
- Fluid resuscitation in hypovolaemia.
- Glucose replacement in hypoglycaemia.
- Direct treatment of a primary arrhythmia.

Life-threatening features in patients with arrhythmia

The first thing to do when you see a fast heart rhythm is to establish the patient's clinical status. In the patient presenting with palpitations and underlying arrhythmia, there are a number of life-threatening (previously called 'adverse') features that, if identified, should be of particular concern:

- Shock – in this context, shock is used to indicate hypotension with a systolic blood pressure of <90 mmHg, symptoms of increased sympathetic activity (pallor, sweatiness and being peripherally shut down), and decreased cerebral perfusion (including confusion or altered consciousness). Cardiogenic shock and arrhythmia may also occur together as the result of other cardiac problems, such as myocardial infarction.
- Syncope – transient loss of consciousness due to a global reduction in cerebral blood flow.
- Myocardial ischaemia – either as chest pain, electrocardiographic evidence of ischaemia or from biochemical markers (e.g., elevation of troponin).
- Severe heart failure – pulmonary oedema (left ventricular failure) +/− raised JVP (right ventricular failure).

These adverse features in conjunction with either a bradyarrhythmia or tachyarrhythmia represent a periarrest situation requiring rapid diagnosis and treatment to avoid deterioration.

CLINICAL NOTES

Many causes of shock are treated with fluid resuscitation. Fluid resuscitation in *cardiogenic* shock may, however, be detrimental, as the heart is already struggling to pump the existing intravascular volume around the body. Additional fluid may predispose to pulmonary oedema.

Management of arrhythmia

If adverse features occur in the context of arrhythmia, management is focused on treating the underlying arrhythmia.

For tachyarrhythmias in the unstable patient with a pulse, treatment usually involves synchronized direct current (DC) cardioversion. For bradyarrhythmias, the primary treatment is generally with chronotropes or pacing. Supportive treatments, such as oxygen, should always be given if indicated.

For more information about the treatment of arrhythmia (including in arrest and periarrest situations), see Chapter 14.

● Chapter Summary

- History taking should be tailored to establish the nature of palpitations, the likely underlying cause and whether palpitations are serious or life-threatening.
- There are a number of different causes of palpitations; most are benign but some are life-threatening.
- It can often be difficult to document episodes of arrhythmia if they occur very infrequently.
- Sometimes simple vagal manoeuvres can revert patients with tachyarrhythmias back to sinus rhythm and avoid the use of medical interventions.
- Patients presenting with palpitations and evidence of myocardial ischaemia, severe heart failure, shock or syncope are potentially periarrest and warrant urgent treatment.

UKMLA Conditions
Arrhythmias

UKMLA Presentations
Palpitations

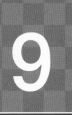
Syncope is a loss of consciousness, usually due to a reduction in perfusion of the brain.

Presyncope is a feeling of light-headedness or that syncope is imminent, but loss of consciousness does not occur.

DIFFERENTIAL DIAGNOSIS OF SYNCOPE

Syncope can occur due to numerous different pathologies (Table 9.1).

There are also a number of other conditions that may cause reduced (or loss of) consciousness but are not true syncope, as they are not due to a reduction in cerebral perfusion. These conditions include:

- Hypoglycaemia.
- Hypoxia.
- Epilepsy.
- Intoxication.

Certain other conditions may also resemble syncope, but there is no loss of consciousness, including psychogenic 'syncope', drop attacks, cataplexy, etc.

It is worth remembering these mimics of syncope in the patient who presents complaining of a faint or collapse.

> **CLINICAL NOTES**
>
> The term 'Stokes-Adams attack' is sometimes used to refer to a reduction in (or loss of) cardiac output and loss of consciousness due to transient arrhythmia (e.g., asystole, ventricular fibrillation, atrioventricular block).

HISTORY

The first differentiation to be made is between cardiac and non-cardiac (usually neurological) syncope (and to decide whether the event is syncope at all)!

> **COMMUNICATION**
>
> Patients may describe syncopal episodes in a number of different ways. Syncopal episodes may be referred to as fits, faints, funny turns, collapses, blackouts – it is important to pin down exactly what they mean!

It is often difficult to definitively diagnose the cause of collapse, but differentiation depends upon a detailed history of the episode of collapse with particular emphasis on the features outlined here. The events preceding the collapse should be elucidated:

- Exertion – can precipitate syncope in hypertrophic cardiomyopathy (HCM) or aortic stenosis.
- Pain, anxiety or prolonged standing – in vasovagal syncope.
- Soon after standing – postural hypotension.
- Neck movements – aggravate vertebrobasilar attacks or carotid sinus hypersensitivity.

Speed of onset of collapse might be:

- Immediate with no warning – classic presentation of arrhythmia.
- Rapid with warning – preceded either by light-headedness (vasovagal) or by an aura (epilepsy).
- Gradual with warning – hypoglycaemia preceded by light-headedness, nausea and sweating.

A collateral history of the syncope itself is vital:

- Patient lies still, breathing regularly – classic of arrhythmia (a prolonged episode can cause epileptiform movements secondary to cerebral hypoxia).
- Patient shakes limbs or has facial twitching, possibly associated with urinary incontinence and tongue biting – suggestive of epilepsy, but myoclonus can occur with vasovagal syncope.
- Patient becomes very pale and grey immediately before collapsing – vasovagal syncope.
- Patient becomes very pale and white following collapse and flushes red when regains consciousness – suggests a cardiac cause such as arrhythmia.

Table 9.1 Differential diagnosis of syncope (more acutely life-threatening conditions are highlighted in red)

Classification	Examples	Notes
Cardiac arrhythmias	• Paroxysmal supraventricular or ventricular tachycardia • Bradyarrhythmia – sinus bradycardia, complete or second-degree heart block, sinus arrest • Pacemaker/implantable cardioverter defibrillator dysfunction	Usually sudden onset and unprovoked, sometimes preceded by palpitations. There may be a personal or family history of cardiac disease. There may be abnormalities seen on a resting electrocardiogram.
Structural cardiac disease	• Valve disease causing obstruction (e.g., aortic stenosis or pulmonary stenosis (rare)) • Hypertrophic cardiomyopathy (HCM) causing obstruction	May have associated murmur. Symptoms generally dependent on severity of underlying condition. May be associated with exertion. May have coexisting signs of heart failure.
	• Acute coronary syndrome	Chest pain, nausea, sweating, or breathlessness may be present. ECG may show ST segment or T wave changes.
	• Atrial myxoma	Most often due to mitral valve obstruction. May have an audible tumour 'plop'.
Cardiopulmonary disease	• Pulmonary embolus	Acute breathlessness, chest pain, hypoxia. ECG may show sinus tachycardia +/– evidence of right heart strain.
	• Acute aortic dissection	Severe tearing chest pain may radiate to the back, may be hypotensive/shocked.
	• Pulmonary hypertension	Often asymptomatic, may cause breathlessness/lethargy.
Neurally mediated (reflex)	• Vasovagal (e.g., due to stress, noxious stimuli, heat, etc.) • Situational (e.g., micturition, defaecation, postexercise, needle phobia, sight of blood, etc.)	Very common, there may be preceding symptoms (dizziness, nausea, flushing, etc.) or obvious precipitant. Often history of previous similar episodes.
	• Carotid sinus hypersensitivity	May occur when rotating head, shaving, etc. May be precipitated by carotid sinus massage.
Orthostatic (postural) hypotension	• Volume depletion (e.g., vomiting, diarrhoea, poor intake, blood loss) • Autonomic failure (e.g., due to drugs, alcohol, multisystem atrophy, diabetic neuropathy, etc.)	Syncope occurs shortly after standing up. History may reveal underlying predisposing factors.
Cerebrovascular/ miscellaneous	• Vascular steal syndromes	Precipitated by arm exercises.
	• Neurogenic (transient ischaemic attack (TIA)/cerebrovascular accident (CVA)/ subarachnoid haemorrhage/ vertebrobasilar disease)	Patient neurological examination may be abnormal. May be severe headache in subarachnoid haemorrhage. It is rare for TIA to cause syncope.

The recovery of consciousness can also be characteristic. In general, if the patient:

- Feels normal soon after the episode – a cardiac cause is more likely.
- Feels washed out and nauseated and takes a few minutes to return to normal – probably vasovagal.
- Feels very drowsy/confused and falls asleep soon after regaining consciousness – epilepsy (postictal state) is probable.

Past medical history

Any cardiac history is important – ischaemia may precipitate arrhythmias.

A history of stroke or transient ischaemic attack (TIA) may suggest a cerebrovascular cause (rare).

Diabetes mellitus may cause autonomic neuropathy and postural hypotension, whereas antihyperglycaemic medications increase risk of hypoglycaemia.

Previous head injury may suggest posttraumatic epilepsy.

Hypotension

Patients experiencing syncopal episodes often have a history of hypotension. This may be either primary (or idiopathic) hypotension or secondary hypotension. Secondary hypotension has many possible causes including medication side effects, hypovolaemia, cardiac disorders, endocrine disorders and neurological disorders; therefore, in patients with hypotension, a detailed history (and later examination) is vital to establish the cause.

Drug history

Important points include the following:

- Antihypertensives and diuretic agents predispose to postural hypotension.
- Class I and class III antiarrhythmics may cause long QT syndrome and predispose to torsades de pointes. All antiarrhythmic agents may cause bradycardia leading to syncope.
- Vasodilators precipitate syncope in pulmonary hypertension.

HINTS AND TIPS

A long list of drugs prolongs the QT interval. Many of these classes begin with 'anti-', e.g., antiarrhythmics, antibiotics, antiemetics, antipsychotics, antidepressants, antihistamines and antimigraine.

Family history

A family history of sudden death or recurrent syncope may occur in patients who have HCM or Brugada syndrome and also in rare familial long QT syndromes.

Social history

Note that:

- Alcohol/benzodiazepine withdrawal (on a background of previous excess) is a risk factor for withdrawal fits.
- Smoking is a risk factor for ischaemic heart disease.
- Occupation is important in terms of diagnostic implications – for instance, certain diagnoses may prohibit driving (discussed later).

EXAMINATION

Points to note on examination are summarized in Fig. 9.1 and discussed below.

On inspection, look for any:

- Signs of shock – such as pallor or sweating.
- Neurological deficit suggestive of a cerebrovascular cause.

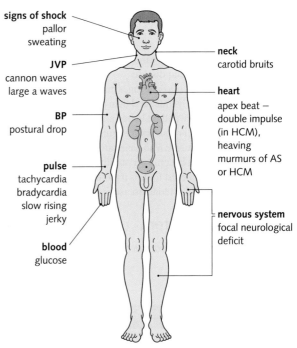

Fig. 9.1 Points to note on examination of a patient presenting with syncope. *AS*, aortic stenosis; *BP*, blood pressure; *HCM*, hypertrophic cardiomyopathy; *JVP*, jugular venous pressure.

COMMON PITFALLS

Remember that fitting whilst unconscious is not always epileptic – it can occur in any patient who has cerebral hypoperfusion or a metabolic disorder (e.g., a patient with vasovagal syncope alone may convulse if held upright!).

Cardiovascular system

Note the following:

- Pulse – any irregularity in rhythm and character of pulse (slow rising in aortic stenosis, jerky in HCM).
- Erect and supine blood pressures (>20 mmHg drop in systolic blood pressure from lying to standing is diagnostic of postural hypotension).
- Jugular venous pulse – cannon waves in complete heart block (due to atrial contraction against a closed tricuspid valve); prominent 'a' wave in pulmonary hypertension.

- Apex beat– double impulse (HCM), heaving (aortic stenosis).
- Any murmurs.
- Carotid bruits – indicating carotid artery stenosis and possible cerebrovascular disease.
- Response to carotid sinus massage (may be indicated in some patients) – apply unilateral firm pressure over the carotid sinus with the patient in bed and attached to a cardiac monitor. Full resuscitative equipment should be easily accessible. Patients who have carotid sinus hypersensitivity will become very bradycardic or asystolic (sinus arrest). Do not test for this if patient has a carotid bruit, known carotid arterial disease or previous stroke.

Neurological system

This system should be fully examined for residual neurological deficit.

INVESTIGATIONS

First-line tests to exclude emergencies are shown in Table 9.2.

Blood tests

The following tests should be performed:

- Full blood count – anaemia may be secondary to haemorrhage, which will cause postural hypotension; leucocytosis is seen in sepsis and following seizure.

Table 9.2 First-line tests to exclude an emergency cause of syncope

Test	Diagnoses
Electrocardiogram (ECG)	Arrhythmia, myocardial infarction, pulmonary embolism.
Blood tests	Haemorrhage, sepsis, electrolyte disturbance leading to arrhythmia, hypoglycaemia.
Continuous cardiac monitoring (e.g., on coronary care unit)	If paroxysmal arrhythmia is suspected or patient at high risk of cardiac arrest.
Chest X-ray	Pulmonary embolism, tension pneumothorax, aortic dissection, cardiomyopathy or heart failure.
CT scan	CT pulmonary angiography if pulmonary embolus is suspected. CT head if possible cerebral infarct/intracranial haemorrhage.

- Electrolytes and renal function – hypo/hyperkalaemia predisposes towards arrhythmias.
- Calcium – hypocalcaemia is a cause of long QT syndrome.
- Cardiac biomarkers if suspicion of acute coronary syndrome – myocardial infarction may cause sudden arrhythmia. Note that arrhythmia itself may cause moderate elevation in cardiac biomarkers.
- Blood glucose – particularly useful if demonstrates hypoglycaemia at the time of syncope. Finger prick testing is quick to perform, but formal laboratory measurement can be useful confirmation.
- Lactate – raised in seizure and ischaemia.

Electrocardiography

This may provide rapid evidence of:

- Bradyarrhythmia or tachyarrhythmia – may be either overt ongoing arrhythmia or evidence that supports presence of paroxysmal rhythm disturbance (e.g., short PR interval and delta waves in Wolff-Parkinson-White syndrome).
- Heart block.
- A long QT interval.
- Ischaemia.
- Pulmonary embolus – sinus tachycardia is the most common finding. Other potential findings include ST depression/T wave inversion in V1–V4, II, III and aVF, right bundle branch block, right axis deviation or an 'S1Q3T3' pattern.

Ambulatory ECG monitoring

Outpatient ambulatory ECG monitoring (Holter monitoring) is used to provide a continuous ECG trace (usually for 24 or 48 hours) to detect paroxysmal episodes of arrhythmia. Longer cardiac monitoring can be performed using implantable loop recorders.

Chest radiography

On the chest radiograph, there may be:

- Cardiomegaly – may suggest cardiomyopathy or heart failure (potentially secondary to valvular abnormality).
- Oligaemic lung fields – suggestive of pulmonary embolus.
- Widened mediastinum – may indicate aortic dissection.

Echocardiography

This may reveal:

- Aortic stenosis or other valvular abnormalities.
- HCM.
- Atrial dilatation in supraventricular tachycardia.

- Ventricular abnormalities in ventricular arrhythmias or as the result of valvular abnormalities. Right ventricular abnormalities may be seen in pulmonary hypertension.
- Pericardial tamponade.

Other investigations

Other investigations that may be considered include:

- Tilt table testing – a noninvasive test where the patient is strapped to a table lying flat and then tilted to an angle of almost upright. Symptoms, blood pressure, and heart rate are measured throughout this process. Simple tilt produces hypotension and possibly syncope in autonomic denervation. Prolonged tilt may provoke vasovagal syncope with bradycardia and hypotension.
- Electrophysiological (EP) study of the heart – consider if arrhythmia is strongly suspected but not revealed by Holter monitoring.
- Electroencephalography (EEG) – if epilepsy is suspected.

REFLEX (NEURALLY MEDIATED) SYNCOPE

Reflex or neurally mediated syncope is a group of conditions that occur as the result of increased activity of the parasympathetic nervous system (increased vagal tone) and reduced sympathetic nervous system activity. This is triggered by activation of the nucleus tractus solitarius in the medulla oblongata. This results in a reduction in heart rate and/or blood pressure.

This causes a reduction in cardiac output and cerebral perfusion, with a resultant presyncope or syncope, dependent on the degree of reduction in cerebral perfusion.

Types of reflex syncope include vasovagal syncope, situational syncope and carotid sinus hypersensitivity. Although perhaps less concerning than some of the causes of syncope discussed later in this chapter, with reflex syncope, injury or death may result from associated fall/collapse, etc.

Before syncope occurs, patients may report feeling hot, sweaty, clammy or nauseated and may report impaired vision or hearing. Loss of consciousness is usually brief. Following the episode, the patient may be nauseated, sweaty and clammy for several minutes afterwards.

Vasovagal syncope

This is the most common cause of syncope (and is what many young people are describing when they report 'fainting'). Vasovagal syncope is often triggered by prolonged standing (especially in warm weather), pain, the sight of blood or psychological/emotional stress.

Situational syncope

Syncope occurs as the result of certain situations, including upon urination, defaecation, coughing, swallowing, etc.

Carotid sinus hypersensitivity

Syncope occurs as the result of increased pressure upon the carotid sinus (located at the carotid bifurcation in the neck). Pressure required may be relatively minor and syncope may occur due to tight collars or even turning the head to the side.

SYNCOPE OF RECENT ONSET IN THE UNWELL PATIENT

It is important to distinguish between benign causes of syncope and life-threatening causes that represent a medical emergency requiring rapid diagnosis and treatment.

Cardiac causes

Aortic stenosis

Syncope is effort-induced as the left ventricular output is restricted by the outflow obstruction. Patients may have an ejection systolic murmur ('tight' or high frequency in critical stenosis), a slow-rising carotid pulse and a heaving apex beat.

Electrocardiography may show left ventricular hypertrophy. Echocardiography reveals the stenotic valve, and assessment by Doppler velocity change through the valve may indicate severity.

Tachyarrhythmias

Syncope due to supraventricular tachyarrhythmia (SVT) tends to occur only if the heart rate is extremely fast. Ventricular tachycardia is more likely than SVT to cause syncope because it is accompanied by asynchronous ventricular contraction. If these arrhythmias are not prominent on ambulatory monitoring, they may be induced during EP testing.

Bradyarrhythmias

Syncope may occur secondary to a bradyarrhythmia if the cardiac output falls markedly as a consequence of the drop in rate. An ongoing bradyarrhythmia is easily detected on ECG (e.g., sinus bradycardia and second-degree or complete heart block). Some conditions, however, occur intermittently and the ECG may be normal after the syncopal episode; for example, heart block may occur intermittently with normal sinus rhythm between episodes.

Ambulatory ECG monitoring may capture these episodes but can be difficult if they are separated by long periods of time.

Acute coronary syndromes

Acute coronary syndromes may lead to syncope due to reduced cardiac output and hypotension as a result of impaired myocardial function or arrhythmia. Patients may also complain of chest pain, sweating, breathlessness and nausea. ECG may show evidence of ischaemia/infarction.

Cardiomyopathies

Hypertrophic obstructive cardiomyopathy can give rise to syncope by obstructing left ventricular outflow on exercise or as a result of ventricular tachycardia or fibrillation. This 'sudden death syndrome' can also commonly occur in patients who have cardiomyopathy of other aetiologies (including arrhythmogenic ventricular dysplasia and dilated cardiomyopathy).

Prolonged QT interval

This may be congenital or drug-induced, usually by psychiatric or class III antiarrhythmic drugs (e.g., amiodarone, sotalol). The syncope is caused by a self-limiting ventricular tachycardia characterized by a systematically rotating QRS vector (torsades de pointes). Tachycardia and syncope may be relieved by rapid ('overdrive') pacing or pharmacological sinus tachycardia (e.g., using isoprenaline). The resting nonarrhythmic ECG shows QT prolongation.

Brugada syndrome

Brugada syndrome is caused by a mutation in the gene coding for cardiac sodium channels. It is generally inherited in an autosomal dominant fashion so there may be a family history of syncope or sudden death. The typical finding is ST elevation followed by T wave inversion in leads V1–V3 of the resting ECG (Brugada sign). The patient presents with episodes of syncope caused by polymorphic VT, which may progress to VF and death if not terminated.

Circulatory causes

Hypovolaemia

This can present as postural hypotension (i.e., loss of consciousness on standing, relieved by lying flat). This occurs because the blood volume is inadequate, even with an intact baroreflex, to maintain arterial blood pressure in the face of gravity-dependent blood pooling. If this is due to acute haemorrhage, there are usually other obvious manifestations, such as trauma or GI blood loss. However, large-volume internal bleeding can sometimes be difficult to detect. With acute blood loss, the haemoglobin may initially be normal because there may not have been time for haemodilution to occur.

Septic shock

This causes similar effects by excessive vasodilatation, which prevents baroreflex compensation for postural-dependent blood pooling. However, the patient is usually obviously septic and febrile.

Aortic dissection

Injury to the innermost layer of the aorta (the intima) allows blood to enter and flow between the layers of the vessel wall, creating a false lumen. Patients may experience a severe, sudden onset, stabbing or tearing pain that sometimes radiates to the back. A widened mediastinum on chest X-ray with this type of pain should raise suspicion of aortic dissection; a computed tomography (CT) scan can confirm the diagnosis. There are a number of complications that may coexist with aortic dissection, including myocardial infarction (involvement of coronary arteries), aortic regurgitation, heart failure, ischaemia or infarction of other organs (e.g., stroke, mesenteric/renal ischaemia). This is an emergency and, in some cases, warrants urgent surgery.

Pulmonary embolism

Obstruction of pulmonary arteries by embolus enters into the differential diagnosis of all cardiovascular emergencies in which syncope is a feature. Chronic thromboembolism or primary pulmonary hypertension can also lead to postural hypotension because the resistance to right ventricular ejection is too high to allow adequate cardiac output when the filling pressure drops on standing. This results in reduced blood flow reaching the left side of the heart from the pulmonary artery and reduced left ventricular output as a result. CT pulmonary angiography (CTPA) may demonstrate pulmonary embolus if suspected.

HINTS AND TIPS

Cardiovascular syncope is always accompanied by hypotension. Syncope with normal blood pressure is likely to have a neurological, cerebrovascular or metabolic cause.

Neurological/cerebrovascular causes

For full explanation of these conditions, consult *Crash Course: Neurology and Ophthalmology*, 6th Edition.

Seizure

A seizure is a sudden abnormal electrical activity in the brain. This can be focal (affecting only one region of the brain) or generalized (causing loss of consciousness), or there can be secondary generalization of a focal onset seizure. The classic history of a generalized tonic–clonic seizure is of a sudden stiffening of the body (the tonic phase), followed by rhythmic jerking (the clonic phase), and then a prolonged recovery whilst the patient is drowsy. They may have muscle aches and a raised lactate due to the muscle contractions. There may be a sense of premonition (aura), and there may be tongue biting (lateral biting is more specific) or urinary/faecal incontinence associated (less specific to seizure).

Stroke and transient cerebral ischaemia

TIA very rarely causes loss of consciousness, whereas the patient is unlikely to regain consciousness quickly after a large territory infarct or haemorrhage. You should be cautious about offering TIA as part of your differential diagnosis for syncope. Severe headache and/or neurological deficit in association with syncope may be indicative of subarachnoid haemorrhage.

Vertebrobasilar syndrome

This is caused by obstruction of the arteries to the posterior part of the brain (brain stem and cerebellum). The syncope may be preceded by vertigo or dizziness. This syndrome is often associated with cervical spondylosis. The vertebral artery becomes kinked on head movement as it travels through the distorted cervical vertebra, interrupting circulation.

Metabolic causes

In the common situation of insulin-dependent diabetes mellitus, most patients are inadequately controlled, which leads to more rapid development of heart disease and autonomic neuropathy. Some patients will have overly tight control; these patients are more likely to experience episodes of loss of consciousness due to hypoglycaemia. However, hypoglycaemia can occur in any treated diabetic patient and may be precipitated by exercise, a reduction in food intake or alcohol.

For more on metabolic causes of syncope, see *Crash Course: Metabolism and Nutrition, 5th edition.*

DRIVING REGULATIONS IN SYNCOPAL PATIENTS

Various diagnoses may disqualify the patient from driving for a period of time (see Table 9.3 for examples). This may have serious occupational implications.

Table 9.3 Overview of current DVLA guidelines on driving after syncope/collapse/seizure

	Group 1 (cars, motorcycles)	Group 2 (HGVs, buses)
Arrhythmia (either atrial or ventricular), sinoatrial node disease, atrioventricular conduction defect	Must not drive if arrhythmia has caused or is likely to cause incapacity. May drive after condition is diagnosed and has been adequately treated for 4 weeks.	Must not drive if arrhythmia has caused or is likely to cause incapacity. May drive after condition is diagnosed, adequately treated for 3 months and left ventricular ejection fraction is >40%.
Congenital complete heart block	No restriction if asymptomatic. Must not drive if symptomatic until pacemaker implanted.	Must not drive until pacemaker implanted.
Pacemaker implantation (including box change)	Must not drive for 1 week.	Must not drive for 6 weeks.
Implantable defibrillator for arrhythmia associated with incapacity	Must not drive for 6 months post-implantation and after any shock, or for 2 years if appropriate shock results in incapacity (and unable to take preventative steps to stop further shock).	Permanently bars from driving group 2 vehicles.
First seizure	Must not drive for 6 months (12 months if presence of underlying causative factor that may increase risk).	Must not drive for 5 years (off of antiepileptics) or longer if further seizure is deemed medically likely.
Epilepsy	May qualify for relicensing if remains seizure-free for 1 year.	Must not drive until seizure-free for 10 years (without antiepileptics) before relicensing considered.

DVLA guidelines on fitness to drive are extensive and regularly updated. To fully describe current guidelines is outside of the scope of this book – for full guidelines visit: https://www.gov.uk/guidance/assessing-fitness-to-drive-a-guide-for-medical-professionals. [Accurate as of Dec 2022.]

● Chapter Summary

- Syncope is a transient loss of consciousness that is the result of reduced perfusion to the brain.
- The differential diagnosis of syncope is extensive and a detailed history (including a collateral history) is vital for diagnosis.
- There are a number of conditions that may mimic syncope or presyncope, including hypoglycaemia, seizure, hypoxia, etc.
- Syncope may be the presenting complaint for a number of different life-threatening pathologies, including episodes of arrhythmia (e.g., ventricular tachycardia/fibrillation/asystole), pulmonary embolism, myocardial infarction, stroke, etc.
- Episodes of syncope may have severe implications for an individual's eligibility to drive (and therefore also their livelihood).

UKMLA Conditions
Arrhythmias
Vasovagal syncope

UKMLA Presentations
Blackouts and faints
Dizziness
Driving advice
Low blood pressure

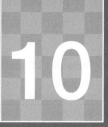

Heart murmurs 10

A heart murmur is a sound caused by turbulent blood flow, when the velocity of blood is disproportionate to the size of the lumen it is moving through. Murmurs are not always pathological.

DIFFERENTIAL DIAGNOSIS

Murmurs may occur due to:

- Valve defects (either stenosis or regurgitation).
- Left ventricular outflow obstruction – an example is hypertrophic cardiomyopathy (HCM).
- Septal defects – ventricular or atrial septal defects.
- Vascular disorders – coarctation of the aorta, patent ductus arteriosus, arteriovenous malformations (pulmonary or intercostal) and venous hum (cervical or hepatic).
- Increased cardiac output with normal anatomy (benign or innocent 'flow' murmur) – high-output states (e.g., anaemia, pregnancy, thyrotoxicosis).
- Increased flow across a normal pulmonary valve with septal defects.

HINTS AND TIPS

Cardiac sounds can be mistaken for murmurs. These include third and fourth heart sounds, midsystolic clicks (heard in mitral valve prolapse), metallic heart sounds and pericardial friction rubs. Other noncardiac sounds (e.g., pleural rubs, venous hums) may be similarly confused.

Differential diagnoses of heart murmurs are shown in Table 10.1.

HISTORY

Focus on:

- Possible aetiology of the murmur (e.g., infective endocarditis, valve lesion secondary to rheumatic heart disease, high-output state, etc.)

- Complications of valve disease (e.g., cardiac failure, exacerbation of ischaemic heart disease, arrhythmias, syncope, etc.)

Presenting complaint

Many patients with murmurs may be asymptomatic. However, patients may present with a variety of symptoms, including:

- Shortness of breath – suggestive of cardiac failure; other features include orthopnoea, paroxysmal nocturnal dyspnoea, peripheral oedema and fatigue.
- Chest pain – may be due to left ventricular outflow obstruction in aortic stenosis or hypertrophic obstructive cardiomyopathy (HOCM), atypical chest pain (a feature of mitral valve prolapse), or coexistent ischaemic heart disease.
- Syncope – especially in left ventricular outflow obstruction (e.g., aortic stenosis or HOCM).
- Fever, rigors and malaise – common presenting complaints in infective endocarditis.
- Palpitations – for example, mitral valve disease is associated with atrial fibrillation.

Past medical history

Focus on possible causes of a murmur:

- Rheumatic fever in childhood.
- Previous cardiac surgery – mechanical prosthetic valves cause a metallic first or second heart sound. Both metal and tissue prosthetic valves frequently cause flow murmurs and can also be complicated by regurgitation, thrombosis/stenosis or infective endocarditis.
- Previous myocardial infarction – may cause ventricular dilatation and consequent functional valve regurgitation, dysfunction of papillary muscle leading to valve regurgitation or a ventricular septal defect.
- Recent dental procedures or operations – may be a cause of infective endocarditis.
- Other medical conditions associated with valvular heart disease (see Table 10.1).

Remember that atrial fibrillation can cause decompensation from stable valvular disease or may be a consequence of valvular disease.

Table 10.1 Differential diagnosis of heart murmurs

Phase of cardiac cycle	Nature of murmur	Lesion	Causes
Systolic	Ejection systolic	Aortic stenosis (AS)	Senile degenerative calcification, calcification of congenital bicuspid valve, rheumatic fever, congenital valvular abnormality, congenital subvalvular stenosis, congenital supravalvular stenosis.
		Aortic sclerosis	Hardening of the valve without causing obstruction to flow. A precursor of aortic stenosis.
		Hypertrophic obstructive cardiomyopathy (HOCM)	Genetic mutations causing myocardial hypertrophy, which can, in some cases, lead to left ventricular outflow tract (subvalvular) stenosis. Without obstruction, it is known as HCM.
		Increased flow across normal valve	Increased cardiac output (e.g., anaemia, pregnancy, thyrotoxicosis, sepsis, athletes, hypertension, large AV fistula, Paget disease, beriberi).
		Pulmonary stenosis (PS)	Congenital malformations (e.g., tetralogy of Fallot, Noonan syndrome, congenital rubella syndrome). Carcinoid syndrome.
		ASD	Congenital.
	Pansystolic	Mitral regurgitation (MR)	Functional MR due to dilatation of the MV annulus such as with LV aneurysm, dilated cardiomyopathy. Valvular: rheumatic fever, infective endocarditis, MV prolapse, chordal rupture (e.g., connective tissue disorder, such as Marfan syndrome), papillary muscle infarction, SLE (Libman-Sacks lesion).
		Tricuspid regurgitation (TR)	Functional due to RV dilatation (most common): chronic LV failure, RV infarction, pulmonary hypertension (e.g., cor pulmonale), Marfan syndrome. Valvular: rheumatic fever, infective endocarditis, congenital malformations (e.g., Ebstein's anomaly), carcinoid syndrome.
		VSD with left-to-right shunt	Congenital, acquired (e.g., septal infarct).
Diastolic	Early diastolic	Aortic regurgitation (AR)	Functional due to dilatation of valve ring or aortic root: cystic medial necrosis (Marfan syndrome), aneurysm, aortic dissection, syphilitic aortitis, hypertension, ankylosing spondylitis. Valvular: rheumatic fever, infective endocarditis, bicuspid aortic valve, degenerative, RA, SLE.
		Pulmonary regurgitation (PR)	Functional due to dilatation of valve ring: pulmonary hypertension, complication of MS (Graham Steell murmur), Marfan syndrome. Valvular: infective endocarditis, rheumatic fever, carcinoid, tetralogy of Fallot.
	Mid-diastolic	Mitral stenosis (MS)	Rheumatic fever (almost always), calcification, congenital.
		Tricuspid stenosis (TS)	Rheumatic fever (almost always), carcinoid syndrome, congenital.
		Austin Flint murmur	Regurgitant jet from AR impinges opening of mitral valve anterior leaflet.
		Left and right atrial myxomas	Tumour obstruction of valve orifice in diastole.
Continuous		PDA	Congenital (physiological in newborns, otherwise pathological).
		AV fistula	Usually iatrogenic (for dialysis).
		Cervical venous hum	Normal/benign finding.
		Mixed AS and AR	As above.

ASD, atrial septal defect; *AV,* arteriovenous; *LV,* left ventricular; *MV,* mitral valve; *PDA,* patent ductus arteriosus; *RA,* rheumatoid arthritis; *RV,* right ventricular; *SLE,* systemic lupus erythematosus; *VSD,* ventricular septal defect.

Family history

Ask about a family history of cardiac problems or sudden death, as may occur in patients with HCM.

Social history

Ask in particular about:

- Smoking – an important risk factor for atherosclerosis.
- Alcohol intake – if excessive, may result in dilated cardiomyopathy.
- History of drug abuse – intravenous use increases infective endocarditis risk (especially right heart involvement), and prolonged MDMA use can induce valve fibrosis.

EXAMINATION

General observation

Fig. 10.1 summarizes potential examination findings in patients with heart murmurs.

Look for clues indicating the cause of the murmur:

- Anaemia – may cause a high-output state or result from infective endocarditis.
- Cyanosis – murmurs are common in congenital heart disease.
- Scars of previous cardiac surgery – median sternotomy, valvulotomy or other thoracotomy scars. These may indicate previous valve replacement or surgery for congenital cardiac disease. If surgery is recent and murmur is new, then consider infective endocarditis.

Look for signs of cardiac failure (e.g., dyspnoea or oedema).

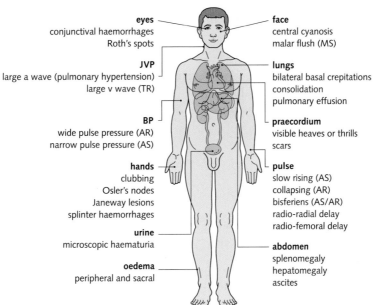

eyes
conjunctival haemorrhages
Roth's spots

JVP
large a wave (pulmonary hypertension)
large v wave (TR)

BP
wide pulse pressure (AR)
narrow pulse pressure (AS)

hands
clubbing
Osler's nodes
Janeway lesions
splinter haemorrhages

urine
microscopic haematuria

oedema
peripheral and sacral

face
central cyanosis
malar flush (MS)

lungs
bilateral basal crepitations
consolidation
pulmonary effusion

praecordium
visible heaves or thrills
scars

pulse
slow rising (AS)
collapsing (AR)
bisferiens (AS/AR)
radio-radial delay
radio-femoral delay

abdomen
splenomegaly
hepatomegaly
ascites

Fig. 10.1 Possible findings in a patient who has a heart murmur. *AS,* aortic stenosis; *AR,* aortic regurgitation; *MS,* mitral stenosis; *TR,* tricuspid regurgitation.

Cardiovascular system

Hands

Look for peripheral stigmata of infective endocarditis:

- Splinter haemorrhages (small linear longitudinal haemorrhages under the nail or in the nailbed). More than five is considered pathological.
- Osler nodes (painful red-purple papules on pulps of fingers/ toes, classically at the tips).
- Janeway lesions (nontender erythematous or haemorrhagic flat lesions on the palms and soles, classically on the thenar eminence).
- Finger clubbing – develops late.

Pulse

Examine both the radial and carotid arteries. Abnormalities due to valvular diseases include:

- Slow rising or plateau pulse in aortic stenosis.
- Collapsing or waterhammer pulse in aortic regurgitation or patent ductus arteriosus.
- Bisferiens pulse in severe mixed aortic valve disease.
- A jerky pulse in HOCM.

Radio-radial and radio-femoral delay can be found in aortic coarctation. This may be associated with a bruit heard over the back, which can be confused for a murmur.

Blood pressure

This may also give important clues:

- A narrow pulse pressure is a sign of severe aortic stenosis.
- A wide pulse pressure may be seen in aortic regurgitation, patent ductus arteriosus or high-output states.

Jugular venous pressure

Possible findings include:

- An elevated jugular venous pressure in congestive cardiac failure.
- Large 'a' waves (see Chapter 2) in pulmonary stenosis and pulmonary hypertension.
- Absent 'a' wave in atrial fibrillation.
- Cannon 'a' waves in complete heart block.
- Large 'v' waves in tricuspid regurgitation.

Precordium

Remember to look for surgical scars.

On palpation, possible abnormalities of apex beat include:

- Double apical impulse – due to HOCM or left ventricular aneurysm.
- Tapping apex beat – due to mitral stenosis.
- Heaving apex beat – due to aortic stenosis, HOCM or left ventricular hypertrophy.
- Displaced thrusting apex beat – due to aortic or mitral regurgitation or any sustained high-output state.

CLINICAL NOTES

It is easier to remember the correct association between murmurs and apex beat character if you bear in mind a heave is due to pressure overload and a thrust is due to volume overload.

A parasternal heave can be felt with the hand along the left sternal edge and is a sign of right ventricular hypertrophy or strain. It may be felt in patients with mitral valve disease, pulmonary hypertension or lung disease (cor pulmonale).

If flow is very turbulent, a thrill (loud palpable murmur) may be felt with the fingertips on the chest wall in any of the areas where the corresponding murmurs are best heard. For locations of valve areas, see Fig. 5.5.

When describing murmurs, consider:

1. Where in the cardiac cycle does it occur (systolic, diastolic or continuous)?
2. How loud is the murmur?
3. Does it produce a 'thrill'?
4. What quality does it have?
5. In which location is it best heard?
6. Does it radiate?
7. In which respiration phase is the murmur loudest?
8. Accentuation manoeuvres?
9. Are there any associated features?

COMMON PITFALLS

The volume of a murmur does not correlate with the severity of the lesion. For example, if left ventricular failure results from severe aortic stenosis, the ejection systolic murmur can become much quieter due to reduced cardiac output. However, the pitch of a murmur correlates with pressure gradient across the orifice – the higher the pressure, the higher the pitch.

After auscultating at the four main valve areas, if a systolic murmur is heard, the axilla and the carotid arteries should be auscultated with the diaphragm of the stethoscope for radiation. The murmur of mitral regurgitation often radiates to the axilla and the murmur of aortic stenosis classically radiates to the carotid arteries, although loud murmurs can sometimes be heard all over the precordium and in the axilla.

Diastolic murmurs (never innocent) can be quiet and difficult to hear and so may be augmented with certain manoeuvres:

- Rolling the patient onto his or her left-hand side brings the apex of the heart into contact with the chest wall and may make the murmur of mitral stenosis audible. Brief exercise by the patient can also make a mitral stenotic murmur louder.

- By asking the patient to sit forward and hold his or her breath in expiration, a murmur of aortic regurgitation can be heard better at the left sternal edge.

HINTS AND TIPS

Murmurs from valves on the left side of the heart (mitral and aortic) are louder on expiration. Those from the right side of the heart (tricuspid and pulmonary) are accentuated by inspiration.

A summary of murmur characteristics is shown in Table 10.2. The most commonly heard murmurs are aortic stenosis and mitral regurgitation.

CLINICAL NOTES

There are a number of eponymous signs that may be seen with aortic regurgitation:

- Quincke's sign – visible nailbed pulsation of blood. Sometimes called the 'lighthouse' sign because it almost flashes.
- Corrigan's sign – exaggerated carotid pulsation.
- De Musset's sign – head nodding.
- Duroziez's sign – diastolic femoral murmur.
- Traube's sign – 'pistol shot' femorals.
- Müller's sign – uvula pulsations.

The intensity of murmurs is graded from 1 to 6, from very quiet to very loud. It may not be wise to describe yourself as an expert in finals by describing a murmur as grade 1!

- Grade 1 – only audible in ideal conditions by an expert.
- Grade 2 – only audible in ideal conditions by a nonexpert.
- Grade 3 – easily audible, no palpable thrill.
- Grade 4 – loud, associated with a thrill.
- Grade 5 – very loud with a thrill, audible with edge of the stethoscope partly off the chest.
- Grade 6 – audible without a stethoscope.

HINTS AND TIPS

Many students (and doctors!) find auscultation and interpretation of murmurs difficult. Don't worry – if you listen carefully to the cardiac cycle of every patient that you examine, you will get a feel for what is normal, and you will pick up abnormalities more easily.

Peripheral pulses

All peripheral pulses should be palpated. Radio-femoral (and occasionally radio-radial) delay may be found with aortic coarctation, and lower limb pulses may be reduced. There may be discrepancy in the blood pressure taken in each arm or between the right arm and either leg.

Peripheral oedema

Pitting oedema may be elicited by applying firm pressure (for at least 10 seconds) with a finger. Be careful, this can be painful for the patient. Observe the patient's face as you press.

Respiratory system

Possible findings include:

- Bilateral basal fine end-inspiratory crepitations – suggests left ventricular failure and pulmonary oedema.
- Evidence of respiratory tract infection – sepsis may cause a high-output state; septic emboli from right-sided infective endocarditis can cause pneumonia.

Gastrointestinal system

Important findings include:

- Hepatomegaly or ascites, seen in right ventricular failure or biventricular failure.
- Splenomegaly, a feature of infective endocarditis.

INVESTIGATIONS

Blood tests

These include:

1. Full blood count – anaemia may be seen as a sign of chronic disease in infective endocarditis and is also a cause of hyperdynamic state; a leucocytosis is also a feature of infective endocarditis.
2. Urea, creatinine and electrolytes – may be deranged in patients with cardiac failure (due to poor renal perfusion or diuretic therapy).
3. Liver function tests – may be abnormal in patients with hepatic congestion secondary to cardiac failure.
4. Erythrocyte sedimentation rate (ESR) and C-reactive protein (CRP) – these are markers of inflammation or infection and are useful in monitoring in infective endocarditis.
5. Blood cultures – crucial if infective endocarditis is suspected, in which case at least three sets should be taken before starting antibiotics.

Table 10.2 Characteristics of murmurs

Timing	Lesion	Best heard (valve area) / Radiates to / Accentuate with / Quality	Possible systemic features
Ejection systolic (crescendo-decrescendo)	Aortic stenosis	B Aortic R Carotids (often all over precordium including axilla) Q Harsh; high pitch if severe	Slow rising pulse Narrow pulse pressure Heaving nondisplaced apex beat Ejection click Quiet or absent S2 (if severe) Reversed splitting of S2 (prolonged LV emptying) S4 May have LVF (S3, pulmonary oedema)
	Aortic sclerosis (*Asymptomatic*)	B Aortic R Classically does not radiate Q Harsh	No slow rising pulse Normal pulse pressure S2 normal or loud
	Hypertrophic obstructive cardiomyopathy	B Aortic and tricuspid for ESM, apex and tricuspid for PSM A Standing from squatting or Valsalva (↑ gradient by emptying LV) Q High pitch	Pulse jerky or normal upstroke Double apical impulse
	Increased flow across normal valve	B Aortic R No radiation Q Soft	No other cardiovascular abnormalities
	Pulmonary stenosis (PS)	B Pulmonary and tricuspid Q High pitch	Ejection click Wide splitting of or quiet S2 RV heave
	Atrial septal defect	B Pulmonary Q Very similar to PS	Fixed splitting of S2
Pansystolic	Mitral regurgitation	B Apex R Left axilla A Exercise Q Blowing	Quiet S1 Obliterated S2 S3 Thrusting, displaced apex beat Often AF Midsystolic 'click' and late systolic murmur in mitral valve prolapse
	Tricuspid regurgitation	B Tricuspid Q High pitched, blowing	Giant 'v' waves in jugular venous pressure (JVP) Pulsatile hepatomegaly May have thrusting RV impulse May have signs of RVF
	Ventricular septal defect	B Tricuspid R Right lower sternal border Q Loud and rough	Wide splitting of S2 Prominent RV impulse May have signs of cardiac failure or Eisenmenger syndrome

Early diastolic	Aortic regurgitation	**B** Tricuspid **A** Leaning forward, breath held in expiration **Q** High pitch	Bounding and collapsing pulse Wide pulse pressure S3 Thrusting, displaced apex Eponymous signs (see clinical notes box) Systolic flow murmur (high flow) Austin Flint (mid-diastolic) murmur Bisferiens pulse (if severe)
	Pulmonary regurgitation	**B** Tricuspid and pulmonary **Q** High pitch	Wide splitting of S2 Hyperdynamic thrusting RV impulse
Mid-diastolic	Mitral stenosis	**B** Apex (bell) **A** Roll onto left side, breath held in expiration the murmur of mitral stenosis will be accentuated by exercise **Q** Rumbling, low-pitch, presystolic accentuation if in sinus rhythm	Tapping nondisplaced apex (palpable S1) Loud S1 Opening snap Often AF Pulmonary oedema If associated pulmonary hypertension, mitral facies/parasternal heave/loud P2/Graham Steell murmur (PR due to MS) May develop signs of RVF
	Tricuspid stenosis	**B** Tricuspid	Elevated JVP, with giant 'a' waves and slow 'y' descent May develop signs of RVF and pulsatile liver Often associated with other valvular lesions
Continuous	Patent ductus arteriosus	**B** Second intercostal space below left clavicle; pulmonary and tricuspid **R** Left scapula **Q** Machinery-like, with late systolic accentuation	Large volume peripheral pulses Prominent apex beat May develop signs of cardiac failure or Eisenmenger syndrome

AF, atrial fibrillation; *JVP*, jugular venous pressure; *LV*, left ventricle; *LVF*, left ventricular failure; *MS*, mitral stenosis; *P2*, pulmonary valve closure; *PR*, pulmonary regurgitation; *RV*, right ventricular; *RVF*, right ventricular failure; *S1*, first heart sound; *S2*, second heart sound; *S3*, third heart sound; *S4*, fourth heart sound.

Urinalysis

This should always be performed with new murmurs. Microscopic haematuria is common in patients with infective endocarditis.

Chest radiography

This may reveal an abnormal cardiac shadow (e.g., large left atrium and prominent pulmonary vessels in mitral stenosis, enlarged left ventricle in mitral or aortic regurgitation or the abnormal aortic shadow in coarctation).

Pulmonary abnormalities (e.g., pulmonary oedema, pleural effusion) may also be seen as a complication of left-sided valvular disease.

Electrocardiography

The 12-lead ECG may give useful information, including:

1. Atrial fibrillation may be a sign of mitral valve disease.
2. P mitrale (broad bifid P waves) may be seen in left atrial enlargement as a result of mitral stenosis, and if this is severe, it may also result in pulmonary hypertension and P pulmonale (peaked P waves) due to right atrial enlargement.
3. Left ventricular hypertrophy and strain pattern may be seen in aortic stenosis, HCM, aortic regurgitation or mitral regurgitation.
4. Right ventricular hypertrophy may be a sign of mitral or pulmonary stenosis.
5. AV block may be seen in infective endocarditis due to aortic root abscess formation.

Echocardiography

Transthoracic echocardiography

Transthoracic echocardiography is the most widely used imaging technique for murmurs and is frequently the key investigation for valvular disease. It enables valves to be visualized, and Doppler echocardiography assesses the direction and velocity of flow (used to derive pressures) across valves. Vegetations may be seen, although infective endocarditis cannot be ruled out without more sensitive transoesophageal echocardiography. Left ventricular function and pulmonary artery pressure can be estimated. The presence of a ventricular septal defect or patent ductus arteriosus may be visualized but may rarely require cardiac catheterization to more accurately assess the abnormality and shunt volume.

Transoesophageal echocardiography

Transoesophageal echocardiography can be very useful because it gives detailed information on structures that are difficult to see using transthoracic echocardiography. Examples of its uses include:

1. Detection of vegetations.
2. Assessment of prosthetic valves.
3. Detailed evaluation of the mitral valve before mitral valve repair.

Cardiac magnetic resonance imaging

This can be useful to more accurately delineate anatomy. It can outline the size of aortic root in aortic regurgitation to demonstrate congenital malformations (e.g., aortic coarctation) and flow across valves can be used to assess valvular stenosis and regurgitation.

Cardiac catheterization

Before valve replacement, this is performed to obtain information about the:

1. Presence of coexisting coronary artery disease.
2. Direct measurement of the degree of pulmonary hypertension in patients who have mitral valve disease.

Catherization can directly measure the severity of the left-to-right shunt in patients who have septal defects.

PRESENTING YOUR FINDINGS

Murmurs crop up regularly in exams. The most frequently tested scenarios in OSCEs are patients with aortic stenosis, mitral regurgitation, infective endocarditis, prosthetic valves, aortic regurgitation and adult congenital heart diseases; however, other murmurs may be examined.

When presenting a murmur, describe it using a system such as below.

- Timing.
- Intensity.
- Position (of stethoscope AND patient) where heard loudest.
- Radiation.
- Quality.
- Systemic features – include complications, such as heart failure, infective endocarditis or prosthetic valve failure.

For example, you might say, 'The most obvious abnormality is an early diastolic murmur of grade 2 intensity. It is heard loudest in the tricuspid area with the patient sitting forward and does not radiate. The murmur is accentuated by the patient holding his breath in expiration. It is a decrescendo high-pitched murmur and is associated with a collapsing pulse, a displaced thrusting apex beat, a third heart sound and bibasal crepitations. There are no stigmata of infective endocarditis, and he is a tall, thin gentleman with a high-arched palate. These features are consistent with aortic regurgitation potentially due to Marfan syndrome and complicated by a degree of left ventricular failure. However, the patient does not look distressed or unwell'.

Chapter Summary

- When taking a history with murmurs in mind, remember to look for potential causes.
- Examination of murmurs includes the entire cardiovascular system and other systems that may explain noncardiac causes of murmurs.
- Remember to take three to six sets of blood cultures before administering antibiotics if infective endocarditis is suspected.
- If a cardiac cause of murmur is suspected, echocardiography is the first imaging investigation of choice and frequently the only imaging required.
- Using a systematic approach will assist in diagnosing the most likely causes of a murmur and help you with a polished presentation.

UKMLA Conditions
Aortic valve disease
Infective endocarditis
Mitral valve disease
Right heart valve disease

UKMLA Presentations
Cyanosis
Fever
Heart murmurs

Section 3

CLINICAL CONDITIONS

Atherosclerosis and its risk factors 11

Atherosclerosis is a progressive, inflammatory disease of large- and medium-sized arteries characterized by focal accumulation of lipid in the vessel intima with associated inflammatory and smooth muscle infiltrate. Atherosclerosis is likely present to some degree in all adults. The consequences of atherosclerosis (including ischaemic heart disease (IHD), peripheral vascular disease and cerebrovascular disease) are estimated to account for 45% of deaths in Europe and 31% of global deaths in 2015.

PATHOGENESIS OF ATHEROSCLEROSIS

The pathogenesis of atherosclerosis is often described by the response to injury hypothesis. This states that chronic vascular endothelial damage and subsequent dysfunction are key in initiating the process. The steps involved in this process (see Fig. 11.1) include:

1. Endothelial dysfunction: chronic endothelial cell injury can occur as a result of smoking and high cholesterol (particularly LDL), leading to metabolic dysfunction and structural changes. Damage activates endothelial cells, upregulating inflammatory adhesion molecules (e.g., ICAM-1) and promoting monocyte and platelet adhesion. This upregulation is also caused by altered gene expression at sites where the pattern of blood flow is altered, such as bends and bifurcations in vessels. Injury increases permeability to lipids and LDL, allowing accumulation in the intima.
2. Formation of a fatty streak: monocytes adhere to the endothelium, migrate into the intima and differentiate into macrophages. Local LDL oxidation attracts macrophages, which, once in the intima, take up the oxidized LDL and become foam cells. Platelets adhere to activated endothelial cells or areas of denuded matrix and become activated. Activated platelets, endothelial cells and macrophages release platelet-derived growth factor, stimulating smooth muscle cell migration from the media to the intima.
3. Development of lipid plaque: smooth muscle proliferation and an increase in extracellular matrix occur in the intima. Additional cytokines and growth factors produced by activated macrophages and platelets promote additional monocyte and smooth muscle infiltration. Lipid may also be released from dying foam cells, contributing to extracellular free lipid pools.
4. Advanced plaques: an advanced atherosclerotic plaque consists of a lipid-rich 'core' and a fibrous (primarily

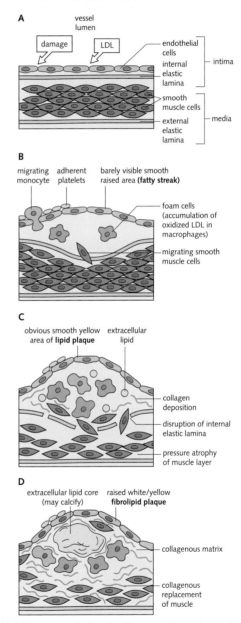

Fig. 11.1 The stages in the development of an atherosclerotic plaque, from the initial endothelial damage through to an advanced plaque. (A) Endothelial dysfunction. (B) Formation of the fatty streak. (C) Development of a lipid plaque. (D) Advanced atherosclerotic plaque. *LDL*, low-density lipoprotein.

collagenous) 'cap'. The core of the lesion (which can become necrotic) consists of free lipid, macrophages, smooth muscle cells and cellular debris. The fibrous cap lies over the core beneath the endothelium.

A stable advanced atherosclerotic plaque is likely to remain asymptomatic for years. Initially, as the plaque expands, it causes remodelling of the media, allowing the vessel to increase its diameter and accommodating the plaque without compromising the vessel lumen. The degree to which this occurs varies greatly. In the absence of this remodelling, the plaque will grow, protrude into the lumen and progressively decrease lumen size. It will only become apparent when the luminal diameter is not sufficient to allow adequate organ perfusion.

CLINICAL NOTES

Clinically significant atherosclerosis may remain silent for years, and the first manifestation is often myocardial infarction.

Plaque stability is dependent on the strength and thickness of the fibrous cap, which relies on the balance between inflammation and repair. If inflammation predominates, the cap may become thinner and less stable, and one of the following may occur (Fig. 11.2):

1. Plaque erosion: occurs when there is damage to the endothelium overlying the plaque. This exposes the prothrombotic subendothelial connective tissue, causing platelet adhesion and thrombus formation on the plaque surface, which can occlude the lumen (Fig. 11.3).
2. Plaque rupture/fissure: occurs in advanced plaque when deep fissures form in the plaque allowing blood to flow into

the plaque. A thrombus then forms within the plaque causing it to expand and occlude the vessel lumen.

Atherosclerotic plaques create areas of weakness in vessel walls, which also predisposes to aneurysm formation.

CLASSIFICATION OF ISCHAEMIC HEART DISEASE

IHD is the manifestation of atheromatous disease affecting one or more coronary arteries. Classification is shown in Table 11.1.

If an atherosclerotic plaque grows slowly, over months, collateral vessels may develop and protect the myocardium from acute insult in the original vessel. A faster rate of vessel occlusion and a greater degree of vessel occlusion will increase the severity of clinical presentation.

Stable angina is the chronic manifestation of coronary artery disease and results from coronary artery stenoses due to stable atherosclerotic plaques.

Unstable angina (UA) occurs if occlusion is incomplete or very short-lived. Myocardial infarction occurs when myocytes die due to myocardial ischaemia. Irreversible damage occurs between 20 and 40 minutes after vessel occlusion. The evolution of infarcted myocardium is depicted in Fig. 11.4. The area of myocardium affected depends on the vessel involved. ECG changes allow assessment of the area involved (see Fig. 12.5). The area of infarction following occlusion of each of the major vessels is shown in Fig. 11.5.

Acute plaque changes can manifest as one of three acute coronary syndromes, in order of increasing severity:

1. UA: angina of increasing severity or at rest without myocardial necrosis.

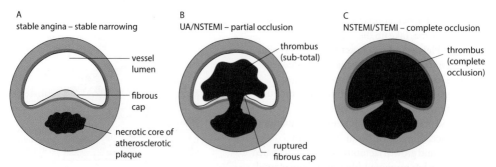

Fig. 11.2 The changes in the atherosclerotic plaque and associated thrombus underlying each of the manifestations of coronary artery disease. (A) Stable angina: atherosclerotic plaque with solid fibrous cap reducing the vessel lumen size. (B) UA/NSTEMI: erosion or rupture of fibrous cap with partially occlusive thrombus formation. (C) NSTEMI/STEMI: erosion or rupture of fibrous cap with complete vessel occlusion by thrombus. *NSTEMI*, non-ST elevation myocardial infarction; *STEMI*, ST-segment elevation myocardial infarction; *UA*, unstable angina.

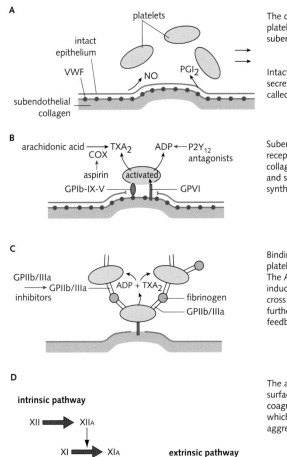

A

The continuous endothelial layer prevents circulating platelets from coming into contact with prothrombotic subendothelial components:
- von-Willebrand factor (VWF)
- Collagen

Intact endothelium prevents activation of platelets by secretion of nitric oxide (NO) and prostacyclin (also called prostaglandin I2, PGI$_2$).

B

Subendothelial VWF tether platelets on platelet surface receptor complex GPIb-IX-V. Firm adhesion to subendothelial collagen via glycoprotein VI (GPVI) activates the platelet and stimulates release of adenosine diphosphate (ADP) and synthesis of thromboxane A$_2$ (TXA$_2$) from arachidonic acid.

C

Binding of GPVI also induces expression and activation of platelet integrin GPIIb/IIIa, which binds to fibrinogen. The ADP and TXA$_2$ released activate other platelets, inducing expression of GPIIb/IIIa and allowing platelet cross linking via fibrinogen. Activation of platelets causes further release of ADP and TXA$_2$, causing a positive feedback effect.

D

The aggregation of platelets provides a prothrombotic surface for the clotting/coagulation cascade. The coagulation cascade (**D**) results in formation of fibrin, which forms a mesh around and between the aggregated platelets. This end result is a clot.

Fig. 11.3 Platelet activation, thrombosis and the coagulation cascade. *ADP*, adenosine diphosphate; *COX*, cyclooxygenase; *GP*, glycoprotein; *NO*, nitric oxide; *PGI$_2$*, prostacyclin; *TXA$_2$*, thromboxane A$_2$; *VWF*, von-Willebrand factor. *Red arrows* – inhibitory action. *Green arrows* – enhancing action.

2. Non-ST-segment elevation myocardial infarction (NSTEMI): new onset chest pain with biochemical evidence of myocardial necrosis but no ST-segment elevation on ECG.
3. ST-segment elevation myocardial infarction (STEMI): acute chest pain, often associated with autonomic symptoms such as sweating or vomiting, with biochemical evidence of myocardial necrosis and ST-segment elevation or new left bundle branch block on ECG. This is usually associated with complete occlusion of the coronary artery and significant myocardial necrosis.

Table 11.1 Classification of ischaemic heart disease in order of increasing severity. This outlines the pathological intracoronary finding, resulting damage, presentation and initial investigation findings

Coronary artery disease			
		Acute coronary syndromes	
		Myocardial infarction	
Stable angina	**Unstable angina**	**NSTEMI**	**STEMI**
Constant stenosis Ischaemia without necrosis	Dynamic stenosis Ischaemia without necrosis	Obstruction to flow Cardiomyocyte necrosis	Obstruction to flow Cardiomyocyte necrosis
Predictable effort-dependent symptoms	Unpredictable/worsening symptoms	Prolonged symptoms, can occur at any time	Prolonged symptoms, can occur at any time
May have reversible ECG changes No biomarker rise	May have reversible ECG changes No biomarker rise	May have irreversible ECG changes Biomarker rise	ST elevation in the distribution of affected coronary artery Biomarker rise

ECG, electrocardiogram; *NSTEMI*, non-ST-segment elevation myocardial infarction; *STEMI*, ST-segment elevation myocardial infarction.

time	macroscopic appearance	microscopic appearance
0–12 hours	not visible	infarcted muscle appears uncoloured on staining with nitroblue tetrazolium due to loss of oxidative enzymes; healthy muscle stains blue
12–24 hours	pale with blotchy discolouration	infarcted muscle is brightly eosinophilic with intercellular oedema
24–72 hours	dead area appears soft and pale with a slight yellow colour	infarcted area excites an acute inflammatory response, neutrophils infiltrate between dead cardiac muscle fibres
3–10 days	hyperaemic border develops around the yellow dead muscle	organization of infarcted area replacement with vascular granulation tissue
weeks– months	white scar	progressive collagen deposition infarct is replaced by a collagenous scar

Fig. 11.4 Morphological changes occurring following myocardial infarction.

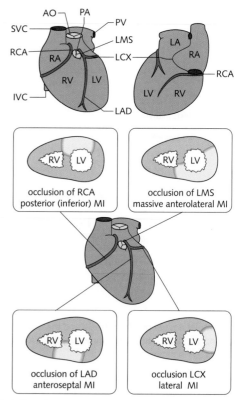

occlusion of RCA posterior (inferior) MI

occlusion of LMS massive anterolateral MI

occlusion of LAD anteroseptal MI

occlusion LCX lateral MI

Fig. 11.5 Site of myocardial infarction and associated vessel involvement. *AO,* aorta; *IVC,* inferior vena cava; *LA,* left atrium; *LAD,* left anterior descending; *LCX,* circumflex coronary artery; *LMS,* left main stem; *LV,* left ventricle; *MI,* myocardial infarction; *PA,* pulmonary artery; *PV,* pulmonary vein; *RA,* right atrium; *RCA,* right coronary artery; *RV,* right ventricle; *SVC,* superior vena cava.

Table 11.2 Nonmodifiable and modifiable risk factors for atherosclerosis

Nonmodifiable	Modifiable
• Age – correlates with number and severity of atherosclerotic lesions • Sex – men are affected to a much greater extent, incidence in women increases after menopause • Genetic predisposition – family history is a strong risk factor, even when known genetic diseases such as familial hypercholesterolaemia are excluded • Known coronary artery disease.	• Smoking • Hypertension • Diabetes mellitus • Dyslipidaemia • Obesity • Sedentary lifestyle • Diet high in saturated fat • Thrombophilias (e.g., antiphospholipid syndrome), other hypercoagulable states (e.g., essential thrombocythaemia) or atrial fibrillation – these are traditionally associated with venous thromboembolism but have a small increased risk of atherosclerosis.

RISK FACTORS FOR ATHEROSCLEROSIS

Risk factors for atherosclerosis and its associated conditions can be broken down into 'modifiable' and 'nonmodifiable'. Some of the more important are in Table 11.2.

RISK PREDICTION AND PRIMARY PREVENTION OF ISCHAEMIC HEART DISEASE

1. Primary prevention aims to reduce a person's risk of developing IHD. It involves treating seemingly healthy individuals, many of whom may never go on to develop the disease.
2. Secondary prevention targets risk factors in a person with known coronary disease, who has a higher risk and will likely receive greater benefit from treatments to prevent progression and future events.

Coronary disease may be asymptomatic for many years but then present unexpectedly with myocardial infarction or sudden death. Primary prevention strategies aim to reduce this risk.

Those with higher risk have potentially more to gain from risk reduction, as the same intervention with fixed relative risk reduction will result in a greater absolute risk reduction. For high-risk patients, lifestyle interventions and pharmacological measures are directed at controlling risk factors such as hypertension, hypercholesterolaemia, poor glycaemic control and obesity.

Although specific approaches to smoking cessation are beyond this book's remit, it is important to encourage cessation both as primary prevention as well as at every stage of coronary artery disease. Opportunistic brief interventions to give advice are shown to be effective, although the most successful may be unfortunately after disease has manifested. Positive encouragement, advice on the complications of smoking and information about self-help groups should all be made available to smokers. Smoking-cessation clinics (which often work on a self-referral basis) are now commonplace.

In-depth information regarding diabetes and its management can be found in *Crash Course: General Medicine*, 6th Edition.

The following sections will concentrate on dyslipidaemias and hypertension.

Risk calculation

To establish who will benefit most from primary prevention measures and pharmacological treatment, various risk stratification models have been developed to estimate an individual's risk of developing cardiovascular disease. This is most pertinently applied to treatment decisions in dyslipidaemia. The first of these was the Framingham risk prediction chart (Fig. 11.6).

The Framingham model was developed in the United States and is less applicable to the UK population. Simple-to-use online risk prediction calculators have been developed and validated in the UK to guide decisions surrounding primary prevention. These take into account many of the major risk factors such as age, sex, smoking, lipid levels and blood pressure (BP), even incorporating postcodes to take into account the index of multiple deprivation score. In England and Wales, the QRISK score (now updated to QRISK3) stratifies risk using a broadened range of factors. In Scotland, the ASSIGN score is used.

Calculators should not be applied if the patient already has other conditions that place them at high risk and would qualify for treatment of these factors in their own right. These include type 1 diabetes, hypertension with target organ damage, chronic kidney disease (CKD) and familial hypercholesterolaemia. Some

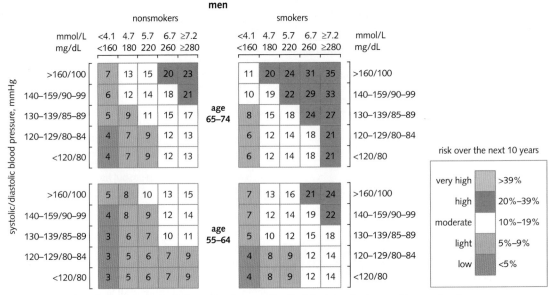

Fig. 11.6 A sample of the Framingham charts for estimating a patient's risk of developing cardiovascular disease.

calculators may also underestimate risk if there are additional risk factors which cannot be inputted (e.g., HIV treatment, serious mental health problems, medications that cause dyslipidaemia, autoimmune and systemic inflammatory disorders).

LIPIDS AND THE CARDIOVASCULAR SYSTEM

Lipid transport and metabolism and targets of lipid-modifying drugs

The insolubility of lipids in plasma means a special transport mechanism is required. This is provided by lipid–protein complexes known as lipoproteins. The apolipoproteins (protein component of lipoproteins) also act as receptors for cell surface proteins, which determine the destination of different lipoproteins. Low-density lipoprotein (LDL) is the main lipoprotein involved in transport of cholesterol. Fig. 11.7 shows the main transport pathways for dietary lipids (exogenous) and for lipids from the body's stores (endogenous).

It is thought that apolipoprotein A is a prothrombotic lipoprotein that is particularly involved in coronary artery disease, while high levels of high-density lipoprotein (HDL) are protective. The classification of lipoproteins is outlined in Table 11.3.

Hyperlipidaemia

Hyperlipidaemia can be classified as hypertriglyceridaemia (raised triglycerides), hypercholesterolaemia (raised cholesterol)

or hyperlipoproteinaemia (raised lipoproteins). In reality, there may be combinations of each. Although these classifications are useful, they must be used with care because, although hypercholesterolaemia is a risk factor for development of atherosclerosis, it is increasingly apparent that the balance between LDL (damaging) and HDL (protective) may be more important than absolute levels. As a result, some people prefer the term 'dyslipidaemia', as it refers to derangement of lipids rather than simply an increase. LDL cholesterol is the most helpful primary treatment target.

HINTS AND TIPS

In patients with high cholesterol, lipids can be deposited in the soft tissues. Common sites include the skin around the eyes (xanthelasma), in tendons (tendon xanthomata), and premature (<45 years) corneal arcus (around the corneal margin).

Management of hyperlipidaemia

Hyperlipidaemia can be treated with lifestyle interventions or pharmacologically. Lifestyle interventions should include reduction of calorie intake, saturated fats and dietary cholesterol. Regular exercise and reduction of alcohol consumption are also beneficial. The efficacy of supplements of omega-3 fat (present in fish oils) is currently unproven.

In patients with known coronary artery disease, the National Institute for Health and Care Excellence (NICE) recommends that

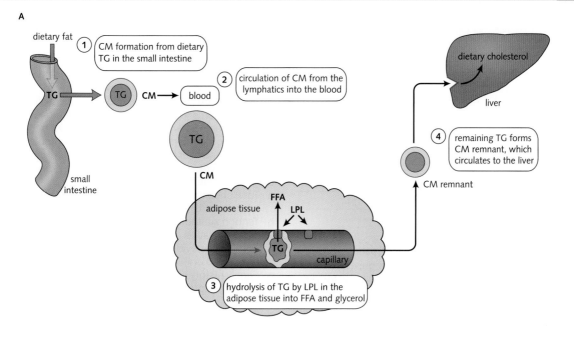

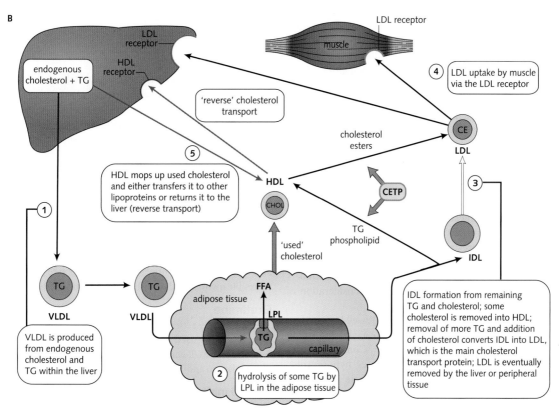

Fig. 11.7 (A) Exogenous and (B) endogenous lipid transport pathways; *CE*, cholesterol esters; *CETP*, cholesterol ester transfer protein; *CM*, chylomicron; *FFA*, free fatty acid; *HDL*, high-density lipoprotein; *IDL*, intermediate-density lipoprotein; *LDL*, low-density lipoprotein; *LPL*, lipoprotein lipase; *TG*, triglyceride; *VLDL*, very low-density lipoprotein.

Table 11.3 Classification of lipoproteins

Particle	Source	Predominantly transports
Chylomicron (CM)	Gut	Trigylcerides
Very low-density lipoprotein (VLDL)	Liver	Triglycerides
Intermediate-density lipoprotein (IDL), low-density lipoprotein (LDL), and high-density lipoprotein (HDL)	Catabolism	Cholesterol
Lipoprotein A	Liver, gut	—

lipid-lowering therapy should be offered to all patients irrespective of their cholesterol as part of a secondary prevention strategy. These patients should be started on a high-intensity statin (e.g., atorvastatin at 80 mg daily if tolerated and no contraindications) aiming for a >40% reduction in non-HDL cholesterol from baseline.

In primary prevention, there is no universally accepted level at which drug therapy should be started and the decision is usually based on assessment of overall risk of cardiovascular disease. NICE guidelines recommend starting atorvastatin 20 mg daily in patients with a 10-year cardiovascular risk of greater than 10% using validated risk calculators (e.g., QRISK3). This recent guidance (May 2023) recognised that although statins are cost effective for people with a 10-year risk of less than 10%, NICE felt that compliance with statin therapy in this lower risk group was likely to be poor. Therefore, focusing on increasing uptake in higher risk patients was felt more likely to be of benefit than reducing treatment threshold. However, NICE have recommended a person-centred approach with an option of 20 mg atorvastatin in any patient who wishes to take statins (regardless of QRISK3 score) or if clinical judgement suggests the patient may be at higher risk than their risk score suggests.

If cholesterol levels are very high, ask about family history and consider familial hypercholesterolaemia. This confers not only increased risk to the individual but also to other family members and should prompt genetic counselling and consideration of treatment.

Secondary causes of dyslipidaemia are less well known than secondary causes of hypertension but make a contribution in a significant proportion of the population. Common causes include excess alcohol, uncontrolled diabetes, hypothyroidism, cholestatic liver disease and nephrotic syndrome. Medication causes include antipsychotic medication, corticosteroids and some immunosuppressant drugs. If treatment of these causes is possible, lipid-lowering treatments may not be required.

Drugs used to lower cholesterol

Statins (e.g., simvastatin, atorvastatin)

Statins are β-hydroxy-β-methylglutaryl coenzyme A (HMG-CoA) reductase inhibitors. HMG-CoA reductase is the rate-limiting step in cholesterol synthesis. When inhibited, the liver compensates for the decreased cholesterol synthesis by increasing LDL receptor expression, decreasing plasma LDL. Statins are the first-line drug for high cholesterol, can reduce cholesterol by more than 50% and have been repeatedly demonstrated to reduce mortality in both primary and secondary prevention of cardiovascular disease. In addition to their cholesterol-lowering effects, statins have an antiatherosclerotic effect, reducing the inflammatory activity within atherosclerotic plaques (and thus strengthening the fibrous cap) and reducing the size of plaques. The main side effects include reversible myositis and disturbed liver function tests.

Ezetimibe

This is an orally acting selective inhibitor of cholesterol absorption. It may be used alone or in combination with a statin in refractory cases. It can lower cholesterol by a further 15% to 20% when taken in addition to a statin.

PCSK9 inhibitors

This class of drugs targets the PCSK9 protein involved in the control of the LDL receptor. The two monoclonal antibodies available, alirocumab and evolocumab, are subcutaneous injections administered usually every 2 weeks. They can lower LDL cholesterol levels by over 50%; however, currently, they are only available for use in certain high-risk cases of familial hypercholesterolaemia or mixed dyslipidaemia where maximal tolerated doses of statins have not achieved sufficient cholesterol reduction. Recently, a small interfering RNA, inclisiran, has been licensed, which inhibits the production of PCSK9. This is administered as a subcutaneous injection every 6 months.

Bile acid binding resins (e.g., colestipol and colestyramine)

Cholesterol is the initial substrate for synthesis of bile acids. These drugs bind bile acids in the intestine, forming insoluble complexes and increasing excretion of bile acids. To replenish bile acid levels, cholesterol is utilized for bile acid synthesis, thus reducing plasma cholesterol levels. This removes LDL cholesterol from circulation; however, these drugs can aggravate hypertriglyceridaemia.

Drugs used to lower triglyceride levels
Fibrates

Gemfibrozil reduces lipolysis of triglycerides in adipose tissue, leading to decreased hepatic production of very low-density lipoprotein (VLDL). Bezafibrate causes decreased VLDL and decreased triglycerides, but it may increase LDL. Fibrates are used mainly in familial hyperlipidaemia. Gemfibrozil does not increase LDL but increases the risk of myopathy from statins; therefore it should not be coprescribed.

HYPERTENSION

Hypertension is not only a major risk factor for myocardial infarction and heart failure but also cerebrovascular disease, peripheral vascular disease, renal failure, cognitive decline and premature death; therefore, it is important to diagnose and adequately treat hypertensive patients.

Definition of hypertension

Normal BP increases with age and varies throughout the day according to factors such as stress and exertion. There is also an underlying diurnal variation, with the lowest BP occurring at around 4 AM. In the population, there is a skewed normal distribution.

The ideal BP for a young, healthy person is considered to be between 90/60 and 120/80 mmHg.

In some people, BP can be consistently higher when measured at their GP or clinic. This is known as 'white coat' hypertension and is defined as a discrepancy of greater than 20/10 mmHg between clinic and average ambulatory/home BP measurement (ABPM/HBPM). When considering a diagnosis of hypertension, multiple BP readings away from the clinical environment are now recommended, as this is shown to correlate better with BP-related clinical outcomes.

The definition of hypertension is somewhat arbitrary, and cardiovascular disease risk increases with increasing BP, even within the normal range. Current NICE/British Hypertension Society guidelines define hypertension as a clinic BP of greater than 140/90 mmHg and an ambulatory/home blood pressure monitoring (ABPM/HBPM) average of 135/85 mmHg or higher. In some patients, diastolic BP may be normal while systolic BP is raised. This is known as isolated systolic hypertension.

Classification and causes

Hypertension is classified according to severity and its underlying cause.

Severity of hypertension

See Table 11.4 for current classification of severity of hypertension.

If BP is greater than 180/120 mmHg, assess for target organ damage as soon as possible:

- If target organ damage, consider antihypertensives immediately without ABPM/HBPM.
- If no target organ damage, confirm diagnosis within 7 days by:
  o Repeat clinic BP measurement, or
  o Consider ambulatory/home monitoring and clinic review.

Essential or secondary hypertension

It is important to establish whether a patient's high BP is due to primary (essential) hypertension or secondary hypertension (hypertension as the result of another disease process).

Table 11.4 Severity of hypertension

Hypertension	Clinic readings (mmHg)		ABPM/HBPM (mmHg)	
	Systolic	Diastolic	Systolic	Diastolic
Stage 1 (Mild)	≥140	≥90	≥135	≥85
Stage 2 (Moderate)	≥160	≥100	≥150	≥95
Stage 3 (Severe)	≥180	≥120	If no target organ damage, consider confirming with ABPM/HBPM and clinic review within 7 days	

ABPM, ambulatory blood pressure monitoring; *HBPM*, home blood pressure monitoring.

Table 11.5 Causes of secondary hypertension

Mechanism	Pathology
Renal	Renal parenchymal disease (e.g., chronic atrophic pyelonephritis, chronic glomerulonephritis, vasculitis). Renal artery atherosclerosis and stenosis decrease renal perfusion, stimulating renin-angiotensin system. Renin-producing tumours.
Endocrine	Adrenal cortex disorders – Conn syndrome (primary hyperaldosteronism), Cushing disease, congenital adrenal hyperplasia – cause salt and water retention, increasing blood volume, preload and thereby cardiac output. Adrenal medulla disorders (e.g., phaeochromocytoma – catecholamine-releasing tumour). Acromegaly. Hypo- and hyperthyroidism. Hypercalcaemia.
Vascular disease	Coarctation (narrowing) of the aorta – usually just distal to the left subclavian artery, increases resistance to aortic blood flow and can result in upper limb hypertension and lower limb normo- or hypotension.
Drugs	Alcohol, oral contraceptives (5% of women), monoamine oxidase inhibitors, glucocorticoids, NSAIDs, stimulants and interestingly liquorice.
Other	Hypertension of pregnancy (in approximately 10% of first pregnancies), carcinoid syndrome, polycythaemia (primary or secondary), psychogenic (stress).

Primary hypertension accounts for around 95% of hypertensive patients; the precise aetiology is unknown, but it is probably multifactorial. Either increased cardiac output or total peripheral resistance will increase BP.

Predisposing factors include:

1. Age (BP rises with age).
2. Genetic susceptibility.
3. High salt intake.
4. Obesity.
5. Physical inactivity.
6. Smoking.
7. Excessive alcohol intake.

Secondary hypertension accounts for the remaining 5% of cases (Table 11.5).

Effects of hypertension of the vessels

Hypertension not only accelerates atherosclerosis but it also results in characteristic changes to arterioles and small arteries known as arteriolosclerosis. All these changes are associated with narrowing of the vessel lumen. Changes in hypertension include:

1. In arteries: muscular hypertrophy of the media, reduplication of the external lamina and intimal thickening.
2. In arterioles: hyaline arteriosclerosis (protein deposits in wall) – this can lead to hypertensive kidney disease.
3. In vessels of the brain: microaneurysms (Charcot–Bouchard aneurysms), thought to increase the risk of haemorrhagic stroke.

Clinical features

History

Most hypertensive patients are entirely asymptomatic, and in essential hypertension, no obvious cause can be found. This can affect compliance with therapy, which may have unwanted side effects. Occasionally in hypertension, patients may complain of headaches, tinnitus, recurrent epistaxis, dizziness, fainting or visual disturbance. It is rare for these to be truly attributable to hypertension.

The aim of history taking is to look for secondary causes (Table 11.6), identify preexisting complications of hypertension and look for other risk factors that increase future risk of complications.

Table 11.6 Summary of the clinical presentation and investigation of several important causes of secondary hypertension

Causes	Renal parenchymal disease	Renal artery stenosis	Primary hyperaldosteronism	Phaeochromocytoma	Cushing syndrome
History	Obstruction or urinary tract infections, haematuria, family history of polycystic kidney disease	Fibromuscular dysplasia: early onset hypertension Atherosclerotic stenosis: hypertension of abrupt onset, resistant to treatment, flash pulmonary oedema	Episodes of muscle weakness, tetany, family history of early onset hypertension and cerebrovascular events	Paroxysmal or persistent hypertension, episodes of headache, sweating, palpitations, pallor, collapse, family history of phaeochromocytoma	Rapid weight gain, polyuria, polydipsia, headache, emotional lability, reproductive dysfunction
Examination	Enlarged palpable kidneys in polycystic kidney disease	Abdominal bruit	Arrhythmias if severe hypokalaemia	Signs of associated neurofibromatosis (e.g., neurofibromas, café-au-lait spots)	Cushingoid features (e.g., acne, hirsutism)
Initial investigation findings	Bloods: decreased eGFR, may have hyperkalaemia. Urinalysis: protein/blood/WCC	Bloods: rapid eGFR decline (spontaneously or in response to ACEi) Ultrasound: size discrepancy between kidneys or abnormal renal artery Doppler waveform	Bloods: hypokalaemia, metabolic alkalosis	Hyperglycaemia, hypercalcaemia, may have increased haemoglobin due to haemoconcentration	Hyperglycaemia
Further diagnostic tests	Renal ultrasound, further renal investigations	CT/MRI: detailed renal artery imaging	Aldosterone-renin ratio, CT/MRI (adrenal masses), selective adrenal venous sampling	Urinary metanephrine collection, CT/MRI (adrenal or extra-adrenal masses)	24-hour urinary cortisol, dexamethasone suppression test, adrenal/pituitary/chest imaging for source

ACEi, angiotensin-converting enzyme inhibitor; *CT,* computed tomography; *eGFR,* estimated glomerular filtration rate; *MRI,* magnetic resonance imaging; *WCC,* white cell count.

CLINICAL NOTES

Both hypothyroidism and hyperthyroidism may lead to hypertension. Weight loss or gain, tremor, hair loss, heat intolerance or feeling cold may suggest the presence of thyroid disease.

Complications of hypertension

1. Atherosclerosis: hypertension increases the risk of developing clinically significant atherosclerotic plaques. Patients may describe angina/myocardial infarction, peripheral vascular disease (ask about intermittent claudication, rest pain and ulceration), or transient ischaemic attack/stroke (ask about previous unilateral motor/sensory deficit, speech disturbance and/or visual disturbance).

2. Cardiac: increased afterload caused by the raised BP increases left ventricular work and causes left ventricular hypertrophy (LVH). This can lead to heart failure. Patients may describe dyspnoea, orthopnoea or ankle oedema.

3. Renal damage: gradual development of renal dysfunction occurs in hypertension, especially if it is poorly controlled. The pattern of renal disease caused by hypertension is often referred to as hypertensive nephrosclerosis. Renal damage is both a cause and consequence of hypertension! The symptoms of renal disease are often nonspecific and there is

some overlap with cardiac disease, including fatigue, poor appetite, oedema, etc.

4. Arrhythmia: the risk of atrial fibrillation is increased in hypertensive individuals. Patients may describe palpitations.
5. Retinal damage: retinal haemorrhages and papilloedema (in advanced stages) can cause visual disturbances.

Past medical history

As hypertension has many varied causes, it is helpful to find out about all previous illnesses and operations, particularly with regards to identifying causes of secondary hypertension and establishing risk factors for hypertension.

Secondary causes of hypertension:

1. Any reason for chronic corticosteroids (such as asthma, chronic obstructive pulmonary disease (COPD), or autoimmune disease).
2. Cushing syndrome (glucocorticoid excess) or Conn (mineralocorticoid excess) syndrome.
3. Renal failure may be caused by recurrent urinary tract infections, especially in childhood, or previous urinary tract obstruction.
4. Hyperthyroidism.
5. Phaeochromocytoma.

Risk factors for hypertension:

1. Dyslipidaemia.
2. Diabetes is a concomitant risk factor for IHD. It can also lead to diabetic nephropathy, which may contribute to hypertension.
3. Renal parenchymal disease, diagnosed or otherwise, is important to identify, as it alone increases risk of cardiovascular conditions and is an indication for BP control without other risks.
4. Myocardial infarction (MI) or stroke in the past – any existing vascular disease will put the patient at much higher risk of future vascular complications.

Drug history

Take a careful history of all drugs being taken, which may increase BP:

1. Prescribed drugs, e.g., oral contraceptives and steroids.
2. Even nasal or eye drops containing vasoconstrictors can cause systemic effects.
3. Over-the-counter analgesics (e.g., NSAIDs).

Ask about previous treatment for hypertension – a high BP reading may be after the patient has decided to stop taking anti-hypertensives or stopped treatment due to side effects (e.g., postural hypotension). If hypertension has been refractory to multiple treatments at a good dose (and patient is compliant with treatments), there should be a search for secondary causes and the patient should be referred for specialist input.

Family history

Primary hypertension is a multifactorial disease with both genetic and environmental inputs. A family history of hypertension is not uncommon. Some genetic secondary causes of hypertension include:

1. Autosomal dominant polycystic kidney disease is associated with hypertension, renal failure and cerebral artery aneurysms.
2. Phaeochromocytoma may occur as part of a multiple endocrine neoplasia syndrome (MEN 2, autosomal dominant) associated with medullary carcinoma of the thyroid and hyperparathyroidism.

A family history of IHD is another risk factor for IHD.

Social history

Social factors that may contribute to hypertension:

- Alcohol.
- Smoking.
- Diet: high salt intake. Unexpected substances such as liquorice can cause apparent mineralocorticoid excess.
- Lack of exercise.
- Stimulants, e.g., cocaine, amphetamine.

Examination

Important points when taking the BP manually:

1. The patient should be seated comfortably – preferably for 5 minutes before measurement in a quiet, warm setting.
2. Use the correct cuff size – if too small, it will cause a spuriously high reading.
3. While palpating the brachial artery, inflate the cuff. The point at which the pulse becomes impalpable is roughly equal to the systolic BP.
4. Deflate the cuff and now place your stethoscope over the brachial artery. Inflate the cuff to 20 mmHg above the estimated systolic pressure.
5. Systolic BP is recorded as the point during bladder deflation where regular sounds start to be heard (Korotkoff phase I).
6. Diastolic BP is recorded as the point at which the sounds disappear (Korotkoff phase V). In children and pregnant women, muffling of the sounds is used as the diastolic BP (Korotkoff phase IV).

HINTS AND TIPS

Remember to measure blood pressure in both arms at initial diagnosis of hypertension.

As with the history, when performing the examination in hypertension (Fig. 11.8), look for signs of:

1. An underlying cause of hypertension.

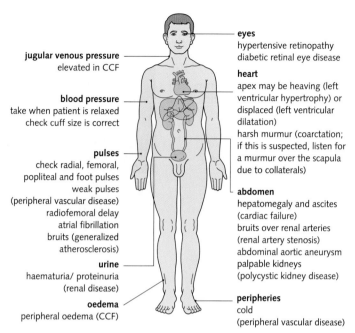

eyes
hypertensive retinopathy
diabetic retinal eye disease

jugular venous pressure
elevated in CCF

blood pressure
take when patient is relaxed
check cuff size is correct

pulses
check radial, femoral,
popliteal and foot pulses
weak pulses
(peripheral vascular disease)
radiofemoral delay
atrial fibrillation
bruits (generalized
atherosclerosis)

urine
haematuria/ proteinuria
(renal disease)

oedema
peripheral oedema (CCF)

heart
apex may be heaving (left
ventricular hypertrophy) or
displaced (left ventricular
dilatation)
harsh murmur (coarctation;
if this is suspected, listen for
a murmur over the scapula
due to collaterals)

abdomen
hepatomegaly and ascites
(cardiac failure)
bruits over renal arteries
(renal artery stenosis)
abdominal aortic aneurysm
palpable kidneys
(polycystic kidney disease)

peripheries
cold
(peripheral vascular disease)

Fig. 11.8 Important clinical findings in hypertensive patients. This illustration is only a guide and there are many other possible findings. *CCF*, congestive cardiac failure.

2. Target-organ/end-organ damage (i.e., LVH, cardiac failure, IHD, peripheral artery disease, cerebrovascular disease, renal impairment and hypertensive retinopathy).
3. Coexistent risk factors for IHD.

Signs consistent with secondary hypertension

- Features of Cushing syndrome: round face, interscapular and supraclavicular fat pads, abdominal obesity, proximal myopathy, easy bruising, striae, acne, hirsutism, acanthosis nigricans.
- Skin stigmata of neurofibromatosis (associated with phaeochromocytoma).
- Polycystic kidneys may be palpable.
- Renal artery bruits may be heard in renovascular hypertension.
- Auscultation of precordial or chest murmurs (aortic coarctation, aortic disease, upper limb arterial disease).
- Diminished and delayed femoral pulses (aortic coarctation, aortic disease, lower limb arterial disease).
- Left-right arm BP difference (subclavian artery stenosis, uncommonly aortic coarctation).
- As secondary hypertension has many possible causes, thoroughly examine all systems and remember to look out for signs of thyroid disease, acromegaly, etc.

Signs of end-organ damage

- Retina: fundoscopic abnormalities as below.
- Brain: motor or sensory deficits, speech disturbance.

- Carotid arteries: disease may cause bruits and is a risk factor for stroke.
- Heart: heart rate, elevated JVP, third or fourth heart sound, heart murmurs, arrhythmias, heaving apical impulse, pulmonary crepitations, peripheral oedema.
- Peripheral arteries: absence, reduction or asymmetry of pulses, poor perfusion and cold extremities, atrophic changes, ischaemic skin lesions.
- Kidneys: peripheral oedema, signs of anaemia or uraemia, fistulae, transplanted kidneys.
- Abdominal aortic aneurysm can be a sign of generalized atherosclerosis.

Signs of other risk factors for ischaemic heart disease

- Diabetes: fingertip black lancet marks, continuous glucose monitor (often placed on the upper arms), lipohypertrophy at insulin injection sites, insulin pump.
- Tendon xanthomata, xanthelasma.
- Obesity.

Additional notes on cardiovascular examination

When examining the pulse, remember:

1. Rate – tachycardia or bradycardia may be found in underlying thyroid disease.
2. Rhythm – atrial fibrillation may occur as a result of hypertensive heart disease.

3. Symmetry – compare the pulses; radial-femoral delay with unequal blood pressures between the upper and lower limbs points towards coarctation.

Bear in mind:

1. In aortic coarctation, continuous or systolic murmurs may be heard in the left infraclavicular area or below the left scapula; however, there may be a continuous hum from collaterals in a range of areas. 85% of cases have an associated bicuspid valve and this may cause an ejection click. There may also be a fourth heart sound (S4) if the heart has become hypertrophied and noncompliant.
2. Hypertensive heart disease – look for LVH (e.g., heaving apex beat) leading onto heart failure, atrial fibrillation or IHD.

COMMON PITFALLS

Left ventricular hypertrophy is due to pressure overload and results in a nondisplaced, heaving apex beat. This should not be confused with the displaced thrusting apex beat secondary to volume overload (e.g., mitral regurgitation) and dilatation of the left ventricle.

Eyes

RED FLAG

Patients exhibiting grade III or IV hypertensive retinopathy have a hypertensive emergency and need urgent treatment.

Fundoscopy looking for features of hypertensive retinopathy provides valuable information about the severity of the hypertension (Fig. 11.9 and Table 11.7).

HINTS AND TIPS

Look for features of both hypertensive and diabetic retinopathy on examination, as diabetes may be undiagnosed.

Investigations

The investigations listed in Table 11.8 should be performed at presentation in all hypertensive patients to look for evidence of end-organ damage, to identify possible secondary hypertension and as a measure of response to treatment. For example, LVH (Fig. 11.10) should gradually regress once hypertension has been successfully controlled.

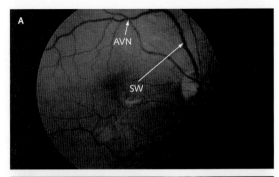
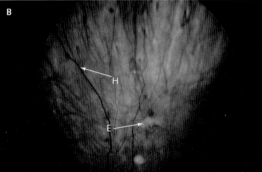
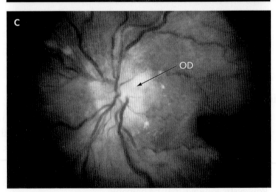

Fig. 11.9 Stages of hypertensive retinopathy. (A) Grade II, showing silver wiring *(SW)* and arteriovenous nipping *(AVN)* where an artery crossing above a vein causes apparent compression of the underlying vein. (B) Grade III, showing evidence of haemorrhages *(H)* and exudates *(E)*. (C) Grade IV, showing papilloedema – the optic disc *(OD)* is swollen and oedematous.

Investigation of secondary hypertension

If the patient is at high risk of having secondary hypertension, then further investigations are indicated. Criteria may include:

1. Younger people (e.g., under 40 years).
2. Symptoms/signs of an underlying cause (Table 11.6).
3. Symptoms and signs of hypertensive emergency (i.e., BP >180/120 mmHg, grade 3 or 4 hypertensive retinopathy or cardiac failure at a young age).

Table 11.7 Grades of hypertensive retinopathy

Grade	Features
I	Narrowing of the arteriolar lumen occurs, giving the classic 'silver wiring' effect
II	Sclerosis of the adventitia and thickening of the muscular wall of the arteries leads to compression of underlying veins and 'arteriovenous nipping'
III	Rupture of small vessels leading to haemorrhages and exudates
IV	Papilloedema (plus signs of grades I–III)

Table 11.8 Investigations for hypertension

Investigations	Notes
Blood tests	Renal function and electrolytes, blood lipid profile, blood glucose/HbA1c
Urine dipstick	Microscopic haematuria or proteinuria
ECG	Can provide evidence of LVH (i.e., R wave in V5 >25 mm, deep S wave in V1 >25 mm, tallest R wave in V5 or V6 added to S wave in V1 >35 mm, R wave in AVL >11 mm, lateral T wave inversion)
Consider echocardiogram	LVH, usually concentric in nature (i.e., left ventricular wall thickness >1.1 cm); performed routinely at some centres because LVH is thought to be a valuable indicator of prognosis

LVH, left ventricular hypertrophy

4. Hypertension refractory to treatment with three different antihypertensives from separate classes.
5. A sharp decline in renal function (reduction in estimated glomerular filtration rate of >25% or increase in creatinine of >30%) after initiation of angiotensin-converting enzyme (ACE) inhibitor or angiotensin II receptor antagonist. The kidney in renal artery stenosis is heavily dependent upon increased levels of angiotensin II to provide adequate BP (and maintain renal perfusion); this is prevented by administration of ACE inhibitors/angiotensin II receptor antagonists.

The following screening tests will exclude most causative conditions:

1. Aldosterone:renin ratio to exclude primary hyperaldosteronism. This may be due to a single adenoma (Conn syndrome) or bilateral adrenal hyperplasia.
2. 24-h urine protein and creatinine clearance to exclude marked renal pathology.
3. Plasma free metanephrines and 24-h urinary fractionated metanephrines to exclude phaeochromocytoma.
4. 24-h urine 5-hydroxy indole acetic acid (5HIAA) or plasma chromogranin A to exclude carcinoid syndrome.
5. 24-h urine cortisol excretion and dexamethasone suppression test to exclude Cushing disease.
6. Renal ultrasound may reveal overt structural abnormality (e.g., bilateral small kidneys in chronic renal parenchymal disease, enlarged polycystic kidneys, phaeochromocytoma, asymmetrical kidneys in renal artery stenosis).
7. CT or MR angiogram to exclude renal artery stenosis if there is a high index of suspicion.
8. If coarctation is suspected, a chest X-ray (CXR) may demonstrate rib notching (specific but often incidental finding) and cardiomegaly. Coarctation may be confirmed on echocardiography or computed tomography (CT)/ magnetic resonance imaging (MRI).

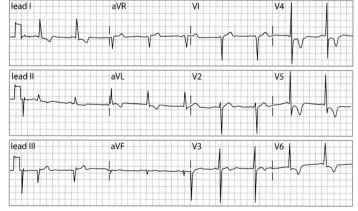

Fig. 11.10 Electrocardiographic features of left ventricular hypertrophy (LVH). Note the cardinal features indicating LVH: R wave in V5 or V6 plus S wave in V1 exceeds seven large squares; T wave inversion in lateral leads V4–V6.

Management

Hypertension is common. If left untreated, multiple organ systems can be damaged; risk of this is reduced by adequate BP control. As patients are often asymptomatic, they sometimes do not comply with medications or medical appointments.

> ### COMMUNICATION
>
> Explain to patients that hypertension can be well treated with medications, but, untreated, hypertension can have serious complications. They may not experience symptoms even if their blood pressure is elevated, so it is important to continue with their treatment even if they feel well. Discuss all treatment options, including lifestyle advice, and if using medicines, discuss their effects and common side effects.

Identifying and stopping contributors to hypertension are important, such as prescribed medicines (e.g., the contraceptive pill, NSAIDs), over-the-counter medicines and drugs of abuse.

All other risk factors for IHD should be sought and treated in these patients.

The 2019 NICE/British and Irish Hypertension Society guidelines (reviewed 2022) for hypertension suggest:

1. Offer and reinforce lifestyle advice to all patients with suspected or known hypertension and continue to offer this periodically.
2. Initiate antihypertensive drug treatment in people with:
   a. Stage 2 or 3 hypertension
   b. Stage 1 hypertension in patients less than 80 years old who have target organ damage, diabetes, cardiovascular disease, renal disease or a 10-year cardiovascular risk score of ≥10%.
3. Optimal BP treatment targets are <140/90 mmHg in patients <80 years (ABPM/HBPM <135/85 mmHg) or <150/90 mmHg in patients ≥80 years (ABPM/HBPM <145/85 mmHg).
4. Use of clinical judgement when considering antihypertensives in patients with frailty or multiple comorbidities.

Nonpharmacological management

Nonpharmacological management may decrease BP sufficiently to prevent the need for drug therapy in patients with mild hypertension or may avoid the need for multiple hypertensives.

Lifestyle interventions may include:

1. Weight loss (losing 10 kg may reduce BP by 10 mmHg).
2. Reduction in salt intake.
3. Reduction in alcohol consumption (maximum recommended weekly intake is 14 units for both men and women).

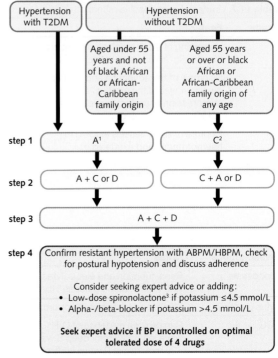

Fig. 11.11 2019 National Institute for Health and Care Excellence (NICE)/British and Irish Hypertension Society (BIHS) guideline for management of hypertension.
[1] Avoid ACE inhibitors and ARBs in pregnancy unless absolutely necessary. Consider an ARB in preference to an ACE inhibitor in patients of Black African or African-Caribbean family origin.
[2] A CCB is preferred but consider a thiazide-like diuretic if a CCB is not tolerated or the person has oedema, evidence of heart failure or a high risk of heart failure.
[3] At the time of publication, not all preparations of spironolactone have a UK marketing authorization for this indication. Informed consent should be obtained and documented.

A: ACE inhibitor or low-cost angiotensin II receptor blocker (ARB)
C: Calcium channel blocker (CCB)
D: Thiazide-like diuretic

4. Smoking cessation.
5. Limiting caffeine intake.
6. Diet low in fat with five portions of fruit and vegetables a day.
7. Regular exercise.

Pharmacological management

The choice of antihypertensive agents in newly diagnosed patients should be guided by the NICE/British and Irish Hypertension Society algorithm, shown in Fig. 11.11.

Choice of therapy may also be influenced by coexisting disease. These agents may be used alone or in combination to

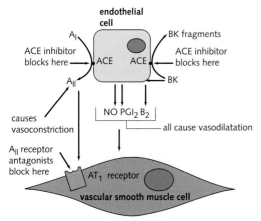

Fig. 11.12 Action of angiotensin-converting enzyme (ACE) inhibitors and angiotensin II (A_{II}) receptor antagonists. A_I, angiotensin I; A_{II}, angiotensin II; AT_1, angiotensin II receptor type 1; B_2, activated bradykinin-activated by endothelial cell; *BK,* bradykinin; *NO,* nitric oxide; *PGI$_2$,* prostacyclin.

achieve good blood-pressure control. Remember, compliance is likely to be better if once-daily preparations are used and polypharmacy is avoided (i.e., the drug regimen is kept as simple as possible by using a higher dose of a single agent before adding another drug).

Angiotensin-converting enzyme inhibitors

ACE inhibitors (e.g., ramipril) inhibit the conversion of angiotensin I to angiotensin II by ACE (Fig. 11.12). They also inhibit breakdown of bradykinin (a vasodilator) by ACE. When started, renal function and electrolytes should be monitored. They should not be used to treat patients with severe renal artery stenosis because inhibition of angiotensin II production will prevent the efferent arteriolar constriction that maintains glomerular filtration in the presence of renal artery stenosis.

Angiotensin II receptor antagonists

Angiotensin II receptor antagonists (e.g., losartan) inhibit angiotensin II from binding to its receptor. They are useful in patients treated with ACE inhibitors who develop a dry cough (due to elevated bradykinin).

Calcium channel blockers

Calcium channel antagonists block voltage-gated calcium channels in myocardium and vascular smooth muscle. This causes a decrease in myocardial contractility, electrical conductance and vascular tone. Calcium antagonists interfere with the action of various vasoconstrictor agonists (e.g., norepinephrine, angiotensin II, thrombin). Due to their negative inotropic effect, they are contraindicated in systolic dysfunction.

The dihydropyridine calcium antagonists, amlodipine and nifedipine, act peripherally on arterioles, relaxing arteriolar vascular smooth muscle and causing vasodilatation. The dihydropyridine calcium channel blockers do not slow the heart rate.

The non–dihydropyridine calcium channel blockers, verapamil and diltiazem, decrease heart rate and therefore are rarely used for hypertension alone.

Diuretics

Usually a thiazide-type diuretic (e.g., bendroflumethiazide) is used. These inhibit sodium reabsorption in the distal renal tubule, which causes increased salt and water excretion, decreasing blood volume and thus decreasing BP. Thiazide diuretics also have a direct vasodilator effect, further reducing BP. Although loop diuretics (e.g., furosemide) produce a more marked diuresis, they are not used in hypertension. The important side effect to be aware of is hypokalaemia (which increases the risk of arrhythmia); if serum potassium is disproportionately low with low drug doses and sodium is high normal, this should raise suspicion of primary hyperaldosteronism. Other side effects include hypercalcaemia, hyperglycaemia and hyperuricaemia. Thiazide-like diuretics (e.g., indapamide, chlorthalidone), which have similar mechanisms of action and side effects to thiazides, are preferred to conventional thiazides by NICE guidelines since 2011.

Spironolactone is a mineralocorticoid receptor antagonist (MRA) and is useful in patients with treatment-resistant hypertension, especially if their potassium is low, as these medications act as potassium-sparing diuretics (will tend to increase serum potassium levels).

α-Blockers

α-Blockers (e.g., doxazosin) are antagonists of α-adrenoceptors. There is postsynaptic blockade of α_1-adrenoceptors, which prevents sympathetically mediated vascular smooth muscle contraction and leads to vasodilatation. They cause a decrease in total peripheral resistance and thus a decrease in BP. Doxazosin is often used for labile (catecholamine-mediated) hypertension. Blockade of α-receptors also prevents sympathetically mediated release of renin in the kidneys.

Side effects of α-blockers include postural hypotension caused by loss of sympathetic vasoconstriction, particularly marked following the first dose.

β-Blockers

β-Blockers were previously first-line but are used rarely for hypertension alone now, as they are less effective and often less well tolerated. If other agents are contraindicated, they may be considered in younger people. β-Blockers are antagonists of β-adrenoceptors. They block sympathetic activity in the heart (β_1), peripheral vasculature (β_2), and other tissues, including the bronchi (β_2). In the heart, this results in a decrease in heart rate and myocardial contractility, which reduces cardiac output and BP.

The effect of β-blockers on the peripheral vasculature leads to a loss of β-mediated vasodilatation, causing an unopposed α-vasoconstriction. This may initially cause an increase in vascular resistance, elevating BP, but in long-term use, the vascular resistance returns to pretreatment levels. Some β-blockers can preferentially act on β_1-adrenoceptors, being more cardioselective; however, even these drugs have some blocking effect on the β_2-adrenoceptor. Types of β-blockers include:

1. Propranolol, atenolol (act on β_1, β_2).
2. Metoprolol, bisoprolol (selective β_1-blockers).

The main side effects of β-blockers are bronchoconstriction and bradycardia. Be cautious in people with asthma or COPD, as β-blockers may exacerbate symptoms.

HINTS AND TIPS

The use of β-blockers alone for phaeochromocytoma can result in severe hypertension due to the unopposed action of noradrenaline on the α-receptors.

A summary of these and other agents is given below (Table 11.9).

Follow-up of hypertensive patients

Follow-up is as important as the initial treatment. Patients should be seen on a yearly basis, involving:

1. Examination to look for evidence of end-organ damage – especially cardiovascular system and retinas.
2. Urinalysis.
3. Blood tests for urea, creatinine and electrolytes – these may be deranged due to renal damage secondary to hypertension, drug therapy or both.
4. ECG and/or echocardiography if there are concerns.
5. Screen for risk factors for IHD (i.e., blood lipid profile, blood glucose) and lifestyle advice if necessary.

Hypertensive emergencies and urgencies

If BP is very quickly raised to extremely high levels, this may result in rapid organ damage over hours to weeks. This is a hypertensive emergency, a rare event that requires same-day hospital assessment and immediate monitored treatment. Hypertensive emergencies are also known as accelerated or malignant hypertension, although these are older and less specific terms. If there is not yet organ damage, this is referred to as hypertensive urgency and should be treated promptly with oral agents.

Any cause of hypertension can cause a hypertensive emergency; however, it is more common with secondary hypertension, especially phaeochromocytoma and renal causes. There are no absolute levels of hypertension associated with symptoms or organ damage; however, levels required are usually beyond the grade 3 hypertension cutoff.

End-organ damage may include hypertensive encephalopathy, cerebrovascular infarct or haemorrhage, acute left ventricular failure, hypertensive retinopathy, aortic dissection, renal failure, microangiopathic haemolytic anaemia and eclampsia.

Symptoms tend to be nonspecific and vary by organ affected and include headache, nausea and vomiting, visual disturbance, altered level of consciousness, seizures, neurological deficit, chest pain and oliguria.

Examination should seek secondary causes of hypertension and look for evidence of end-organ damage (focusing on cardiovascular, neurological examination and fundoscopy predominantly).

Investigations include:

- Blood tests: full blood count (FBC), clotting screen, urea and electrolytes (U&Es), liver function tests (LFTs), thyroid function tests (TFTs).
- Urinalysis: protein, blood.
- ECG: LVH, left atrial (LA) enlargement.
- CXR: LVH, cardiac failure.
- Other tests for organ damage and secondary causes if suspected.

Urgent admission to a high-dependency unit (HDU)/ICU is required for hypertensive emergencies for continuous monitoring of BP and controlled gradual BP reduction. Rare cases may require additional procedures (e.g., intracranial pressure monitoring if intracranial pressure is increased or dialysis in renal failure). The rate of BP reduction and agents used depends on the specific organ damaged. Generally, the goal is to lower BP slowly to prevent sudden drops that may prompt ischaemia. There are two main exceptions: (1) in aortic dissection, if tolerated, rapid BP lowering is preferred to minimize the tendency for dissection to extend, and (2) in acute ischaemic stroke when there should generally be no intervention to BP unless there is a strong indication in case reduction worsens cerebral perfusion and brain injury.

Malignant hypertension is an old term that reflects the historic prognosis that mortality was 80% in the first year and 5-year survival was close to zero. Now, prognosis is markedly improved with better BP control and survival is approximately 80% at 5 years.

Table 11.9 Overview of drugs used to treat hypertension

Class of drug	Examples	Indications	Precautions/ contraindications	Adverse effects
Diuretics	Thiazides (e.g., bendroflumethiazide), thiazide-like diuretics (e.g., indapamide, chlorthalidone)	Mild hypertension or in conjunction with other agents for more severe hypertension	Thiazides exacerbate diabetes mellitus; all diuretics should be avoided in patients who have gout if possible	Hypokalaemia, dehydration, exacerbation of renal impairment, gout
Antiadrenergic agents	β-Blockers (e.g., atenolol, propranolol, bisoprolol, metoprolol)	Moderate to severe hypertension (note that they are antianginal)	Asthma, cardiac failure, severe peripheral vascular disease	Postural hypotension, bradycardia, bronchospasm, fatigue, impotence, cold extremities, nightmares
	α-Blockers (e.g., prazosin, doxazosin)	Moderate to severe hypertension	Postural hypotension	Postural hypotension, headache
	Centrally acting agents (e.g., methyldopa)	Moderate hypertension (safe during pregnancy)	Depression, phaeochromocytoma, acute porphyria	Postural hypotension, allergic reactions, drowsiness, galactorrhoea, gynaecomastia, haemolytic anaemia
Calcium channel blockers	Nifedipine, amlodipine, verapamil, diltiazem*	Moderate hypertension (note that they are antianginal)	Cardiac failure, heart block (second- or third-degree) – these are contraindications mainly for verapamil and diltiazem	Postural hypotension, headache, flushing, ankle oedema
Angiotensin-converting enzyme inhibitors	Ramipril, captopril, enalapril, lisinopril, perindopril	Moderate to severe hypertension, especially with cardiac failure	Renal artery stenosis, pregnancy	Postural hypotension, dry cough (in approx. 10%), rash, angioedema, renal failure, hyperkalaemia, loss of taste
Angiotensin-II receptor blockers	Candesartan, losartan, valsartan	Moderate to severe hypertension, especially with cardiac failure	Renal artery stenosis, pregnancy	Postural hypotension, renal failure, hyperkalaemia
Vasodilators	Hydralazine	Moderate to severe hypertension	Severe tachycardia, systemic lupus erythematosus	Postural hypotension, headache, lupus-like syndrome
	Sodium nitroprusside (as an intravenous infusion)	Hypertensive emergency	Compensatory hypertension, severe vitamin B12 deficiency	Weakness, cyanide toxicity if the drug is not protected from light

* Diltiazem and verapamil are less commonly used for hypertension because they have a more pronounced action on heart muscle and conductive tissues, respectively. Diltiazem is used predominantly for angina; verapamil is used for its antiarrhythmic effects.

Chapter Summary

- Atherosclerosis is a progressive inflammatory disease; early evidence of it can be found even in our twenties. It is the pathological basis of ischaemic heart disease, cerebrovascular disease and peripheral arterial disease, which are major causes of mortality.
- Slow, stable progression of atherosclerosis may lead to collateral vessel formation and a degree of compensation.
- Acute plaque events may lead to acute coronary syndrome, ischaemic stroke, or acute limb/mesenteric ischaemia.
- Early ECG and biomarker measurement will identify and differentiate the acute coronary syndromes.
- Optimal control of the risk factors for ischaemic heart disease is clearly required after ischaemic events (secondary prevention). In primary prevention, the threshold of pharmacological management is best determined by validated online risk calculators in most cases, but these calculators are not used in target organ damage, type 1 diabetes, and CKD and familial hyperlipidaemia, as these are indications for treatment in their own right.
- Effective risk factor management is reliant upon patient education and participation.
- Dyslipidaemia can usually be well-controlled with statins or additional agents, and the mainstay of treatment is statins.
- Hypertension is common and often asymptomatic.
- Ambulatory or home BP monitoring is often important to accurately diagnose hypertension to prevent unnecessary long-term treatment and more frequent primary care follow-up.
- History, examination and investigation aim to identify secondary causes, existing complications of hypertension and coexistent cardiovascular risk factors.
- Pharmacological treatment of cardiovascular risk factors depends on age, ethnicity, comorbidity and tolerance.
- Hypertensive urgencies require urgent assessment and oral treatment, but hypertensive emergencies require ICU or HDU management.

UKMLA Conditions
Acute coronary syndrome
Essential or secondary hypertension
Ischaemic heart disease
Myocardial infarction
Unstable angina

UKMLA Presentations
Hypertension
Low blood pressure

Ischaemic heart disease, also known as coronary artery disease (CAD), is the leading cause of death in the Western world and contributes to significant morbidity. The pathogenesis and clinical classification are described in Chapter 11 and include stable angina and acute coronary syndromes (ACS).

Causes of angina and ACS can be split into causes of reduced perfusion and increased demand. Exacerbating factors include reduced oxygen content of blood reaching the myocardium.

Reduced perfusion:

1. Intracoronary:
   - Atheromatous stenosis of coronary arteries (most common).
   - Thrombosis within coronary arteries.
   - Dissection of coronary arteries (may occur with aortic dissection, during angiography or, rarely, spontaneously).
   - Spasm of epicardial coronary arteries (Prinzmetal angina).
   - Coronary arteritis in vasculitis (e.g., polyarteritis nodosa, Kawasaki syndrome).
   - Emboli as a result of atrial fibrillation (AF)/mechanical valves/infective endocarditis, etc. (rare).
2. Extracoronary:
   - Severe aortic valve stenosis (remember angina is the first of the classic triad of symptoms to present).
   - Hypertrophic cardiomyopathy.
   - Hypertension.
   - Microvascular angina (angina and evidence of exercise-induced ischaemia without obstructive atherosclerotic CAD).

Increased demand:

1. Increased cardiac output – exercise, stress, thyrotoxicosis, tachyarrhythmia, etc.
2. Increased cardiac work required to maintain adequate output (severe aortic stenosis).
3. Increased peripheral vascular resistance (hypertension).
4. Hypertrophy, either secondary to aortic stenosis or hypertension or as a primary defect, as in hypertrophic cardiomyopathy.

Decreased blood oxygen content:

1. Severe anaemia.
2. Decreased oxygen saturations.

STABLE ANGINA

Angina pectoris is a symptom complex, primarily of central chest discomfort on exertion, relieved by rest. This is caused by coronary arterial insufficiency leading to intermittent myocardial ischaemia. Ischaemia occurs when the oxygen and nutrient demand is greater than its supply.

CLINICAL NOTES

Myocardial oxygen demand is very high (about 8 mL O_2/min per 100 g) and can increase up to fivefold during exercise. Even at rest, the coronary circulation receives 3% to 5% of the total cardiac output, 10 times the average blood flow per gram of tissue. In angina, the stenosed vessel is unable to accommodate the necessary increase in blood flow during exertion, causing ischaemia and chest pain that subsides at rest when demand reduces. As a rule of thumb, the stenosis will need to reduce cross-sectional area of the vessel lumen by 70% before it produces symptoms.

The most common cause by far is atherosclerosis in one or more coronary artery, producing predictable reversible ischaemic symptoms, and the rest of this chapter will focus on this.

Clinical features of angina

Angina means 'choking' and pectoris means 'of the chest'. Based on the history, angina is largely a clinical diagnosis.

Angina is classically a 'heavy', 'crushing', 'aching' or 'band-like' pain across the centre of the chest that may radiate to the arm, neck or jaw. Patients may deny pain but describe 'tightness' or 'discomfort'. Other precipitating factors include cold air and after a meal. Dyspnoea is often associated with chest pain. Angina equivalent, described as exertional dyspnoea without pain that is relieved rapidly at rest or with nitrates, is rare but can occur in those at risk of neuropathy (e.g., elderly, diabetics).

Typical angina fulfils all of the following criteria (Diamond classification):

1. Substernal chest discomfort of characteristic quality and duration.
2. Provoked by exertion or emotional stress.
3. Relieved by rest and/or nitrates within minutes.

If only two of these criteria are fulfilled, it is termed *atypical angina*, and if one or none of the criteria are fulfilled, it is classified as nonanginal chest pain.

Important points to note when diagnosing angina:

1. Oesophageal pain can also be relieved by nitrates.
2. Atypical chest discomfort, especially if related to effort, could still be angina.
3. Silent ischaemia is more common in patients with diabetes or the elderly who have autonomic neuropathy.

Typically, stable angina equates to predictable brief symptoms on exertion. However, as the coronary artery narrowing worsens, the amount of exertion required to produce angina reduces and the pain may occur even at rest or on minimal exertion. If this occurs over a short period of time, it may be termed *crescendo* or *unstable angina* (see Acute coronary syndromes, later). If pain continues even beyond rest, consider myocardial infarction (MI).

RED FLAG

A sudden worsening of exertional angina may be due to rupture of an atheromatous plaque in the coronary artery, which causes a steep decrease in its luminal diameter and may even cause intermittent occlusion of the vessel. This condition may progress to myocardial infarction.

Obvious clinical signs are frequently absent in patients with angina alone. Signs to help diagnosis may relate to:

- Risk factors:
  - Hypertension.
  - Hypercholesterolaemia: premature corneal arcus (age <45), xanthelasma, xanthomata. If these are found, consider familial hypercholesterolaemia (see Chapter 11).
  - Diabetes mellitus: fingertip blood glucose measurement marks, lipodystrophy, insulin pump.
  - Smoking: odour, tar staining of the fingers.
- Coexistent arterial disease (increases the likelihood of CAD):
  - Carotid bruits.
  - Peripheral arterial disease.
  - Cerebral vascular disease.
- Conditions that cause decompensation of angina:
  - Anaemia: pallor, including conjunctival.
  - Thyrotoxicosis: fine tremor, eye signs, goitre, AF.
- Heart failure as a result of ischaemic heart disease:
  - Raised jugular venous pressure (JVP) or peripheral oedema.
  - Cardiomegaly or third heart sound.
  - Bibasal crepitations.

- Other causes of angina:
  - Arrhythmia.
  - Aortic valve disease.
  - Hypertrophic cardiomyopathy.

Investigation of angina

The investigation of patients presenting with chest pain is explained in detail in Chapter 6. The following investigations may be considered in a patient with angina:

1. Resting electrocardiogram (ECG): usually normal between episodes. During an attack, there may be ST-segment depression and inverted T waves. Occasionally, evidence of previous infarction may be seen unexpectedly.
2. Computed tomography coronary angiography (CTCA): improvements in the spatial and temporal resolution of CT scanning have allowed it to be used in the assessment of CAD. CTCA can detect atherosclerotic plaques (both calcified and noncalcified) and accurately measure any stenoses in the coronary arteries; it is now arguably the gold standard in the majority of cases. Flow limitation may be calculated.
3. Coronary angiography (Figs. 12.1 and 12.2) assesses the patency of the coronary vasculature by demonstrating the location and extent of coronary artery stenosis. Despite developments in CT scanning, invasive angiography is still the gold standard for dedicated luminal assessment of the coronary arteries (but may miss atherosclerotic plaques that do not narrow the lumen). It is important to remember that coronary angiography is invasive and there is a small risk of morbidity and mortality associated with the procedure. Invasive coronary angiography should be offered when non-invasive imaging is inconclusive (or to enable treatment in patients whose symptoms are not controlled medically).
4. Exercise ECG: current National Institute for Health and Care Excellence (NICE) guidelines recommend that exercise ECG testing should not be used routinely to diagnose or to exclude stable angina in people without known coronary artery disease. However, this may be useful in some situations, particularly in patients with confirmed coronary artery disease, to help establish whether this is the cause of the patient's chest pain- see Chapter 4 for more details. If the patient's symptoms only occur at high workload, exercise testing may not reveal any symptoms or ECG changes. Exercise ECG is not feasible in patients who cannot use the treadmill (e.g., due to severe arthritis).
5. Nuclear perfusion imaging: this relies on the principle that when the myocardium is stressed (either by exercise or pharmacologically with a positive inotrope, such as dobutamine), uptake of a radionucleotide tracer will be increased in line with the increase in perfusion. However,

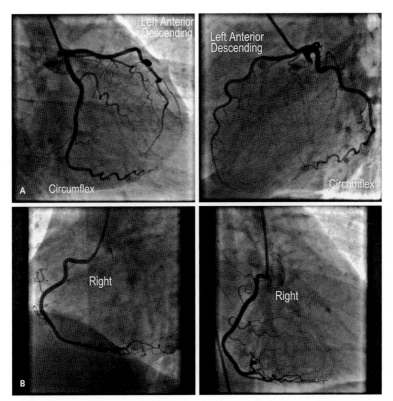

Fig. 12.1 Coronary angiograms of normal (A) left and (B) right coronary arteries, each taken in two perpendicular views. (Courtesy Newby DE, Grubb NR. *Cardiology: An Illustrated Colour Text.* Edinburgh: Elsevier, 2005.)

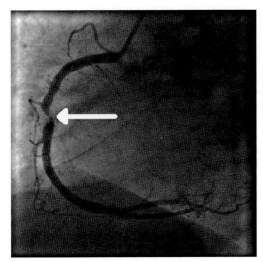

Fig. 12.2 Coronary angiogram of a patient with a severe coronary stenosis *(arrow)*. (Courtesy Newby DE, Grubb NR. *Cardiology: An Illustrated Colour Text.* Edinburgh: Elsevier, 2005.)

areas of myocardium that have impaired perfusion (due to stenosis in the arteries supplying them) will not exhibit increased uptake in response to stress.

6. Stress echocardiography (e.g., with dobutamine): reversible wall motion abnormalities may suggest an area of myocardium that is less well perfused when stressed. Decreased ejection fraction may be found as a complication.

7. Stress perfusion MRI: penetration of gadolinium contrast medium is reduced within the myocardium in areas of impaired perfusion during stress (as for nuclear perfusion imaging).

The choice between investigation modalities may depend on local availability and patient characteristics (including whether the patient is known to have coronary artery disease). Current National Institute for Health and Care Excellence (NICE) guidelines recommend CT coronary angiography as the first-line investigation in patients with suspected angina. Patients with known CAD and possible angina should be assessed by stress imaging (stress echocardiogram, nuclear perfusion scan or magnetic resonance perfusion imaging).

Management of angina pectoris

Angina can be a result of other diseases (e.g., severe aortic stenosis) and treatment should target any underlying cause. Treatment of exacerbating factors, such as severe anaemia, may resolve symptoms. However, management of standard stable angina involves addressing simultaneously:

1. Management of any modifiable risk factors.
2. Secondary prevention.
3. Management of the angina itself.

Management of risk factors

The main risk factors are described in Chapter 11. Any modifiable risk factors should be sought and treated to reduce the risk of disease progression, MI and death. This is also essential for risk stratification, and high-risk patients may benefit from more intensive preventative strategies.

1. Smoking: encourage cessation at every stage of management.
2. Hypertension: diagnose and monitor, encourage lifestyle modification and use medication if required.
3. Diabetes: encourage good glycaemic control with dietary control and medication.
4. Hypercholesterolaemia: medication is part of the secondary prevention strategy and should be offered to all, but lifestyle measures will still make a significant difference.

Secondary prevention

All patients with angina should be treated with:

1. Aspirin: reduces platelet aggregation to lower the risk of future MI and death.
2. Statin: As per NICE CG181 (2023), patients with cardiovascular disease should be started on treatment with a high-intensity statin (typically atorvastatin 80 mg daily).
3. Angiotensin-converting enzyme (ACE) inhibitors: especially important in those with hypertension, left ventricular (LV) dysfunction, prior MI or diabetes mellitus.

Treatment of the angina

Treatment strategies for angina aim to restore the balance between myocardial supply and demand by increasing blood supply, and thereby oxygen supply, to the ischaemic myocardium and by decreasing the oxygen demand of the myocardium (Fig. 12.3).

Increasing blood supply can be achieved by:

1. Decreasing heart rate: coronary artery flow occurs primarily during diastole. Decreasing heart rate prolongs diastole, allowing more time for perfusion of the myocardium.
2. Dilating coronary arteries: this may be of more benefit in angina due to coronary artery spasm, as stenosed coronary arteries are likely to be already maximally vasodilated by endogenous metabolic vasodilators (such as adenosine).

Decreasing heart rate, contractility, preload or afterload will all reduce the oxygen demand of the myocardium.

Antianginal drugs

Organic nitrates. Organic nitrates, such as glyceryl trinitrate (GTN), relax vascular smooth muscle cells by producing nitric oxide, which increases levels of cGMP and brings about vasodilation. Nitrates mediate their effects by:

1. Dilatation of venous capacitance vessels (predominant effect). This causes pooling of blood in the venous system which:
   a) Reduces the preload of the heart and (due to Starling law) decreases cardiac output, thereby decreasing myocardial work.

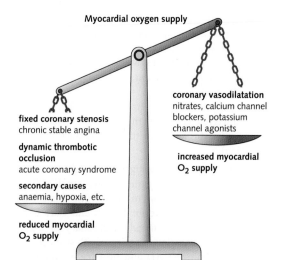
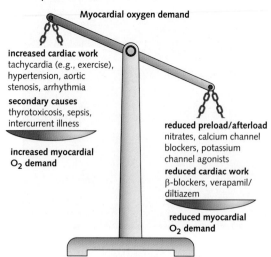

Fig. 12.3 Balance of myocardial oxygen supply and demand in ischaemic heart disease, and the rationale for the use of antianginal therapies. (Courtesy Newby DE, Grubb NR. *Cardiology: An Illustrated Colour Text.* Edinburgh: Elsevier, 2005.)

b) Decreases arterial blood pressure, thus reducing the afterload.
2. Dilatation of coronary arteries: nitrates have a direct vasodilatory effect on coronary arteries at high doses, increasing myocardial perfusion.

GTN is usually administered sublingually to avoid first-pass metabolism and its effects last around 30 minutes. GTN is available as tablets (short shelf-life) or a spray (shelf-life 3 years). Tolerance develops to the effects of GTN if used regularly over 2 or 3 days and patients should be aware of this. It can be used to relieve an attack or can be taken prophylactically to prevent one.

Longer-acting nitrates include isosorbide mononitrate and isosorbide dinitrate, and require a 'nitrate-free' interval overnight to prevent tolerance. These can come in oral tablet form or transdermal patches or cream where the location of application should be varied.

Nitrate side effects include postural hypotension, sometimes a reflex tachycardia (as the body attempts to maintain blood pressure), and very occasionally syncope. More common side effects are headache and facial flushing.

β-Blockers (e.g., atenolol, metoprolol). These drugs block sympathetic stimulation of the heart, leading to:

1. Decreased contractility (negative inotropic effect) and decreased oxygen demand.
2. Decreased heart rate (negative chronotropic effect), decreased oxygen demand and prolonged diastole, increasing duration of coronary blood flow.

They are also effective antihypertensive agents, and in some patients, they can perform a dual role, simplifying drug therapy.

Remember that β-blockers are contraindicated in:

1. Unstable cardiac failure.
2. Bradyarrhythmia.
3. Asthma (blockade of bronchial β_2-receptors causes bronchoconstriction, but chronic obstructive pulmonary disease without bronchospasm may not be a contraindication).

Side effects include:

1. Tiredness.
2. Postural hypotension – especially in elderly patients (who should start on a small dose initially).
3. Loss of sympathetic response to hypoglycaemia – use a more cardioselective agent.
4. Nightmares – use a non–fat-soluble agent (e.g., atenolol).
5. Male impotence.

HINTS AND TIPS

Many drugs of the same class have similar suffixes to their names. For example, most β-blockers end in '-olol' (e.g., propranolol, atenolol, metoprolol). This is useful when identifying the class of an unfamiliar drug.

Calcium channel blockers. These drugs block L-type Ca^{2+} channels in the heart and arteriolar smooth muscle:

1. Blockade of myocardial Ca^{2+} channels (greatest with nondihydropyridine agents, verapamil and diltiazem) decreases heart rate and myocardial contractility, thereby decreasing myocardial oxygen demand. These medications also decrease electrical conductance and therefore are class IV antiarrhythmics.
2. Blockade of Ca^{2+} channels in vascular smooth muscle (greatest with dihydropyridine agents, such as nifedipine and amlodipine):
   a) Peripheral vasodilatation decreases arterial blood pressure, decreasing afterload and myocardial work.
   b) Direct dilatation of coronary arteries, increasing myocardial perfusion.

Nifedipine may be beneficially combined with β-blockers to minimize the side effect of reflex tachycardia. This occurs less with amlodipine and combination with β-blockers is safe. These both have additional antihypertensive effects. As amlodipine and nifedipine mainly affect peripheral vessels, side effects include flushing, headache and ankle oedema, but these are less of a problem with diltiazem and verapamil.

Verapamil predominantly inhibits conduction through the atrioventricular (AV) node, decreasing heart rate. It also exerts a negative inotropic effect, decreasing myocardial contractility. Diltiazem acts both on the heart and on the arterioles, decreasing heart rate and causing vasodilatation. Avoid verapamil or diltiazem in combination with β-blockers because of the risk of heart block and profound bradycardia. However, they may be useful single agents if β-blockers cannot be used due to excessive bronchoconstriction. Diltiazem can be a good antianginal agent, and verapamil can be useful in angina but is mainly used as an antiarrhythmic.

Nicorandil. Nicorandil is a potassium channel agonist that affects adenosine triphosphate (ATP)-dependent K^+ channels in vascular smooth muscle, causing hyperpolarization and vasodilatation. It affects both veins and arteries, thus reducing both preload and afterload. Nicorandil also has a nitrate component in that it is a nitric oxide donor. Nicorandil is not used first-line but is an alternative to nitrates when tolerance occurs and if β-blockers and Ca^{2+} antagonists are contraindicated. Side effects are generally similar to nitrates and include headache and flushing. Other side effects include gastrointestinal ulceration. Tolerance does not occur. They are contraindicated in hypotension or heart failure.

Ivabradine. This is a newer sinoatrial (SA) node modulator. It acts as an antagonist at the I_f ion channel, which inhibits the pacemaker potential in the SA node, slows the rate of depolarization and reduces heart rate (contraindicated in bradycardia). As it does not have the other effects of β-blockers and calcium channel blockers, it has additional benefits in heart failure. It is ineffective in patients with AF.

Ranolazine. This affects late sodium currents in myocardial cells, reducing intracellular calcium through the sodium-calcium exchanger and improving myocardial relaxation and coronary blood flow. This occurs independently of heart rate; therefore it can be used safely in combination with drugs that lower heart rate. It prolongs QT interval and is contraindicated in patients at risk of QT prolongation.

CLINICAL NOTES

Antianginal drugs
Drug choice depends on comorbidities and contra-indications, and the simplest combination sufficient to control symptoms should be used. A possible plan of action is:

1. Prescribe all patients aspirin 75 mg daily and a statin if no contraindication.
2. Prescribe all patients a GTN spray and advise them to use it for the relief of angina or prior to any activity known to bring angina on.
3. Prescribe a β-blocker if not contraindicated.
4. Control hypertension and diabetes (may affect choice of other agents).
5. If β-blockade fails to control the symptoms or is contraindicated, there is a choice to start either a calcium antagonist (be prepared to add a long-acting nitrate if the effect is still insufficient) or to prescribe nicorandil, which has effects similar to those produced by a combination of calcium antagonist and nitrate. Avoid rate-limiting calcium antagonists in combination with β-blockers, as there is a risk of precipitating heart block and bradycardia.
6. However, there is not much evidence that using multiple antianginal drugs is beneficial; therefore revascularization is considered if a combination of two appropriate drugs has not controlled symptoms sufficiently.

Interventional treatments
There are two main ways of mechanically improving myocardial blood supply:

- Percutaneous coronary intervention (PCI).
- Coronary artery bypass graft (CABG).

Coronary angiography is used to help decide which revascularization technique to use.

Percutaneous coronary intervention. PCI describes a number of procedures to relieve stenosis in the coronary arteries performed by insertion of a catheter, via the radial or femoral artery, under local anaesthetic and light sedation.

Percutaneous treatment options for CAD include:

1. Balloon angioplasty: an inflatable balloon is passed into the affected coronary artery and inflated within the stenosis, compressing it and expanding the lumen.

2. Metal stents: a balloon-mounted metallic stent is positioned within the stenosis, expanding the vessel walls and restoring vessel patency. Stents decrease the need for reintervention when compared with balloon angioplasty but the stents can stimulate a proliferative response of the vascular smooth muscle. This proliferative response causes scar tissue deposition that can lead to narrowing of the expanded lumen (termed *restenosis*). This usually occurs within 3 to 6 months of implantation. Attempts to overcome this have led to the use of drug-eluting stents, which are coated with immunosuppressive agents.

Stents are highly thrombogenic and can cause blood clots to form, occluding the artery. This risk of thrombosis is ameliorated by the use of intravenous heparin at the time of PCI and dual antiplatelet therapy, i.e., aspirin indefinitely and a P2Y$_{12}$ receptor (often 3–12 months, length dependent on thrombosis and bleeding risk). Glycoprotein IIb/IIIa receptor inhibitors may also be used in high-risk cases. See Table 12.1 and Chapter 11, Fig. 11.3.

Complications of PCI:

These include major adverse effects such as:

1. MI – secondary to thrombosis, spasm or dissection of the coronary artery.
2. Coronary artery perforation.
3. Stroke.
4. Rarely, death.

Table 12.1 Antiplatelet agents used to prevent thrombosis following angioplasty ± stenting

Class of drug and examples	Action	Side effects
Aspirin	Irreversible inactivation of cyclooxygenase 1 within platelets – potent reduction of platelet aggregation.	Gastritis including ulcer formation and bleeding, bronchospasm, renal impairment, rashes.
P2Y$_{12}$ antagonist (clopidogrel, ticagrelor, prasugrel)	Inhibits the platelet ADP receptor P2Y$_{12}$, preventing initiation of thrombus formation.	Haemorrhage, diarrhoea, nausea, neutropenia, hepatic dysfunction.
Glycoprotein IIb/IIIa receptor inhibitors (tirofiban, eptifibatide, abciximab)	Inhibits the binding of fibrinogen to GP IIb/IIIa receptors, thus inhibiting platelet aggregation. Given as an infusion at the time of the procedure and only usually when thrombotic complications occur.	Thrombocytopenia, haemorrhage.

Less severe but more common adverse effects such as:

1. Arrhythmias.
2. Contrast reactions (allergy and nephrotoxicity).
3. Haemorrhage or infection at the puncture site.

Coronary artery bypass graft. This is a major operation performed under general anaesthesia. Via median sternotomy to access the heart, the patient's own veins and/or arteries are reattached to bypass the stenosis in the coronary arteries. The vessels commonly used include the internal mammary artery, which is directly anastomosed distal to the stenosis, and the radial artery of the forearm and the long saphenous vein of the leg, which are anastomosed proximally to the aorta and distally beyond the stenosis. Arterial grafts have much better long-term patency than vein grafts.

The procedure is traditionally performed with the patients on a cardiopulmonary bypass machine that pumps and oxygenates the blood, and the heart is stopped using cooling and cardioplegic solutions. In recent years, some surgeons have been performing this procedure on beating hearts using a specialized instrument to immobilize the area around the anastomosis (socalled 'off-pump' CABG).

CABG is usually indicated in patients with left main stem disease or triple-vessel disease, while patients with single- or double-vessel disease are usually treated with PCI. Generally, although CABG is associated with higher short-term mortality and morbidity, the need for subsequent reintervention is less than with PCI, and overall long-term mortality is reduced.

Complications of coronary artery bypass grafting:

1. Death – mortality rates of approximately 1%.
2. MI, stroke and peripheral thromboembolism.
3. Wound infection.
4. Complications related to cardiopulmonary bypass – include clotting and pulmonary abnormalities, and impaired cognitive function.

Minimally invasive CABG (MICABG) is a newer technique that involves a smaller incision, usually a left anterior minithoracotomy. The left or right internal mammary artery is used to graft the occluded vessel, which is generally the left anterior descending artery because this is within easy reach. Cardiopulmonary bypass is avoided; instead, the heart is slowed using β-blockers and a small immobilizing instrument.

> **CLINICAL NOTES**
>
> ## PCI vs. CABG
> Advantages of PCI over CABG:
>
> 1. Avoids major surgery, general anaesthesia and cardiopulmonary bypass, and the associated higher initial mortality.
> 2. Quicker healing and shorter hospital stay.

3. Patients who have clotting disorders or recent thrombolysis can be treated in an emergency.
4. If PCI is unsuccessful, CABG can still be performed (whereas a second CABG operation carries a much higher risk).

Disadvantages of PCI compared to CABG:

1. Not all patients will have CAD amenable to PCI. Patients with complex coronary disease, such as stenosis of the left main stem, multivessel disease and chronically occluded vessels, may be better served by CABG.
2. Thrombosis can occur at the site of stenting. Additionally, approximately 10% of patients who have had PCI will develop 'in-stent restenosis' (ISR). This rate is higher in diabetic patients and those with smaller calibre or longer segments of stent. ISR can be treated by further PCI. The rate of early ISR has been reduced by the introduction of drug-eluting stents, but late ISR is increased and requires longer dual antiplatelet therapy, yet the need for revascularization after PCI is still higher than after CABG. Long-term mortality is also lower with CABG.
3. Although it may provide symptomatic relief, there is no clear evidence that PCI confers any prognostic benefit over medical therapy in stable angina.

ACUTE CORONARY SYNDROMES

The pathophysiological basis and classification of ACS are described in full in Chapter 11.

In unstable angina, the patient typically presents with a sudden increase in exertional angina, with symptoms on minimal exertion or at rest; the pain usually subsides with rest and nitrates. In contrast to MI, there is no permanent change to the ECG or biochemical evidence of myocardial damage (normal troponin level).

> **CLINICAL NOTES**
>
> Reminder:
>
> 1. Unstable angina due to coronary arterial thrombosis – there is rupture of an atheromatous plaque in the coronary artery, which causes a marked decrease in luminal diameter. The condition may progress to full infarction without urgent treatment. Patients should be treated as with NSTEMIs (risk assessed, started on NSTEMI treatment and admitted to hospital). This is an increasingly uncommon condition with the advent of high-sensitivity troponin assays (patients who may previously have been diagnosed with unstable angina are now often diagnosed with an NSTEMI).

2. Non-ST-elevation myocardial infarction (NSTEMI) – there is necrosis caused by thrombotic coronary artery occlusion in which the myocardial cell death is confined to the endocardial layers (not full thickness). Usually, this occurs because the occluded artery is relatively small, is a side branch or there is some collateral flow around the occluded vessel.
3. ST-elevation myocardial infarction (STEMI) – this represents a developing full-thickness MI, which can lead to arrhythmia, death or leave the patient with severe heart failure. This is a common ECG to see in final exams, as making the diagnosis and rapidly instigating management is absolutely crucial. Delayed intervention leaves dead muscle, which shows as permanent Q waves on the ECG (see Fig. 12.4). Remember that new LBBB with prolonged cardiac chest pain should also be treated as acute STEMI with urgent primary PCI or thrombolysis.

Clinically, acute MI is defined by acute increase and/or fall of troponin, with at least one value raised above the 99th centile of the upper reference limit and at least one of the following:

- Symptoms consistent with ischaemia (lasting >20 mins).
- New, or presumed new, significant ST-T wave changes or left bundle branch block (LBBB) on 12-lead ECG (Fig. 12.4).
- New, or presumed new, pathological Q waves on ECG.

- New, or presumed new, loss of viable myocardium or regional wall motion abnormality on imaging.
- Intracoronary thrombus on angiography.

Criteria for established MI includes:

- New pathological Q waves in the absence of another cause.
- Imaging findings of regional wall motion abnormality in the absence of another cause.
- Pathological findings of healed or healing MI.

CLINICAL NOTES

As raised troponin can be seen in other conditions, terminology for myocardial infarction has evolved over recent years. MI is now classified as below:

- Type 1: Injury related to primary myocardial ischaemia (spontaneous myocardial infarction, usually secondary to atheroma, STEMI and NSTEMI).
- Type 2: Injury related to supply/demand imbalance of myocardial ischaemia ('troponitis' – caused by myocardial stretch/damage: spasm, embolism, tachycardias, hyper/hypotension, anaemia, pulmonary oedema).
- Type 3: Myocardial infarction resulting in death when biomarker values are unavailable.
- Type 4: (a) Periangioplasty (>5 × upper limit of normal); (b) secondary to stent thrombosis.
- Type 5: related to CABG (>10 × upper limit of normal).

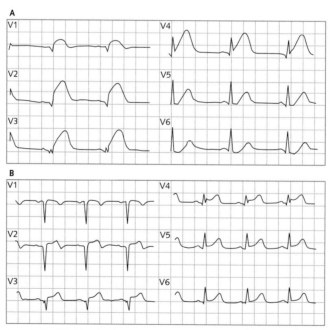

Fig. 12.4 (A) ECG showing acute anterior ST-elevation myocardial infarction. (B) ECG 24 hours after anterior STEMI, showing evolving ST changes and development of Q waves.

Clinical features of ACS

History

In MI, the history provides clues about the likelihood and severity of the infarction. The time of onset is crucial to determine appropriate therapy. Ongoing chest pain suggests ongoing ischaemia and requires urgent treatment.

Classically, the main presenting complaint is of chest pain, usually:

1. Severe.
2. Lasts at least 20 minutes.
3. Tight, crushing, heavy or band-like in nature.
4. Retrosternal in location.
5. May radiate to the left arm, throat or jaw.
6. Associated features include sweating, nausea and breathlessness.

Elderly and diabetic patients may have relatively little pain but may present with features of LV failure (profound breathlessness) or syncope.

Important features include a history of angina or intermittent chest pain, including an increase in severity or frequency in the few weeks preceding this event. The patient may have a history of previous MI or of cardiac intervention, such as angiography, PCI or CABG. Find out if the patient is already on medications for CAD.

Ask about any bleeding risks because this will affect further management.

Determine how many of the risk factors for ischaemic heart disease are present: smoking, hypertension, diabetes mellitus, hypercholesterolaemia and positive family history.

Examination

The patient is often extremely anxious, distressed and restless; they may be in severe pain. Tachypnoea/increased work of breathing suggests pulmonary oedema, as does the presence of pink frothy sputum. The patient may be pale, clammy and sweaty with a reduced capillary refill time or confused and oliguric, suggesting cardiogenic shock. Look for scars of previous surgery.

The pulse may be rapid secondary to anxiety or LV failure. In inferior MIs, there is often bradycardia and AV block as a result of ischaemia of the AV node or due to increased vagal tone secondary to ischaemia.

The blood pressure may be raised (preexisting hypertension or raised due to anxiety). If there is cardiogenic shock, the blood pressure may be low.

The JVP may be elevated in cases of congestive cardiac failure or in pure right-ventricular infarction.

Examination of the precordium may reveal the following:

1. A displaced diffuse apex in cases of LV failure.
2. Rarely with anterior infarction, a paradoxical systolic outward movement of the ventricular wall may be felt parasternally.
3. The murmur of mitral regurgitation or ventricular septal defect – may occur as a new murmur due to rupture of the papillary muscle or ventricular septum, respectively.
4. A pericardial rub – if a delayed presentation, MI may be complicated by pericarditis, which is also a differential diagnosis.
5. Additional heart sounds – third or fourth heart sounds may be heard in MI and suggest LV failure.

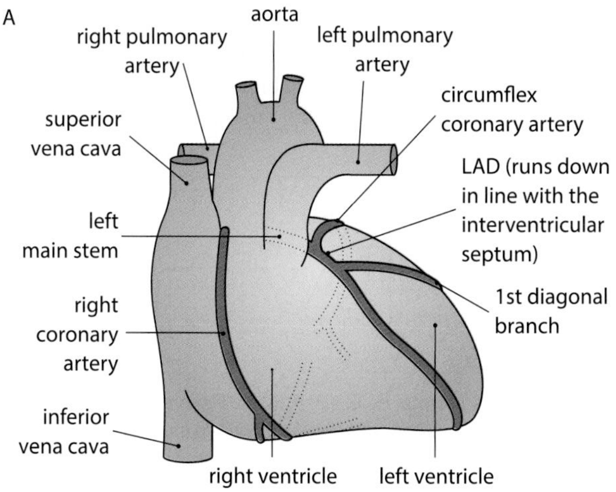

Location of MI	ECG changes
Anteroseptal (LAD)	ST elevation in leads V1–4
Inferior (RCA or circumflex coronary artery)	ST elevation in leads II, III, aVF
Lateral (circumflex coronary artery)	ST elevation in leads I, avL, V5–6
Posterior (RCA or circumflex coronary artery)	Prominent R wave in V1 and V2 with ST depression (mirror image of anterior MI)
Anterolateral (proximal LAD) above diagonal branch	ST elevation I, aVL, V3–6 (V1–V2 may also be involved in extensive anterolateral MI)
Right ventricular infarction (suspect in inferior or posterior MI)	Consider right-sided ECG using lead V1 (as normal), leads V3–6 placed on the right side, limb leads as normal

Fig. 12.5 (A) Location of coronary arteries. Note the left anterior descending (LAD) coronary artery branch supplies the anterior aspect of the heart (the left ventricle and the septum), the right coronary artery (RCA) usually supplies the inferoposterior aspect and the circumflex supplies the lateral part of the left ventricle. (B) Correlation between ECG leads and location of myocardial infarction.

Auscultate the lung bases; bilateral crepitations may suggest LV failure. Peripheral oedema may suggest right ventricular (or bi-ventricular) failure. It is most important to determine if there is any sign of LV impairment or cardiogenic shock, as these require urgent treatment.

Investigation of ACS

As you can see from the definitions, early ECG and measurement of cardiac biomarkers are the most urgent investigations to determine suitable treatment.

Electrocardiography

The ECG is a main diagnostic test in acute MI. It is important to have a thorough knowledge of the ECG appearances of different types of MI (see Chapter 3 and Figs. 12.4–12.6). Treatment should be given as soon as possible for maximum benefit – 'time is muscle'!

> **HINTS AND TIPS**
>
> Posterior MI can be missed and can be seen as ST depression in the anterior leads with a dominant R wave and upright T waves. Flip the ECG upside down, looking through the back of the paper – the anterior ST depression of posterior MI looks like an anterior STEMI when looked at from behind.

In ST elevation MI (STEMI), ST elevation or new LBBB must be present to make the diagnosis. Fig. 12.6 shows ST-segment elevation and the subsequent changes seen on ECG in the days/weeks following a STEMI:

1. ST-segment elevation – this is due to full-thickness myocardial injury and may appear within minutes of the onset of infarction; it is almost always present by 24 hours. The criteria for acute reperfusion therapy (primary percutaneous coronary intervention or thrombolysis) are a good history and

ST-segment elevation >1 mm in two or more consecutive limb leads, or >2 mm in two or more consecutive chest leads. Reciprocal ST-segment depression may be present at the same time and represents the mirror image of the ST elevation as seen from the opposite side of the heart.

2. The ST elevation resolves and the T waves begin to invert.
3. Q waves develop within 24–72 hours.

> **HINTS AND TIPS**
>
> Persistent elevation of ST-segments after 1 week is unusual and usually indicates either re-infarction or left ventricular aneurysm.

> **COMMON PITFALLS**
>
> A patient with a recent MI presenting with chest pain and ST elevation usually causes concern regarding another MI. Be aware that sharp chest pain, worse on lying and improved on sitting forward, with saddle-shaped ST elevation across all the leads is likely to be pericarditis.

If there is LBBB, it is important to find an old ECG to compare – if it is new, this may represent an MI.

In unstable angina/non-STEMI (NSTEMI), ST-segment depression and T wave inversion (similar to during an attack of angina) may be present. Be aware that in these cases, the ECG may also be completely normal.

Blood tests
Biochemical markers of myocyte necrosis

Myocyte necrosis can be detected biochemically; the diagnosis is nearly universally made by measuring high-sensitivity

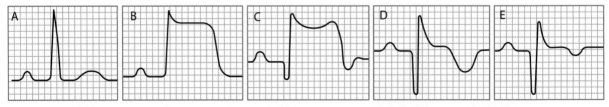

Fig. 12.6 Evolution of ECG changes following transmural myocardial infarction. (A) Normal ECG. (B) Acute ST elevation ('the current of injury'). (C) Progressive loss of R wave, developing Q wave, resolution of the ST elevation and terminal T-wave inversion. (D) Deep Q waves and T-wave inversion. (E) Old or established infarct pattern; the Q wave tends to persist but the T-wave changes become less marked. The rate of evolution is variable but, in general, stage B appears within minutes, stage C within hours, stage D within days and stage E after several weeks or months. (Adapted from *figure courtesy of Newby DE, from Penman I, Ralston S, Strachan M, Hobson R (eds): Davidson's Principles and Practice of Medicine.* 24th ed. Elsevier; 2022. Figure 16.64.)

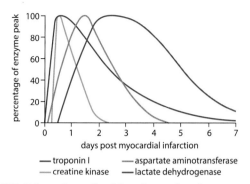

Fig. 12.7 Schematic profile of the release of cardiac enzymes and markers. (Courtesy Newby DE, Grubb NR. *Cardiology: An Illustrated Colour Text.* Edinburgh: Elsevier, 2005, p. 93.)

cardiac troponin T or I, but creatine kinase-MB and lactate dehydrogenase will also be elevated. A rise in these markers suggests myocardial necrosis and therefore infarction (Fig. 12.7). NSTEMI may suggest a smaller area of infarction than STEMI; however, markers can be significantly elevated in NSTEMI. This is in contrast to unstable angina, where dynamic ischaemia does not result in cell injury or loss.

Other causes of myocardial injury can cause a raised troponin level, such as:

1. Myocarditis.
2. Takotsubo cardiomyopathy.
3. Tachyarrhythmia.
4. Massive pulmonary embolism.
5. Critical illness (e.g., shock, sepsis).
6. Renal failure.

Renal function and electrolytes
These are important in all patients who have MI. Renal function may be deranged or may worsen due to poor renal perfusion in cardiogenic shock. Hypokalaemia/hyperkalaemia may predispose to arrhythmias and may need to be corrected because acute MI is in itself a proarrhythmogenic condition.

Blood glucose
Diabetes mellitus should be controlled intensively after MI and all patients who have diabetes mellitus benefit from close blood glucose monitoring and management. However, hypoglycaemia should be avoided, as this is associated with worse outcomes.

Full blood count
Anaemia may worsen angina. There is often a leucocytosis after acute MI.

Serum cholesterol
This should be measured within 24 hours of an MI; hypercholesterolaemia is a risk factor for MI and needs to be treated. Cholesterol level falls to an artificially low level 24 hours after MI, so after this time, a true reading can only be obtained 2 months after the MI.

Chest radiography
This should be performed on all patients who have acute MI. Points to note are:

1. Signs of pulmonary oedema – signify the need for heart failure treatment.
2. An enlarged heart – suggests chronic cardiac failure or tamponade.
3. Widening of the mediastinum – suggests possible aortic dissection, either as a differential diagnosis or in conjunction with MI, and an absolute contraindication for thrombolysis.

Echocardiography
Echocardiography is not an urgent investigation, but it is important to evaluate ventricular function following an acute MI. Complications of MI may be found which may alter management, such as mural thrombus, mitral regurgitation as a result of papillary muscle infarction, myocardial/septal rupture and pericardial effusion. It may occasionally demonstrate signs of right heart strain, which could alternatively suggest that a large volume pulmonary embolus is the cause of the chest pain and associated troponin rise.

Management of ACS
ACS is a medical emergency. You must know its acute management, and it is one of the few occasions in an exam when you will be expected to know the doses of drugs given.

Immediate management of all patients with ACS should be the administration of analgesia (usually morphine titrated to effect), aspirin 300 mg, a $P2Y_{12}$ antagonist (clopidogrel 300 mg, prasugrel 60 mg or ticagrelor 180 mg), and a β-blocker (explained later). It is important to treat hypoxia with oxygen, but oxygen is not currently recommended for nonhypoxic patients routinely, as there is evidence of possible harm. Morphine reduces pain and anxiety, which is not only important in making the patient more comfortable but may indirectly decrease O_2 demand by reducing heart rate and blood pressure. Remember to give an antiemetic together with morphine to prevent the common side effect of nausea/vomiting; this is also a common symptom of ACS. The subsequent management is dependent on the presence of ST elevation and is shown in the algorithm in Fig. 12.8; however, remember to follow the guidelines in your local hospital.

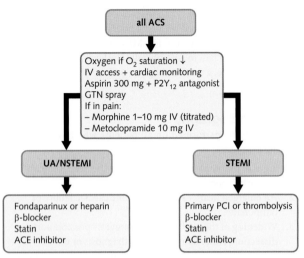

all ACS

Oxygen if O_2 saturation ↓
IV access + cardiac monitoring
Aspirin 300 mg + $P2Y_{12}$ antagonist
GTN spray
If in pain:
– Morphine 1–10 mg IV (titrated)
– Metoclopramide 10 mg IV

UA/NSTEMI

STEMI

Fondaparinux or heparin
β-blocker
Statin
ACE inhibitor

Primary PCI or thrombolysis
β-blocker
Statin
ACE inhibitor

Fig. 12.8 Algorithm for the treatment of acute coronary syndromes.

In the context of cardiac chest pain, ST-segment elevation on the 12-lead ECG usually signifies complete occlusion of a proximal coronary artery. If untreated, myocardial necrosis commences within 30 minutes, affecting full myocardial thickness within 6 hours. Forty percent of patients die before reaching the hospital. Once ECG confirms STEMI, arrange urgent cardiology review for primary angioplasty where available and give additional antiplatelet/anticoagulant agents as recommended; otherwise, consider thrombolysis if there are no contraindications and admission to the coronary care unit. Treat new LBBB with cardiac chest pain as STEMI.

In NSTEMI or unstable angina, arrange a cardiology review and admit for ongoing specialist care and likely inpatient coronary angiography.

Drugs used in the immediate treatment of ACS

Preventing thrombus extension

Antiplatelet agents aim to prevent further activation and aggregation of platelets, reducing the likelihood of expansion of the thrombus occluding the affected coronary artery. A number of agents are available (see Table. 12.1).

Aspirin. Aspirin is the most important antiplatelet drug in the treatment of CAD and reduces mortality in ACS. It irreversibly inhibits the enzyme cyclooxygenase (COX), which is involved in the synthesis of the potent platelet activator thromboxane A_2 from arachidonic acid. Inhibiting COX also blocks the synthesis of prostaglandin I_2 (PGI_2), an inhibitor of platelet function. However, endothelial cells produce PGI_2 and are able to produce more COX enzyme (which platelets are unable to do, as they have no nucleus). This leads to the balance shifting towards production of the antiplatelet PGI_2. In ACS, 300 mg aspirin should be given initially and 75 mg daily thereafter. Side effects are relatively few and include an increased risk of bleeding due to inhibited platelet function and gastric irritation leading to stomach ulcers.

$P2Y_{12}$ antagonists. Clopidogrel is a thienopyridine derivative that blocks the $P2Y_{12}$ component of the adenosine diphosphate (ADP) receptor on platelet cell membranes. The blockade of this receptor prevents fibrinogen binding to the platelet and inhibits platelet aggregation. This is irreversibly modified by clopidogrel and prasugrel and reversibly modified by ticagrelor. Clopidogrel has been the standard addition to aspirin for years for all ACS patients (300 mg loading dose for NSTEMI or 600 mg for STEMI, then 75 mg daily); however, newer agents have been developed. Ticagrelor (180 mg loading dose, then 90 mg twice daily) is now recommended as an initial treatment with aspirin in most situations (e.g., NICE guideline from 2020), and prasugrel (60 mg loading dose, then 10 mg once daily) may be considered as an alternative in some high-risk groups.

GPIIb/IIIa inhibitors. The glycoprotein IIb/IIIa platelet receptor on activated platelet membranes binds fibrinogen, von Willebrand factor and other adhesive molecules. GPIIb/IIIa inhibitors inhibit this binding and thereby inhibit platelet aggregation and thrombus formation. Examples include tirofiban, abciximab and eptifibatide. These drugs are only used in ACS for high-risk patients and those undergoing urgent PCI.

Anticoagulant agents. All patients with unstable angina or NSTEMI should receive a pentasaccharide (fondaparinux 2.5 mg subcutaneously once daily for up to 8 days or until discharge), low-molecular-weight heparin, or if renal function does not allow these, unfractionated heparin.

Immediate antianginal therapy

Nitrates. Nitrates are a useful early ACS treatment; they decrease cardiac workload (through venodilatation and peripheral artery vasodilatation) as well as directly cause coronary artery vasodilatation. In ongoing ischaemia, IV nitrate infusions can be a helpful bridge to coronary angiography. Remember that as they can reduce blood pressure, hypotension is a contraindication and close monitoring should be provided.

β-Blockers. Administration of β-blockers decreases heart rate and myocardial work. They have been demonstrated to be beneficial in patients following ACS and should be continued long term. Commencement is contraindicated if the patient has acute heart failure, slow heart rate (<65/min), low blood pressure (<110 mmHg) or cardiogenic shock. Avoid if the patient has asthma.

Calcium channel blockers. These decrease myocardial work and dihydropyridines can be added to a β-blocker if chest pain is ongoing. If β-blockers are not tolerated, verapamil or diltiazem would be a better choice, as they reduce the heart rate and do not cause rebound tachycardia.

Urgent reperfusion therapies

Urgent restoration of coronary blood flow (reperfusion) prevents further LV damage and improves prognosis in STEMI. The amount of myocardium that can be salvaged falls exponentially with time, the greatest benefit being within 3 hours of symptom onset and modest benefit beyond 12 hours.

Primary PCI

Primary PCI describes the situation when PCI is the initial definitive therapy to relieve the blockage and allow reperfusion of the myocardium and thrombolytic agents have not been administered. There is no benefit from primary PCI for NSTEMI. For STEMI, immediate angioplasty with stenting leads to better outcomes than thrombolysis, and it should be considered if within 12 hours of chest pain onset and it can be delivered within 2 hours (if this is not feasible, immediate thrombolysis should be considered). When thrombolysis has been unsuccessful and PCI is performed, this is called rescue PCI.

Thrombolytic therapy

Thrombolytic (fibrinolytic) therapy is used to break down the thrombi that cause MI and allow reperfusion of the affected area. These agents achieve this by converting plasminogen to the fibrinolytic enzyme plasmin, which breaks down the fibrin mesh that binds a thrombus together (fibrinolysis). They are only used in STEMI within 12 hours of onset when primary PCI is not available within 2 hours and must be administered by a senior doctor after careful assessment for contraindications. The administration of thrombolytic agents (except streptokinase) should be followed by an infusion of heparin for 48 hours to prevent recurrent thrombus formation and ischaemic events.

Thrombolytic agents include:

1. Tissue plasminogen activators (tPA), e.g., alteplase, tenecteplase, reteplase (these are the primary agents of choice for thrombolysis).
2. Streptokinase: rarely used in clinical practice now. Streptokinase cannot be used repeatedly, as antibodies are generated which may induce anaphylaxis on subsequent exposure.

Important contraindications to thrombolysis (discuss each case with a senior clinician):

1. Previous intracranial haemorrhage or stroke of unknown origin at any time.
2. Recent ischaemic stroke (within 6 months).
3. Central nervous system damage/tumour/AV malformation.
4. Recent head injury/major trauma/surgery/bleeding.
5. Known bleeding disorder.
6. Suspected aortic dissection.
7. Noncompressible vascular punctures in the last 24 hours.
8. Relative contraindications include prolonged or traumatic resuscitation, pregnancy and refractory hypertension.

Nonacute management
Complications after MI

After the patient is admitted, daily history, examination and observations aim to identify the development of complications. Cardiogenic shock would indicate a severe complication, such as myocardial rupture, unstable arrhythmia or significant heart failure. Patients with recurrent angina after ACS are at high risk, and timely angiography should be considered. Symptoms or signs of heart failure are treated, and any deterioration should prompt reconsideration of the cause and a search for new complications.

Sudden death (within 6 hours of symptom onset) occurs in up to 25% of patients following STEMI, usually as a result of arrhythmia. Many of these patients die before reaching the hospital. For the patients that reach the hospital, mortality is much lower, approximately 5% at 7 days. Cardiac monitoring

Table 12.2 Complications of acute myocardial infarction

Time frame	Complication
Early (0–48 hours)	Arrhythmias – VT, VF, SVT, heart block Cardiogenic shock due to left or right ventricular failure
Medium term (2–7 days)	Arrhythmias – VT, VF, SVT, heart block Pulmonary embolus (4–7 days) Rupture of papillary muscle (3–5 days) Rupture of interventricular septum (3–5 days) Free wall rupture (3–5 days) Note: Rupture of the above structures usually presents with acute cardiac failure and progresses rapidly to death; some patients may survive after surgery.
Late (weeks to months)	Arrhythmias – VT, VF, SVT, heart block Cardiac failure Dressler's syndrome (3–8 weeks) Left ventricular aneurysm (after several weeks to months) Mural thrombus and systemic embolization

SVT, supraventricular tachycardia; VF, ventricular fibrillation; VT, ventricular tachycardia.

is applied to all patients initially and is continued until the patient is deemed stable. In those who survive this initial period, MI can lead to a number of acute and chronic complications, detailed in Table. 12.2. The major ones include:

1. Heart failure: infarcted myocardium is unable to contract effectively.
2. Arrhythmia: this can be any arrhythmia, although ventricular fibrillation (VF) is likely the cause in many patients who die suddenly following STEMI. Arrhythmias are also common immediately following myocardial reperfusion.
3. Myocardial rupture: this can be either the free wall of a ventricle or the interventricular septum and can be rapidly fatal without emergency surgical intervention.
4. Mitral regurgitation: owing to infarction and subsequent rupture of the papillary muscles.
5. Pericarditis: this can occur a few days after infarction (periinfarction) and weeks to months later as an immunological phenomenon called Dressler syndrome.

Heart block after MI. Ischaemic injury can occur at any point in the conducting system – the SA node, the AV node or anywhere from the bundle of His downwards.

AV block is commonly associated with inferior MI. This is due to ischaemia of the AV node and usually recovers with reperfusion. However, if there is high-degree AV block with clinical compromise, temporary pacing may be required.

Anterior MI may cause heart block if there is marked septal necrosis (indicating a large anterior MI) and will usually require a permanent pacemaker (see Chapter 14).

Cardiogenic shock after myocardial infarction. Patients with cardiogenic shock due to a reversible cause such as MI may be treated with an intraaortic balloon pump. This is an infrequent bridging measure. The balloon sits in the descending aorta and, using the ECG for timing, inflates during diastole. This forces blood back to the coronary arteries and forward to the renal arteries, increasing perfusion of the heart and kidneys. The benefit of this treatment is unclear and the priority is usually to perform an angiogram and revascularize the patient as soon as possible.

Secondary prevention

- Antiplatelet therapies are continued. Usually this is lifelong aspirin, and in patients who have had a drug-eluting stent, this is generally a $P2Y_{12}$ antagonist for between 3 months and 1 year.
- High intensity statin (regardless of measured cholesterol), as statins give benefit to MI regardless of cholesterol level.
- Long-term β-blockers potentially reduce recurrent infarction and may improve mortality, especially if there is significant LV dysfunction.
- ACE inhibitors confer greatest benefit in those with LV dysfunction but can have an effect on ventricular remodelling, prevent heart failure and improve mortality. Additional benefit may be gained from aldosterone antagonists (e.g., spironolactone, eplerenone) if there is reduced ejection fraction after an MI.

Further management

Implantable cardioverter defibrillators are beneficial in patients with severely reduced ejection fraction after MI.

Early mobilization (after 48 hours) is instituted to prevent venous stasis.

Follow-up care with a cardiologist and access to cardiac rehabilitation is provided. This consists of:

1. Smoking cessation. This reduces the rate of recurrent MI by two-thirds to three-quarters. It is the single most important intervention (including medication) in reducing risk of recurrent MI. Where necessary, psychological and pharmaceutical support should be provided.
2. Dietary advice, particularly emphasizing the value of fish and olive oil and fresh fruit and vegetables. Carbohydrate restriction for non–insulin-dependent diabetes mellitus and insulin resistance. Calorie restriction for patients who have diabetes mellitus or who are obese.
3. Advice on medications, their role in improving prognosis, and the importance of compliance.
4. Progressively increasing exercise level to incorporate rapid walking on a daily basis if possible. Group gym sessions may

help some patients by encouraging exercise and giving psychological support to each other.

5. Advice from a clinical psychologist on how to cope with the illness.

6. A subsequent support group may be continued as long as each individual patient finds it helpful.

DVLA guidelines state that Group 1 drivers (most drivers) cannot drive for at least 1 week if they have been successfully treated with angioplasty or 4 weeks if not (as long as ejection fraction is >40%). Group 2 drivers (large goods vehicles or passenger-carrying vehicles) cannot drive for 6 weeks, will require assessment before relicensing, and cannot renew a Group 2 license if ejection fraction is <40%.

Chapter Summary

- Stable angina occurs due to myocardial demand exceeding supply as a result of a fixed stenosis. There are many possible exacerbating factors.
- CT coronary angiography is recommended as the first-line investigation in patients with suspected angina. If patients have known coronary artery disease and possible angina, then stress imaging should be offered. In practice, local availability of investigations may affect investigation pathways.
- If two antianginal drugs have not sufficiently controlled symptoms of stable angina, consider revascularization.
- Acute coronary syndrome is a medical emergency.
- Urgent ECG is essential to identify STEMI early, and troponin should be sent quickly, as the result will take time to return.
- Manage ACS with an A–E approach and remember to apply the cardiac monitor early, as many deaths occur due to early arrhythmia.
- STEMI is treated with emergency primary PCI, if possible, or thrombolysis if the patient cannot be transferred to a PCI centre within 2 hours.
- In ACS, give antiplatelets as soon as possible to reduce mortality rates.

UKMLA Conditions
Acute coronary syndromes
Cardiac arrest
Ischaemic heart disease
Myocardial infarction
Unstable angina

UKMLA Presentations
Cardiorespiratory arrest
Chest pain

Heart failure (cardiac failure) is the clinical syndrome that arises when the heart is unable to maintain sufficient tissue perfusion to meet the metabolic demands of the body's tissues, despite normal filling pressures. This leads to inadequate cardiac output and/or increased intracardiac pressures.

Heart failure is a serious condition with a very poor prognosis: 20% to 30% of patients will die within 1 year and 60% will be dead within 5 years. This is a worse prognosis than many cancers.

Heart failure can affect the left and right ventricles individually or both together. If left untreated, left-ventricular failure (LVF) will lead to right-ventricular failure (RVF) due to high right-ventricular pressure load.

COMMUNICATION

Patients may find the term 'heart failure' frightening, and it is important to address any concerns as they arise. It may help to explain the term means that the heart is not pumping as effectively as it should; patients sometimes interpret 'heart failure' to mean their heart will stop beating.

PATHOPHYSIOLOGY OF HEART FAILURE

In the normal heart, during exercise and other stresses, there is an increased adrenergic stimulation of the myocardium and cardiac pacemaker tissue resulting in tachycardia and increased myocardial contractility.

Venoconstriction shifts blood to the central compartment resulting in increased end-diastolic volume (EDV) of the left ventricle and stretching of the myocytes. This stretch usually causes an increase in myocardial performance – as predicted by the Frank-Starling law (Fig. 13.1).

In most patients with heart failure, impairment of systolic function (contractility) of the left ventricle means the Starling curve is shifted downwards such that stroke volume is reduced for any given end-diastolic pressure (EDP). Together with concurrent symptoms and signs of heart failure, ejection fraction <40% is referred to as heart failure with reduced ejection fraction (HFrEF), and ejection fraction 41% to 49% is termed heart failure with minimally reduced ejection fraction (HFmrEF), although these conditions should be seen as being on a continuum.

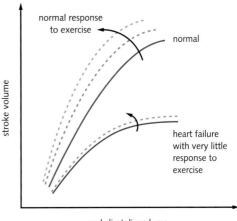

Fig. 13.1 Relationship between end-diastolic volume and stroke volume in normal and failing myocardium (Frank-Starling relationship). In heart failure, reduced contractility reduces stroke volume for a given filling volume.

Low-output heart failure can also be caused by diastolic dysfunction in situations where ventricular filling is impaired. This limits the EDV and thus stroke volume and cardiac output. In diastolic dysfunction, ventricular compliance usually decreases and the relationship between EDV and EDP becomes nonlinear. As a result, the Starling curve is no longer valid. The relationship between EDV and stroke volume, however, is still valid. In this situation, EDV is reduced, restricting stroke volume, but the ejection fraction is preserved (>50%). This is referred to as heart failure with preserved ejection fraction (HFpEF). Simplistically, this is a situation where enough blood cannot get into the heart to be pumped around the body to maintain a satisfactory cardiac output.

High-output heart failure occurs when there is excessive demand on a normal heart. Although cardiac output is increased, it cannot keep up with the volume overload. This may be either acute or chronic.

Causes of heart failure

The most common cause of heart failure (in high-income countries) is systolic failure as the result of myocardial damage, due to:

- Ischaemic heart disease – an infarcted segment of ventricle is unable to contract effectively, decreasing systolic function; see Chapter 12.
- Myocarditis/cardiomyopathy – see Chapter 16.

Sometimes there is no initial abnormality of myocardial function, but cardiac failure occurs due to increased cardiac workload, as seen in:

- Hypertension – chronically increased afterload leads to compensatory left ventricular hypertrophy. This increases myocardial oxygen demand and impairs diastolic filling due to decreased ventricular compliance.
- Valvular heart disease – can cause both pressure overload (aortic stenosis) and volume overload (aortic or mitral regurgitation) in the left ventricle, decreasing efficiency.
- High-output cardiac failure – common causes include thyrotoxicosis, sepsis and chronic anaemia. Rarer causes include Paget disease of bone, arteriovenous malformations, high-flow arteriovenous dialysis fistulae, phaeochromocytoma and beriberi.

These processes most commonly affect the left ventricle (LV), but isolated failure of the right ventricle (RV) can occur in some circumstances. Remember that the most common cause of RVF is LVF, resulting in biventricular failure. Causes of isolated RVF include:

- Right ventricular myocardial infarction (MI).
- Cor pulmonale: this is RVF due to disease of the pulmonary vasculature. It can be caused by recurrent pulmonary emboli, primary pulmonary hypertension or any respiratory disease in which there is persistent widespread hypoxic pulmonary vasoconstriction, such as chronic obstructive pulmonary disease (COPD). All of these conditions increase pulmonary vascular resistance, causing pressure and volume overload of the right ventricle.

Decreased RV output limits LV preload and thus LV stroke volume – this can bring about the same signs and symptoms as those that occur when the LV is primarily affected.

HINTS AND TIPS

Remember, it is always necessary to identify the underlying pathology responsible for heart failure so that a targeted treatment regimen can be employed.

Compensatory mechanisms

When stroke volume and cardiac output are reduced due to either systolic or diastolic dysfunction, there are a number of compensatory changes (Fig. 13.2) that occur to attempt to restore cardiac output and maintain tissue perfusion. These changes are successful initially and can be useful, e.g., in athletes. The decrease in stroke volume reduces arterial blood pressure, causing unloading of the arterial baroreceptors. This brings about a number of changes including:

- Increased sympathetic and decreased parasympathetic outflow to the heart, increasing heart rate and contractility (this process is limited in a diseased myocardium).
- Increased sympathetic outflow to peripheral vasculature causing vasoconstriction to increase total peripheral resistance (TPR), limiting venous pooling and increasing venous return.
- Decreased renal blood flow and increased sympathetic outflow to the kidneys increase the release of renin. Renin-angiotensin-aldosterone system (RAAS) activation causes further peripheral vasoconstriction and promotes salt and water retention in the kidneys.
- Antidiuretic hormone (ADH) secretion is increased from the posterior pituitary, increasing renal water reabsorption.

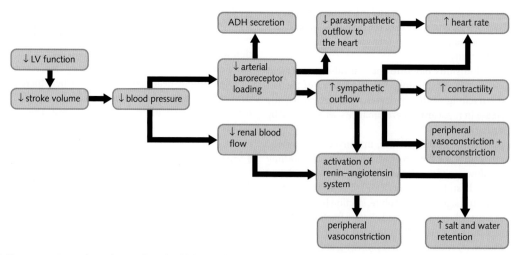

Fig. 13.2 Compensatory adaptations to impaired left ventricular function. *ADH*, antidiuretic hormone; *LV*, left ventricular.

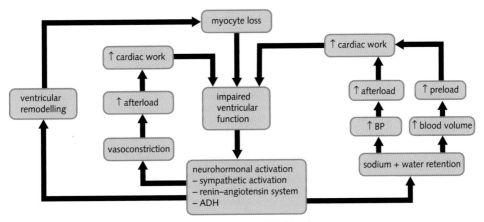

Fig. 13.3 The vicious cycle of heart failure. *ADH*, antidiuretic hormone; *BP*, blood pressure.

These changes increase circulating volume and cardiac filling pressures, which increase stroke volume (by virtue of Starling law), as well as increase heart rate and TPR, which together maintain arterial blood pressure and tissue perfusion. In the early stages, these changes compensate for impaired cardiac function and the clinical features of heart failure may be minimal.

The vicious cycle of heart failure

As systolic dysfunction progresses and these compensatory mechanisms persist and intensify, they become maladaptive, accelerate disease progression and bring about the clinical syndrome of heart failure (Fig. 13.3):

- Persistent RAAS activation and ADH release cause further fluid retention. Initially in place to increase filling pressures to maximize stroke volume, filling pressures become excessive and stroke volume decreases due to excessive stretch of the myocytes. This moves the heart onto the downward part of the Starling curve.
- Increased filling pressures and ventricular pressures cause congestion in the pulmonary circulation and alveolar oedema (due to LV backpressure) and in the systemic veins causing peripheral oedema (due to RV backpressure).
- Excessive filling pressures cause dilatation of the ventricular walls. As the ventricles distend, afterload increases. Dilatation can also cause disruption of the atrioventricular (mitral and tricuspid) valve annulus, leading to valvular regurgitation.
- The persistent tachycardia reduces the duration of diastole and thus the duration of coronary blood flow. With the increase in contractility, myocardial oxygen demand is increased while oxygen delivery is reduced. These two

factors combined may cause myocardial ischaemia, further impairing function.
- Persistently high levels of angiotensin II, aldosterone and catecholamines leads to LV remodelling, with changes in cardiac metabolism, myocardial thinning and fibrosis.

HINTS AND TIPS

A dilated heart is generally indicative of chronic rather than acute heart failure. The dilation does not have time to occur if failure is a purely acute process.

CLINICAL FEATURES

The symptoms and signs of cardiac failure vary depending upon a number of factors:

- Severity of heart failure.
- Chronicity and cause of heart failure.
- Which ventricle is involved (isolated right heart failure is less common and a pulmonary cause should be excluded).
- Age of the patient.

In acute heart failure (e.g., caused by MI), onset is rapid due to lack of time to fully develop compensatory mechanisms. In chronic heart failure (e.g., due to valvular heart disease), compensation may limit overt clinical features initially, but any new insult (e.g., atrial fibrillation) can lead to rapid decompensation and acute-on-chronic heart failure.

Regardless of the cause of heart failure, it is possible to predict the effects if the mechanics of pump failure are

Table 13.1 Signs and symptoms of left and right ventricular failure and general signs and symptoms that might be seen in either. Often patients have a combination of left AND right ventricular impairment

	Left ventricular (LV) failure	Right ventricular (RV) failure	General
Symptoms	• Dyspnoea due to pulmonary oedema. • Orthopnoea. • Paroxysmal nocturnal dyspnoea. • Wheeze (due to pulmonary oedema).	• Dyspnoea due to poor pulmonary perfusion. • Ankle swelling. • Anorexia, nausea, abdominal discomfort (due to hepatic congestion). • Nocturia.	• Fatigue. • Palpitations. • Exercise intolerance. • Dizziness.
Signs	• Bibasal pulmonary crackles. • Pleural effusions (usually bilateral but if unilateral, tends to be right sided). • Slow capillary refill +/− peripheral cyanosis. • Murmur of mitral regurgitation.	• Elevated jugular venous pressure. • Pitting bilateral peripheral oedema (ankle +/− sacral). • Hepatic enlargement and ascites. • Murmur of tricuspid regurgitation.	• Pale peripheries. • Tachycardia (either sinus tachycardia or arrhythmia). • Low-volume pulse. • Hypotension. • Additional heart sounds (S3 +/− S4). • Cachexia.

considered. The effects can be divided into forward and backward effects.

Forward effects

Forward effects refer to the failure of the pump to provide an adequate output. This applies to the LV resulting in:

- Poor renal perfusion predisposing to prerenal failure.
- Poor perfusion of extremities resulting in cold extremities.
- Secondary changes in skeletal muscle structure leading to weakness and fatigue.
- Hypotension (cardiogenic shock).

Forward failure of the RV results in reduced pulmonary flow leading to dyspnoea and underfilling of the LV resulting in hypotension and so on (as above).

Backward effects

Failure of the RV and LV results in congestion of the systemic and pulmonary venous systems, respectively, leading to systemic and pulmonary oedema. In the case of systemic oedema, this tends to be dependent (legs if walking, sacrum if bed-bound) but liver congestion and ascites may also occur.

HINTS AND TIPS

Although dividing heart failure into LVF and RVF seems complicated, it is worth taking the time to learn, as it makes it much easier to work out logically the cause of a given set of signs and symptoms.

Symptoms and signs of heart failure

Many of the symptoms and signs of heart failure are due to reduced cardiac output, volume overload and increased venous pressures within the circulation. LVF will result in increased congestion into the pulmonary circulation and can cause further backpressure and congestion into the systemic venous circulation. RVF, on the other hand, does not cause pulmonary congestion but does cause congestion of the systemic veins.

Because of this, right and left ventricular failure tend to present differently (Table 13.1). One or the other may be dominant and the clinical picture varies accordingly. Often there are signs of both.

The severity of the symptoms and functional capacity of patients are often described using the New York Heart Association (NYHA) classification (Table 13.2).

Dyspnoea may result from pulmonary oedema, impaired skeletal muscle function, depressed respiratory muscle function and reduced lung function. It can present in a number of ways:

- Exertional dyspnoea – as cardiac failure worsens, the level of exertion required to cause dyspnoea decreases until the

Table 13.2 NYHA functional classification for heart failure

NYHA Class	Features
Class I (mild)	No limitation of physical activity by symptoms
Class II (mild)	Symptoms with ordinary activity
Class III (moderate)	Symptoms with minimal activity
Class IV (severe)	Symptoms at rest

patient is breathless at minimal exertion (e.g., when dressing or even when speaking).

- Orthopnoea – the increased central blood volume when the patient lies flat is often too much for the failing heart to pump, resulting in the development of pulmonary oedema. Patients who have severe LVF often sleep with several pillows to prop them up.
- Paroxysmal nocturnal dyspnoea (PND) – after being asleep for some time, the patient is awakened by severe breathlessness, which is relieved only after standing or sitting upright. This is due to pulmonary oedema from gradual resorption of interstitial fluid overnight and nocturnal depression of respiratory function.

Fatigue and weakness result from reduced perfusion of skeletal muscles, which can lead to loss of muscle mass and cachexia in chronic heart failure. Nocturia is due to peripheral oedema being reabsorbed into the circulation when supine. This results in increased circulating volume, increased renal perfusion and thus increased urine output.

Cough may be:

- A nocturnal dry cough due to bronchial oedema or cardiac asthma (bronchospasm secondary to oedema).
- Productive of pink frothy sputum due to pulmonary oedema.
- Dry cough as a side effect of angiotensin-converting enzyme (ACE) inhibitor therapy.

Epigastric discomfort occurs in cases of hepatic congestion. Anorexia (due to oedema of the gut), ankle swelling (due to peripheral oedema), and shortness of breath (due to inadequate pulmonary perfusion) may occur in a patient who has predominantly right-sided heart failure.

See Fig. 13.4 and Chapter 7 for a summary of clinical examination in patients suspected of heart failure.

HINTS AND TIPS

If a raised JVP is nonpulsatile, consider superior vena cava obstruction.

When examining the patient with heart failure, for the patient's comfort remember that:

- Dyspnoea secondary to pulmonary oedema is worse on lying flat and in severe cases, the patient has to sit upright. In this situation, it may be unreasonable to ask the patient to sit at a 45-degree angle; therefore conduct the examination in the upright position.
- Take care when palpating the liver or attempting to elicit hepatojugular reflux because congestive cardiac failure can result in tender hepatomegaly.

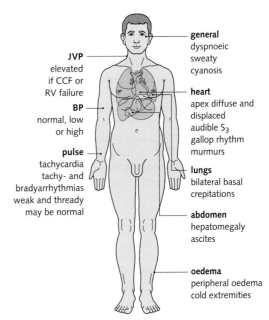

Fig. 13.4 Clinical findings in a patient who has heart failure. *BP*, blood pressure; *CCF*, congestive cardiac failure; *JVP*, jugular venous pressure; *RV*, right ventricular.

INVESTIGATIONS

Blood tests

Electrolytes and renal function

Hypokalaemia and hyponatraemia are common findings in patients on diuretic therapy. There may also be renal impairment due to hypoperfusion or diuretic therapy. Hyponatraemia is common in heart failure and due to high circulating ADH levels (dilutional hyponatraemia).

Hyperkalaemia may be seen in patients treated with potassium-sparing diuretics (e.g., amiloride or spironolactone), ACE inhibitors (e.g., ramipril or lisinopril), or angiotensin II receptor blockers (ARBs), such as losartan or candesartan.

Full blood count

Severe anaemia may lead to heart failure. Conversely, chronic heart failure (irrespective of aetiology) frequently leads to mild anaemia. Leucocytosis may suggest infection, which may exacerbate failure.

Thyroid function tests

Hypothyroidism and hyperthyroidism can both precipitate heart failure.

Cardiac biomarkers in heart failure

Mild or moderate elevations in troponin are seen in patients with ongoing heart failure. It may be significantly raised if there is ongoing (or recent) ischaemia or infarction. A trend in troponin levels can be useful to assess for an acute event (in the context of history, ECG findings, etc.).

Serum natriuretic peptides can be measured to diagnose or to monitor heart failure. Brain natriuretic peptide (BNP) and N-terminal (NT) proBNP (a biologically inactive peptide split from the prohormone of BNP) are released into the bloodstream by the ventricular myocardium when excess stretch of cardiomyocytes occurs. NT-proBNP is preferred, as it is more stable than BNP.

CLINICAL NOTES

Another natriuretic peptide known as *atrial natriuretic peptide* (ANP) is secreted by the cardiomyocytes in the atria in response to increased stretch. Assessment of ANP is less useful as a diagnostic test due to a shorter half-life.

Levels of BNP are significantly raised in patients with heart failure and there is evidence to suggest the levels correlate with symptom severity (with a very high level indicative of poor prognosis). However, BNP can be raised for many noncardiac causes and can be normal in heart failure, especially when the patient has well-compensated treated heart failure without fluid overload.

BNP (and ANP) act to:

- Increase natriuresis – with loss of sodium, fluid is also lost. This helps to combat fluid overload, reducing cardiac preload.
- Vasodilate – this helps to lower TPR and therefore afterload.

BNP <100 pg/mL or NT-proBNP <300 pg/mL should rule out acute heart failure.

In the nonacute setting, the National Institute for Health and Care Excellence (NICE) guidelines (updated 2017) recommend that patients with a suspected diagnosis of heart failure and an NT-proBNP of 400 to 2000 ng/L should be referred for specialist assessment and echocardiogram within 6 weeks. Very high levels of natriuretic peptides are correlated with poor prognosis and patients with a BNP of over 2000 ng/L should be referred for urgent assessment within 2 weeks. The more recent European Society of Cardiology (ESC) guidelines (2021) recommend that a BNP <35 ng/L or an NT-proBNP <125 ng/L should rule out chronic heart failure.

BNP and NT-proBNP have very high negative predictive values and are useful to rule out heart failure (and identify those who do not require echocardiography and specialist assessment). However, they have poorer positive predictive values (false positives are common) and are therefore less useful in establishing a diagnosis of heart failure. They can also be used to assess the response to diuretic treatment: as the fluid overload falls, so does the BNP level.

Other blood tests

Other blood tests may be useful:

- Liver function tests – may be impaired due to liver congestion.
- Arterial blood gases – may show hypoxia, hypocapnoea and metabolic acidosis. Profoundly hypoxic patients may require artificial ventilation.
- Fasting lipids – may demonstrate hyperlipidaemia.
- Glucose – may identify coexisting diabetes or poor diabetic control.
- Iron studies – haemochromatosis may cause cardiomyopathy; iron deficiency is common in heart failure.

Electrocardiography

This is rarely normal and may show ischaemic or hypertensive changes. Q waves may indicate previous MI. Arrhythmias such as atrial fibrillation may precipitate heart failure. If arrhythmia is suspected, a 24-hour ECG may be of diagnostic benefit.

Chest radiography

This may identify other causes of the patient's symptoms. Typical findings in the patient with heart failure (see Fig. 13.5, also Fig. 7.2) include:

- Diffuse **A**lveolar oedema – classically in a bat's-wing distribution (bilateral and peri-hilar).

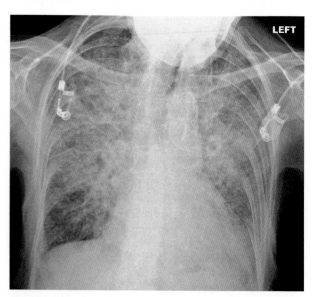

Fig. 13.5 Chest X-ray showing extensive alveolar pulmonary oedema with classic 'bats-wing' perihilar opacification.

- Fluid in the fissures and Kerley **B** lines (interstitial oedema causing horizontal lines of fluid-filled interlobular septa at the peripheries of the lungs, usually at the bases).
- **C**ardiomegaly – seen as increased cardiothoracic ratio. This indicates ventricular hypertrophy/dilatation.
- Upper lobe venous **D**iversion (prominent veins in upper lobes).
- Pleural **E**ffusions.

These findings are easy to remember using an **ABCDE** mnemonic.

Echocardiography

This is essential in heart failure; it is noninvasive and can be performed at the bedside if necessary. It can help to determine:

- Left and right ventricular dimensions and function.
- Regional wall motion abnormalities – usually indicating coronary artery disease (hypokinetic/akinetic areas may indicate ischaemia or infarction).
- Valvular structural/functional abnormalities.
- Pressure gradients across narrowed valves and estimation of pulmonary artery pressure.
- Intracardiac thrombus – may be the result of arrhythmia or previous infarction. Note transoesophageal echocardiography is more sensitive.
- Intracardiac shunts (e.g., due to septal defect).

Cardiac catheterization

Cardiac catheterization may be of use if coronary artery disease is suspected as a cause of heart failure. Coronary revascularization (where necessary) *may* improve the pumping ability of the heart. This is generally not performed acutely unless there is objective evidence of acute ischaemia (e.g., ongoing ischaemic chest pain and new elevation in cardiac biomarkers).

Other investigations

Other investigations may be of use, dependent on suspected aetiology of patient's presentation:

- Cardiac magnetic resonance imaging – can very accurately assess ventricular volume and function. Useful for identifying myocardial scarring, infiltration and inflammation.
- Computed tomography (CT) angiography – may be useful if heart failure is precipitated by pulmonary embolus. CT coronary angiography may be used in an attempt to rule out significant coronary artery disease.
- Pulmonary function tests, urinalysis, etc. – to rule out other causes of patient's symptoms.

MANAGEMENT

Management is divided into management of acute heart failure and chronic heart failure.

Acute left ventricular failure

Acute LVF with pulmonary oedema is very common and a medical emergency. Patients with acute LVF require rapid treatment and it is important to have good knowledge about necessary treatments (Table 13.3). Patients may be extremely unwell and it is therefore important to call for help at an early stage.

CLINICAL NOTES

If the patient presenting with acute heart failure is already taking β-blockers (e.g., bisoprolol), NICE recommends continuing this treatment unless the patient has a heart rate of <50 beats per minute or second/third-degree atrioventricular block or shock.

Additional treatments

There are a number of other treatments for heart failure that may be considered in patients presenting with acute heart failure, dependent on the situation:

- Noninvasive ventilation (NIV)/continuous positive airways pressure (CPAP) – consider if the patient has severe dyspnoea and acidaemia, either at the acute presentation or as a later addition to other therapies if the patient fails to improve.
- Invasive ventilation – consider in patients who, despite other treatments, are heading towards (or develop) respiratory failure, reduced consciousness or physical exhaustion.
- Nitrate therapy – There is lack of clinical trial evidence of benefit, although nitrates reduce preload and afterload and can improve stroke volume. NICE recommends nitrates should not routinely be offered in acute heart failure (as they were sometimes used in the past) and that intravenous nitrates may be used in certain circumstances, e.g., if there is coexisting evidence of myocardial ischaemia, severe hypertension or aortic/mitral valve regurgitation. The ESC states that nitrates can be considered in acute heart failure where SBP >100 mmHg for symptomatic relief. Titrated infusion or repeated boluses may be used; blood pressure should be closely monitored.
- Ultrafiltration (extracorporeal removal of fluid from the blood) – may sometimes be considered in patients with diuretic resistance.

Table 13.3 Algorithm for management of patient with acute left ventricular failure

Management	Notes
A. Sit the patient up.	Reduces venous return to the heart and therefore reduces accumulation of pulmonary oedema.
B. Administer high-flow (15 L/min) oxygen via non–rebreathe mask.	Improvement of arterial oxygenation will reduce myocardial oxygen debt and hopefully improve myocardial function.
C. Establish peripheral intravenous access and administer IV furosemide (either as a bolus or infusion).	Furosemide acts as both a venodilator and a powerful diuretic. Its initial action as a venodilator reduces load on the heart before diuresis occurs. Furosemide's diuretic action results in increased excretion of water and salt, reducing circulating volume. This allows resorption of fluid from the interstitial to intravascular space. Patients who are already on diuretic therapy will generally need a higher dose than that which they were prescribed preadmission. If oedema is resistant to increased loop diuretic doses, consider adding a thiazide-like diuretic.
D. Closely monitor urine output.	Furosemide will cause diuresis and the patient will generally be unwell, making use of a bedpan difficult. A urinary catheter may be useful. It is crucial to accurately monitor fluid output to help identify oliguria and renal impairment early.
E. Consider additional treatments.	Various other treatments may be of benefit but these would generally require more intensive monitoring and potentially higher-level care (e.g., cardiac care unit, high dependency unit, intensive care unit).

- Inotropes or vasopressors – consider if there is acute heart failure with a potentially reversible cause of cardiogenic shock.
- Intraaortic balloon counterpulsation – especially where there is a reversible cause and cardiogenic shock.

COMMON PITFALLS

Opiates (e.g., morphine) are no longer routinely recommended to patients with acute LVF (as per NICE guidelines). There is limited evidence for benefit and some evidence of increased harm due to respiratory depression and the need for mechanical ventilation, intensive care unit admission, etc.

Acute right ventricular failure

Acute RVF is a relatively uncommon situation but may be the result of an inferior or posterior MI. If RV systolic function is impaired, this results in low RV stroke volume and therefore poor LV filling and hypotension.

A patient who has an inferior MI and hypotension should be assessed carefully.

Hypotension after inferior MI may be secondary to the combination of RVF and relative underfilling of the RV (due to nitrates, dehydration, diuretics, etc.). Provided that there is no evidence of pulmonary oedema (suggesting presence of significant LV impairment), treatment is with careful fluid challenges and central venous pressure monitoring.

Chronic management of heart failure

The general aims when treating heart failure include the following:

- Decrease preload.
- Decrease afterload by reducing both ventricular volume and blood pressure.
- Reverse or limit ventricular remodelling.
- Limit heart rate.

General measures

Patients with heart failure should restrict their intake of salt and, if they are volume overloaded, fluid restriction may also be useful. Alcohol should be avoided due to its toxic effects on the heart. Exercise improves exercise tolerance and quality of life. Multidisciplinary care optimizes treatment throughout all stages of heart failure. Patients should also have other comorbidities (such as hypertension, ischaemic heart disease, diabetes, etc.) effectively managed.

Pharmacological treatments

The main agents used in the treatment of heart cardiac failure are summarized in Table 13.4.

Angiotensin-converting enzyme inhibitors

ACE inhibitors (e.g., enalapril, lisinopril, ramipril) inhibit production of angiotensin II by ACE. Inhibition of angiotensin II in heart failure limits the degree of ventricular remodelling, reduces the afterload on the heart (by removing its vasoconstrictor effect), and limits salt and water retention.

Table 13.4 The main pharmacological treatment options in patients with heart failure

For all patients with reduced ejection fraction (if not contraindicated). All four categories improve survival and work synergistically; therefore, it is recommended to commence each as early as possible, at lower doses to be titrated up to their target doses.			
• Angiotensin-converting enzyme (ACE) inhibitors OR sacubitril/valsartan combination. • Angiotensin II receptor antagonists (ARBs) if ACE inhibitor/ARNI not tolerated.	• β-Blockers.	• Mineralocorticoid receptor antagonists (MRA).	• Sodium-glucose cotransporter 2 (SGLT2) inhibitors.
These medications may be useful in specific situations: • Diuretic therapy as required for symptomatic relief in volume overload. • Ivabradine. • Hydralazine and nitrates in combination. • Digoxin.			

ACE inhibitors have been repeatedly demonstrated to improve survival and symptoms in heart failure. They should be offered to everyone with heart failure secondary to LV systolic dysfunction, whether symptomatic or not (unless not tolerated or if there is a specific contraindication). Patients taking ACE inhibitors should have regular checks of renal function and electrolytes, as they may cause renal impairment and hyperkalaemia.

Around 10% of patients taking ACE inhibitors will experience a dry cough. This is caused by inhibition of the metabolism of bradykinin (another function of ACE). Cough usually appears in the first few weeks of treatment. In these cases, switch to an ARB. Other common side effects include rashes, angioedema and loss of taste (or a metallic taste).

Angiotensin II receptor blockers

ARBs (e.g., candesartan, valsartan) have the same benefits as ACE inhibitors in heart failure, but the main advantage is that these drugs do not prevent breakdown of bradykinin, so cough does not occur as a side effect and angioedema is less common.

Angiotensin receptor-neprilysin inhibitor

Angiotensin receptor-neprilysin inhibitor (ARNI) is a newer drug, a combination of sacubitril and valsartan (an ARB). Sacubitril acts to inhibit an enzyme called neprilysin or neutral endopeptidase; this enzyme is responsible for breakdown of several vasoactive peptides, including ANP, BNP and bradykinin. These peptides work to reduce blood volume by causing natriuresis and diuresis when the myocardium is under excessive stretch. Sacubitril therefore promotes the action of ANP and BNP and helps to reduce circulating volume. There is some recent evidence to suggest this combination may be more effective (in terms of reducing cardiovascular mortality and heart failure admissions) than an ACE inhibitor alone. However, there are concerns about long-term safety (and increased risk of symptomatic hypotension and angioedema). The ESC recommends replacing the ACE inhibitor with an ARNI in patients with heart failure with reduced ejection fraction due to their superior mortality benefit; this should be started under specialist advice. When switching to an ARNI, the ACE inhibitor should be withdrawn 48 hours before to avoid a theoretical increased risk of angio-oedema.

β-Blockers

The benefits of β-blockers (also known as β-adrenoreceptor antagonists) in heart failure include reduction in heart rate, which increases coronary blood flow and also decreases the metabolic demand of the myocardium. In combination with ACE inhibitors, β-blockers improve survival and reverse ventricular remodelling. β-blockers (e.g., bisoprolol, atenolol) should be offered to all patients with heart failure secondary to left ventricular systolic dysfunction (including the elderly, those with peripheral vascular disease, COPD without reversibility, etc.)

In some cases, the decreased contractility and heart rate may worsen symptoms, so they should be introduced at low doses and the dose increased slowly ('start low, go slow'). In the patient who presents with acute heart failure, β-blockers should not be started (or restarted) until their condition is stable (when they are no longer requiring intravenous diuretics, for instance).

Mineralocorticoid receptor antagonists

Mineralocorticoid receptor antagonists (MRAs) (e.g., spironolactone, eplerenone) act to reduce preload by blocking aldosterone receptors in the distal convoluted tubule of the nephron.

Aldosterone promotes sodium retention and potassium excretion; it also has a number of unfavourable extra-renal effects, including sympathetic stimulation, parasympathetic inhibition, vascular damage and impairment of arterial compliance, all of which adversely affect cardiac function. It promotes fibrosis and adverse remodelling of the heart.

Patients with severe heart failure receiving both ACE inhibitors and MRAs have a 30% lower mortality rate than patients receiving ACE inhibitors plus a placebo. MRAs do, however, increase the risk of life-threatening hyperkalaemia, especially when used in combination with an ACE inhibitor, so electrolyte levels must be closely monitored.

HINTS AND TIPS

Other side effects of spironolactone include gynaecomastia and breast pain/tenderness. Eplerenone does not have the same effect.

Sodium-glucose cotransporter 2 inhibitors

Sodium-glucose cotransporter 2 (SGLT2) inhibitors (empagliflozin, dapagliflozin) block the SGLT2 receptor in the proximal convoluted tubule, reducing glucose reabsorption markedly. This results in glycosuria, osmotic diuresis, BP reduction and weight loss. They were developed initially for use in type 2 diabetes mellitus; however, they have recently been shown to reduce heart failure hospitalization and death in heart failure significantly, even in the absence of diabetes. Very recent evidence suggests that this benefit may even be seen in heart failure with mildly reduced ejection fraction and potentially in those with preserved ejection fraction. This has overhauled the treatment guidelines.

SGLT2 inhibitors increase risk of ketoacidosis and are contraindicated in type 1 diabetes and those with a history of ketoacidosis; they are recommended to be withheld when the ketosis risk is higher (e.g., fasting for surgery). Caution should be used in patients with increased risk of genital infections – this is uncommon but can be severe (e.g., Fournier gangrene). They can be initiated when eGFR ≥20 mL/min per 1.73 m²; renal function

should be monitored; there is usually an initial dip in renal function, but SGLT2 inhibitors have actually been shown to reduce chronic kidney disease progression in the long term.

Diuretics

Diuretics (Table 13.5) increase salt and water excretion in the kidneys. Loop diuretics are the class most widely used in heart failure to reduce circulating volume (and thus preload), reducing pulmonary congestion and peripheral oedema. Combination with thiazide-like diuretics should be considered if loop diuretics alone are not effective in relieving symptoms. Unlike many of the other drugs used in heart failure, diuretics do not improve survival; they do, however, provide effective symptomatic relief and improve exercise tolerance. The exception to this statement is MRAs, which have both diuretic function and act to improve prognosis.

COMMUNICATION

Communication and patient education are especially important in heart failure. The patient should be advised to monitor for acute weight changes (which may be indicative of fluid retention/loss) and advised what to do if this changes or if they deteriorate clinically. They should be aware of what to do if they become unwell (sick day rules), as ongoing treatment with certain drugs (e.g., furosemide, spironolactone and ACE inhibitors) in this setting may result in acute kidney injury and electrolyte abnormalities.

Ivabradine

Ivabradine acts to reduce heart rate via inhibition of the I_f ('funny') channel in the sinus node; therefore, it only works during sinus rhythm. Ivabradine was initially used in the treatment of angina pectoris but has more recently entered heart failure guidelines. The ESC recommends ivabradine treatment in symptomatic heart failure with ejection fraction ≤35%, in sinus rhythm at

Table 13.5 Site of action (in the nephron) and adverse effects associated with commonly used diuretics

Class of diuretic	Site of action	Adverse effects
Loop diuretics (e.g., furosemide, bumetanide).	Thick ascending loop of Henle.	Electrolyte abnormalities (e.g., hypokalaemia), gout.
Thiazide diuretics (e.g., bendroflumethiazide) and thiazide-like diuretics (e.g., indapamide, chlortalidone, metolazone).	Distal convoluted tubule.	Hyperglycaemia, gout, electrolyte abnormalities (e.g., hypokalaemia, hyponatraemia), elevated triglycerides/low-density lipoproteins (LDL).
Potassium-sparing diuretics (e.g., spironolactone, amiloride).	Collecting duct and distal convoluted tubule.	Hyperkalaemia (use with caution with angiotensin-converting enzyme inhibitors), gynaecomastia with spironolactone.

≥70 beats per minute at rest, and when already on treatment with a maximally tolerated dose of β-blocker (or if β-blocker is contraindicated) as well as an ACE inhibitor and an MRA.

Nitrates

Glyceryl trinitrate (GTN) increases levels of cyclic guanosine monophosphate (cGMP), which acts to relax vascular smooth muscle. It preferentially dilates venous vessels, thereby decreasing preload and reducing the degree of ventricular volume overload. Nitrate use in heart failure is somewhat limited to the acute setting because tolerance to its effects develops over 1 or 2 days. However, asymmetric regular dosing can be used in combination with hydralazine.

Hydralazine

Hydralazine is a potent vasodilator, predominantly of arterioles; therefore it reduces afterload, which acts to improve cardiac function. Side effects include flushing and a lupus-like syndrome. It is prescribed in combination with a nitrate medication in patients who cannot tolerate an ACE inhibitor, ARNI or ARB (particularly if these medications induce renal failure), and also sometimes as an additional therapy in severe heart failure, especially where there is pulmonary hypertension.

Digoxin

Digoxin is an inhibitor of the sodium/potassium pump on the sarcolemmal and cell membranes. This adenosine triphosphate (ATP)-dependent pump plays a role in transporting calcium out of the cell. Its inhibition, therefore, prevents this, resulting in increased intracellular calcium concentration, which in cardiac muscle, results in a positive inotropic effect. Digoxin also acts on the atrioventricular node to prolong the refractory period and decrease conduction velocity, thereby slowing conduction of the cardiac impulse and reducing ventricular rate – a negative chronotropic effect. The use of digoxin is recommended in patients with heart failure and atrial fibrillation to control the heart rate. It is also used in patients with heart failure (secondary to left ventricular systolic dysfunction) that is severe or worsening despite first- and second-line treatments (those mentioned previously).

Retrospective analysis showed that patients with low therapeutic digoxin levels saw a mortality benefit, whereas those with high levels saw an increase in sudden cardiac death; therefore, digoxin therapy is probably best used with monitoring of drug levels.

CLINICAL NOTES

Inotropic drugs increase the contractility of the myocardium. Other than digoxin, their principal role should be restricted to the management of acute heart failure, as they are associated with increased mortality with long-term use.

Implantable devices

Roughly one-third of patients with heart failure have left bundle branch block. As the conduction system in these individuals is abnormal, the ventricles do not contract simultaneously. In patients without heart failure, the effects of this are generally not noticed. However, in dilated, poorly functioning hearts, it has a significant effect in reducing stroke volume and cardiac output and can lead to mitral regurgitation.

Cardiac resynchronization therapy (CRT), with a biventricular pacemaker to stimulate both ventricles simultaneously, may be considered in certain patients. This increases cardiac output and is of benefit in patients with heart failure and broad QRS complexes (≥130 ms and especially when ≥150 ms) in terms of improving patients' quality of life, the amount of exercise they are able to perform and reducing both heart failure hospitalizations and mortality. Current NICE guidance recommends CRT in patients who are NYHA class III to IV with an ejection fraction ≤35% and prolonged QRS duration in sinus rhythm. Some patients may also benefit from a CRT device with defibrillator function (known as a *CRT-D*) or an implantable cardioverter defibrillator (ICD), although indications are relatively complex (see **NICE guidance TA314** for further information).

Ventricular assist devices

Mechanical ventricular assist devices (VADs) are implantable devices that take over the work of the failing ventricle(s). They are connected to an external control unit/battery. VADs can be used as a temporary solution until transplantation can be performed or in cases of cardiogenic shock that are expected to recover.

CLINICAL NOTES

Some VADs pump in a pulsatile manner (as per the natural action of the heart) while more recent VADs operate as continuous flow pumps. A patient with a left ventricular assist device that pumps continuously will either have a very low-intensity pulse or often no pulse at all!

Cardiac transplantation

Heart transplantation is the only definitive treatment for severe, intractable heart failure. The procedure requires life-long immunosuppression, which puts patients at increased risk of infection. With good patient selection, the prognosis is good, with 1-year survival rates of 85% to 90% and 3-year survival approaching 75%. The quality of life of the majority of patients is dramatically improved.

Chapter Summary

- Heart failure arises when the heart is unable to maintain sufficient tissue perfusion to meet the body's metabolic demands and is the end result of many pathological processes.
- Heart failure occurs due to a number of adaptive changes that, as they persist and intensify, become maladaptive, accelerate disease progression and bring about the clinical syndrome of heart failure.
- The most common cause of heart failure in high-income countries is systolic failure as the result of myocardial damage, usually due to ischaemic heart disease.
- Myocardial failure can affect the left and right ventricles individually or both together. Isolated right ventricular failure (RVF) is uncommon, as the commonest cause of RVF is left ventricular failure (LVF).
- LVF causes congestion into the pulmonary circulation and presenting complaints include dyspnoea (especially on exertion), orthopnoea and paroxysmal nocturnal dyspnoea.
- RVF causes systemic venous congestion and presenting complaints include dyspnoea, ankle swelling, abdominal discomfort/lethargy and nausea.
- It is important to attempt to clarify the cause of heart failure to tailor management plans appropriately.
- Acute LVF causing pulmonary oedema is a medical emergency; treatment is with intravenous diuretics, oxygen and respiratory support, as necessary. There are a number of other treatments that may be used in certain situations.
- Acute RVF is uncommon but is treated with careful fluid boluses (assuming no pulmonary oedema is present).
- The main aims in chronic heart failure are to decrease preload, decrease afterload, reverse/limit ventricular remodelling and limit heart rate – management includes optimization of comorbidities, pharmacological treatments and device therapy in certain situations.
- In HFrEF, the medications shown to have most benefit are ACE inhibitors/ARNI, β-blockers, MRAs and SGLT2 inhibitors – if there are no contraindications, these should all be introduced as early as possible, at lower doses initially if needed.

UKMLA Condition
Cardiac failure

UKMLA Presentations
Breathlessness
Peripheral oedema and ankle swelling

Normal sinus rhythm is defined as a regular rhythm of normal heart rate (60–100 bpm), with every QRS complex preceded by a P wave in a 1:1 ratio. PR interval remains constant.

Arrhythmia means irregularity in the normal heartbeat or electrical conduction system of the heart, including:

- Bradyarrhythmias – slow heart rhythms.
- Irregular rhythms of normal rate.
- Supraventricular arrhythmias – fast heart rhythms of origin above the ventricles.
- Ventricular arrhythmias – heart rhythms of ventricular origin, usually fast.

Cardiac arrest and resuscitation are covered later in the chapter.

CLINICAL NOTES

Sinus arrhythmia is a normal physiological phenomenon seen in young, healthy individuals where the beat-to-beat heart rate varies during the respiratory cycle due to changes in vagal tone. Inspiration increases the heart rate, and expiration slows it.

BRADYARRHYTHMIAS

Bradyarrhythmias are slow heart rhythms (Table 14.1). Many bradyarrhythmias are due to dysfunction in the heart's electrical conduction pathways, but bradycardia can occur in individuals without underlying heart disease.

Sinus bradycardia

Sinus bradycardia occurs when the heart is in sinus rhythm, but the resting heart rate is less than 60 beats/min. This can be physiological (e.g., during sleep) and is also seen in young, fit individuals. Pathological causes include:

- Sinus node disease (especially in the elderly).
- Raised intracranial pressure (part of the 'Cushing reflex').
- Severe hypoxia.
- Hypothyroidism (myxoedema).
- Hypothermia.
- Tumours (cervical, mediastinal).
- Sepsis.
- Drugs (β-blockers, calcium channel blockers and other antiarrhythmic agents).

Table 14.1 Differential diagnosis of bradyarrhythmia, in order of increasing electrical dysfunction. Red denotes serious/life-threatening arrhythmias (often requiring temporary or permanent pacemaker implantation).

Bradyarrhythmia	Features
Sinus bradycardia	Heart rate <60 beats/min.
Sinoatrial node disease and sick sinus syndrome	Bradycardia, may be associated with tachyarrhythmias and intermittently with tachy-brady syndrome.
First-degree heart block	PR interval >0.20 s.
Second-degree heart block- Mobitz type I	Wenckebach phenomenon – progressive prolongation of PR interval with eventual dropped beat. Generally benign and does not require intervention.
Second-degree heart block-Mobitz type II	Intermittent dropped beats. Nonprolonged, or unchanging, PR interval. Indicative of impending complete heart block and an indication for permanent pacemaker implantation.
Second-degree heart block – 2:1 heart block/3:1 heart block	Fixed ratio of P waves to QRS complexes, e.g., 2:1, 3:1 – result of either Mobitz I or Mobitz II conduction (not always possible to differentiate).
Complete heart block/third-degree heart block	Complete atrioventricular dissociation (no relationship between P waves and QRS complexes). QRS complex is often broad.
Asystole	No beats conducted; no atrial or ventricular activity.
Ventricular standstill/P wave asystole	Visible P waves but no QRS complex.

Patients are usually asymptomatic, and no treatment is required. Occasionally, however, syncope, hypotension or dyspnoea may occur. In these severe acute circumstances, treatment with intravenous (IV) atropine, isoprenaline or insertion of a temporary pacing wire might be required to speed up the heart rate until the underlying condition is treated.

Sinus node disease

The sinoatrial (SA) node is the natural cardiac pacemaker. It is a crescent-shaped cluster of cells approximately 15 mm × 5 mm. The SA node is located just below the epicardial surface at the junction of the right atrium and the superior vena cava.

The rate at which the SA node generates impulses is determined by both vagal and sympathetic tone. Excessive vagal tone (such as during vomiting) can cause marked sinus bradycardia. The impulses are conducted via the atrial myocardium to the atrioventricular (AV) node.

Disease of the SA node may be due to:

- Age-related degeneration and fibrosis.
- Ischaemia and infarction (in 60% of patients, the SA node is supplied by the right coronary artery).
- Myocarditis.
- Genetic (rare).

This can result in pauses between consecutive P waves (>2 s). There are degrees of SA node conduction abnormality:

- SA exit block – an expected P wave is absent, but the following one occurs at the expected time (i.e., the pauses are exact multiples of the basic P-P interval).
- Sinus pause or sinus arrest (Fig. 14.1) – the interval between P waves is longer than 2 s and is not a multiple of the basic P-P interval.

Tachy-brady syndrome (sick sinus syndrome)

This is a combination of sinus node disease and abnormal tachyarrhythmias. It is most commonly caused by degenerative fibrosis of the SA node in the elderly.

Management

Patients with symptomatic or recurrent sinus pauses often require permanent pacing (assuming rate-slowing drugs have been discontinued). Many patients with SA node disease also have more distal conduction disease, so dual- (rather than single-) chamber pacemakers are usually used.

Antiarrhythmic drugs may also be needed if the patient has sick sinus syndrome. Pacemaker insertion should be considered before commencing these drugs because they may worsen the SA node conduction defect. Paroxysmal atrial fibrillation (AF) often coexists, so such patients also need anticoagulation.

Atrioventricular block

The AV node is a complex structure in the right atrial wall on the septal surface between the ostium of the coronary sinus and the septal leaflet of the tricuspid valve. In 90% of patients, the right coronary artery supplies the AV node. The rest are supplied via the circumflex artery.

The AV node conducts impulses from the atria to the ventricular conductive tissue.

First-degree atrioventricular block

In this conduction disturbance (Fig. 14.2), conduction time through the AV node is prolonged, but all impulses are conducted. The PR interval is longer than 0.20 s.

This condition does not require treatment in a healthy patient but should be watched because it can herald greater degrees of block (in approximately 40% of cases). This is particularly important in patients with other conducting tissue disease, e.g., bundle branch block.

CLINICAL NOTES

Progressive prolongation of PR interval on serial ECGs in infective endocarditis carries a poor prognosis. This can occur in patients who develop a para-aortic abscess (the conducting tissue is close to the aortic valve ring). This usually heralds rapid development of complete heart block and valve dehiscence.

Second-degree atrioventricular block

In second-degree block, some impulses are not conducted from the atria to the ventricles.

Mobitz type I heart block – Wenckebach phenomenon

Mobitz type I (also known as Wenckebach) AV block is characterized by progressive prolongation of the PR interval (Fig. 14.2), eventually

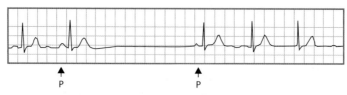

Fig. 14.1 Sinus pause or arrest. Note the interval of more than 2 seconds between P waves.

First-degree block (constantly prolonged PR interval)

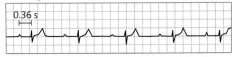

Each QRS complex has a preceding P wave, but the PR interval is prolonged at 0.36 s (normal is 0.12–0.20 s).

Second-degree block (Mobitz type I, Wenkebach) (PR interval increases with each beat and then results in a dropped QRS complex)

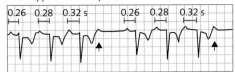

The PR interval progressively increases and then there is one isolated P wave without a following QRS complex; the PR interval then returns to its starting point and increases again.

Second-degree block (Mobitz type II) (PR interval constant, but some P waves have no QRS)

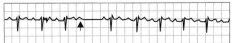

There is a constant, normal PR interval, but there are isolated P waves without following QRS complexes.

Third-degree (complete) block (QRS complexes are independent of P waves)

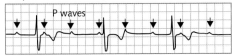

There are 90 P waves/min. There is no relationship between P waves and QRS complexes.

Fig. 14.2 Classification of heart blocks. Only the large squares of the ECG are shown for clarity.

resulting in a nonconducted P wave (dropped QRS complex). The cycle is then repeated.

This process is usually due to a reversible block in electrical conduction at the level of the AV node. Cells in the AV node become progressively fatigued until they fail to conduct an impulse.

This common phenomenon can occur in any cardiac tissue, including the SA node.

Wenckebach phenomenon can occur in athletes and children and is due to high vagal tone. It is usually benign and not usually an indication for pacing.

When it occurs after an inferior myocardial infarction (MI), no treatment is required unless the patient is symptomatic. In symptomatic patients, atropine or temporary pacing may be used.

Mobitz type II heart block

The PR interval remains constant in Mobitz type II AV block, but QRS complexes are dropped intermittently (Fig. 14.2). This usually occurs due to intermittent failure of the conduction system at the level of the AV node or His-Purkinje system and is often due to underlying structural damage. It is a precursor to complete heart block and therefore requires close cardiac monitoring and insertion of a pacemaker.

Mobitz II heart block may be due to idiopathic fibrosis of the conducting system, certain inflammatory conditions or following anterior MI due to septal infarction and necrosis of the conducting system.

2:1 or 3:1 heart block

Fixed ratio heart blocks occur when the ratio of P waves to QRS complexes is fixed at 2:1 or 3:1, etc. This may result from either Mobitz I or Mobitz II conduction, and it can often be challenging to determine the underlying pathophysiology from the ECG. However, there may be clues that can help. Often a rhythm strip or telemetry may help determine the underlying disturbance, as individuals with fixed ratio block may also demonstrate intermittent runs of more characteristic Mobitz I or Mobitz II conduction.

Note that in Mobitz type I or II, every 2nd/3rd/4th QRS complex is dropped. In 2:1 or 3:1 heart block, every 2nd or 3rd QRS complex is conducted.

Third-degree or complete heart block

Third-degree heart block (also known as *complete heart block*) results in complete electrical dissociation of the atria from the ventricles (Fig. 14.2). The P wave and QRS complexes are regular in rhythm but entirely independent and bear no temporal relationship to one another. There is a ventricular 'escape' rhythm, which usually gives rise to wide QRS complexes. Note that the complexes may be narrow if the AV block is proximal ('high'). This often occurs in congenital complete heart block.

Management depends upon the underlying cause:

- After inferior MI, a temporary pacemaker should only be inserted in the event of haemodynamic compromise. Usually, the AV block is high (at the level of the AV node itself), temporary and the escape rate is reasonable. Most of these cases revert to normal conduction within a few weeks, and a permanent pacemaker (PPM) is rarely needed.
- After anterior MI, a PPM will be required and should be inserted promptly (if the patient is unstable, a temporary wire is inserted first, followed by a PPM some days later). The AV block is lower, generally permanent, and the escape rate unsustainably low (the block occurs due to necrosis of the electrical conduction system).
- If heart block is due to drugs (e.g., β-blockers), it may resolve once these are withdrawn.
- In all other patients with complete heart block, the patient should be permanently paced, whether symptomatic or not.

Bundle branch block

Bundle branch block is an interventricular conduction disturbance. The bundle of His arises from the AV node and, at the level of the top of the muscular interventricular septum, it divides into the left and right bundle branches (Fig. 14.3), which supply the left and right ventricles, respectively. The left bundle divides again into anterior and posterior divisions (or hemifascicles).

Damage to one or more of these bundles due to ischaemia or infarction (or other conditions disturbing electrical conduction; see Sinus node disease, earlier) results in a characteristic ECG picture as the ventricular depolarization pattern is altered. When conduction is blocked in one of the bundle branches, affected areas of the myocardium are stimulated later by conduction from unaffected myocardium. This leads to widening and disruption of the QRS complexes (>0.12 s).

Looking at leads V1 and V6 in right bundle branch block, there is:

- A second R wave (R′) in V1 – the last part of the QRS in lead V1 is positive due to delayed right ventricular depolarization.
- A deeper, wider S wave in V6.

In left bundle branch block, there is:

- A Q wave with an S wave in V1 – the last part of the QRS in lead V1 is negative due to delayed left ventricular depolarization.
- A notched R wave in V6.

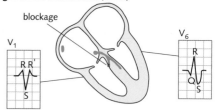

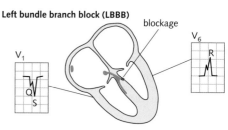

Fig. 14.3 Left and right bundle branch blocks. Disruption of the conduction system delays activation of ventricular muscle, producing a characteristic split peak in the ECG.

Asystole

This is a form of cardiac arrest without ventricular depolarization (and, therefore, cardiac output). See the Cardiac arrest and resuscitation section later in the chapter for more details.

Investigation of bradyarrhythmias

Investigation of bradyarrhythmias includes:

- Electrocardiography (ECG) – may show heart block but may be normal if heart block is intermittent. In a patient with unexplained syncope and apparently normal 12-lead ECG, it is essential to exclude intermittent conduction disturbances using ambulatory ECG monitoring.
- Blood tests – serum electrolytes, liver function and thyroid function tests may reveal causes of sinus bradycardia.
- Chest X-ray – may show cardiomegaly in patients with cardiomyopathy. Pulmonary oedema may result from bradycardia.
- Echocardiography – may show regional wall hypokinesia due to areas of ischaemia or infarction. This is especially relevant if it involves the septum.

Pacemakers

Indications for permanent pacing

A pacemaker delivers electrical stimuli via leads in contact with the heart. The leads not only deliver energy but can also sense

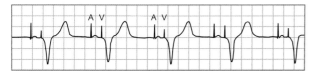

Fig. 14.4 A paced rhythm showing both atrial (A) and ventricular (V) pacing spikes. Not all paced rhythms will show both of these and not all heartbeats will be preceded by pacing spikes. Appearance will depend on pacemaker type, number of leads and underlying rhythm. Paced ventricular beats often have a wide QRS complex/bundle branch block morphology.

Table 14.2 Indications for a permanent pacemaker

Complete AV block – should be paced whether symptomatic or not unless following recent inferior MI (may recover).
Mobitz type II AV block.
Persistent AV block post anterior MI.
Persistent AV block post inferior MI after trial with temporary pacing wire (may recover).
Persisting symptomatic bradycardia or sinus node pauses.

spontaneous electrical activity from the heart. The aim of inserting a pacemaker is to mimic as closely as possible the heart's normal electrical activity in patients with potentially life-threatening conduction disturbances – for example, ECG of a patient with a paced rhythm is in Fig. 14.4. PPM indications are listed in Table 14.2.

Indications for temporary pacing

The following indications for temporary pacing are appropriate:

- Indications in Table 14.2 if permanent pacing is not immediately available.
- Symptomatic drug-induced bradyarrhythmias – until the drug's effect has worn off, e.g., after a trial or overdose of a β-blocker.
- Heart block after inferior MI (if haemodynamic compromise).

Pacemaker insertion

Temporary pacing wires are inserted via a major vein (usually the right subclavian, right internal jugular or right femoral vein). The wire is advanced until it reaches the right ventricular apex and then it is secured in place. The end of the wire is connected to an external pulse generator, which is then set appropriately to achieve adequate pacing.

PPM implantation is generally carried out under local anaesthetic and often conscious sedation. Insertion rarely requires general anaesthesia. The pacemaker box is implanted in a pocket formed overlying the pectoral muscle, inferior to the clavicle, usually on the side of the nondominant arm. The pacemaker lead(s) are inserted into a major vein (usually subclavian or cephalic) and advanced until secured in the appropriate region(s)

of the heart muscle. The other end of the lead(s) are then attached to the pacemaker box.

Complications of pacemaker insertion

The following are recognized complications of pacemaker insertion:

- Complications of wire insertion, including pneumothorax, haemorrhage, brachial plexus injury (during subclavian vein puncture), arrhythmia and infection (may progress to infective endocarditis).
- Complications of PPM box positioning (e.g., haematoma formation, pocket infection and erosion of the box through the skin).
- Difficulties with the wire, such as wire displacement and loss of ability to pace or sense (need to reposition wire), fracture of the wire insulation (usually due to tight sutures or friction against the clavicle – need to replace wire), and perforation of the myocardium (uncommon unless after MI when the myocardium is friable – need to reposition wire).

Types of pacemaker

Pacemakers can be classified as:

- Single chamber – a single wire into either the ventricles (most commonly) or atria (less common). A single ventricular lead might be used in AF when the atrium cannot be appropriately sensed.
- Dual chamber – one wire into the atria and one into the ventricles. This more closely resembles the normal activities of the heart. The atrial contribution may be up to 25% of total cardiac output, and a dual chamber pacemaker should be fitted in patients in whom the atrium can be sensed and paced.
- Biventricular pacemakers – leads into the right atrium, right ventricle and left ventricle. This is useful in treating patients with heart failure and ventricular conduction abnormalities, such as left bundle branch block. This is also called *cardiac resynchronization therapy,* as pacing both ventricles helps to 'resynchronize' the ventricles and may improve efficiency of heart contraction.

CLINICAL NOTES

Evidence has shown that pacemaker leads implanted in the right ventricular apex worsen left ventricular function and increase the risk of heart failure; therefore, leads are now placed away from this area.

Pacemaker syndrome

Permanent single-chamber right ventricular pacing in a patient with intact atrial function can lead to atrial activation by retrograde conduction from the ventricle – so-called *pacemaker syndrome*. There is a cannon wave with every beat, pulmonary arterial pressure rises, and cardiac output is impaired. This is managed by replacing the pacemaker with a dual-chamber device.

> **CLINICAL COMMUNICATION**
>
> Patients must be informed of the need to notify the DVLA following pacemaker insertion. Car drivers may drive after 1 week, but bus/HGV drivers must wait 6 weeks before driving. Patients must also promise to attend follow-up pacemaker checks.

SUPRAVENTRICULAR TACHYARRHYTHMIAS

Supraventricular tachyarrhythmias are fast rhythms characterized by narrow QRS complexes (unless aberrant conduction is present). The arrhythmogenic focus is supraventricular. None of these are generally immediately life-threatening (except in AF if an accessory pathway is present).

Tachycardia is a rate of 100 beats/min or greater. In order of increasing atrial electrical dysfunction, these are:

- Sinus tachycardia.
- Atrial ectopics.
- Nodal ectopics.
- Atrial tachycardia.
- Junctional tachycardia and supraventricular reentry tachycardia.
- Atrial flutter.
- Atrial fibrillation.

Sinus tachycardia

Sinus tachycardia (Fig. 14.5) is defined by:

- Heart rate of over 100 beats/min.
- A normal P wave precedes every QRS complex.
- The PR interval is within normal limits and remains stable.

There are numerous physiological causes of sinus tachycardia, including:

- Fever.
- Thyrotoxicosis.
- Hypotension.
- Hypoxia.
- Any form of stress (e.g., pain, anxiety and exertion).

Occasionally, an inappropriate resting sinus tachycardia occurs. This is due to an abnormality of sinus node discharge or another atrial focus of activity near the sinus node.

Premature atrial complexes

These are seen on the ECG as a premature P wave (may be normal or abnormal in appearance) followed by a PR interval, which may be prolonged or short depending upon where in the atrium the impulse arises (Fig. 14.6). The QRS complex should be of normal morphology. A pause often follows this because the AV node is refractory and cannot conduct. In contrast to ventricular premature complexes, this pause is not fully compensatory (i.e., the next sinus beat occurs earlier than it otherwise would have done; after premature ventricular complexes, the sinus beats continue as normal).

Premature atrial complexes can be precipitated by many conditions, including:

- Stress.
- Alcohol.
- Myocardial ischaemia/inflammation.

Treatment is not indicated unless the patient is very symptomatic, in which case β-blockers may be of benefit.

Nodal and junctional ectopics

These abnormal beats arise from the AV node or adjacent AV junctional area. These structures can fire autonomously but are usually suppressed, as their firing rate is slower than the SA node.

If impulses arise ectopically from these areas, the impulse is conducted to the atrium, producing a retrograde ('inverted') P wave, and also to the ventricles, where a narrow QRS complex is produced (Fig. 14.7). The P wave may occur before, after, or simultaneously with the QRS complex depending on relative conduction speeds. As with atrial ectopics, treatment is not usually indicated.

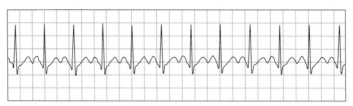

Fig. 14.5 Sinus tachycardia.

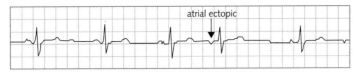

Fig. 14.6 ECG illustrating an ectopic atrial beat. Note the abnormally shaped P wave and normal QRS complex. A compensatory pause follows.

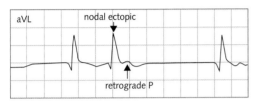

Fig. 14.7 A nodal ectopic. The ectopic complex is similar to the normal QRS, suggesting it originates from the atrioventricular or junctional region. The P wave is retrograde and seen after the ectopic QRS superimposed on the T wave. A compensatory pause follows the ectopic beat.

Atrial tachycardia

Atrial tachycardia is a tachyarrhythmia generated in the atrial tissue. The atrial rate is usually 150 to 200 beats/min. Because the origin of the tachycardia is not the SA node, the P-wave morphology and axis may differ from normal (Fig. 14.8).

Causes of atrial tachycardia
The following may lead to atrial tachycardia:

- Structural heart abnormality.
- Coronary artery disease.
- Digitalis toxicity.

Investigation and diagnosis
On examination, the pulse is usually rapid and of variable intensity. The jugular venous pulse may reveal many a waves to each v wave if a degree of AV block is present.

ECG may show either 1:1 conduction or variable degrees of AV block. It is sometimes difficult to differentiate atrial tachycardia from atrial flutter. Diagnosis may be aided by enhancing AV block to more easily visualize underlying atrial activity (P wave rate and morphology). This may be done by:

- Valsalva manoeuvre or carotid sinus massage – increases vagal stimulation of the SA and AV node.
- IV adenosine – results in transient complete AV block.

HINTS AND TIPS

Remember that atrial flutter usually has an atrial rate of 300 beats/min with a degree of AV block (e.g., 2:1, 3:1, etc.) and a 'saw-tooth' pattern. Atrial tachycardia has a slightly slower atrial rate with abnormal P waves.

Management
The underlying cause should be treated (for instance, check digoxin levels and stop the drug if appropriate). Drugs used to treat atrial tachycardia include:

- AV blocking drugs, such as digoxin, β-blockers and calcium channel blockers (e.g., verapamil) slow the ventricular response rate but do not affect the atrial tachycardia itself.
- Class IA (e.g., disopyramide), IC (e.g., flecainide), or III (e.g., amiodarone) drugs can be used to try to terminate the atrial tachycardia.

Electrical cardioversion is often successful.

Atrioventricular junctional tachycardia

This is a tachycardia arising from the junctional area when there is a focus of activity with a discharge rate faster than the SA node. This is abnormal and usually due to ischaemic heart disease or digitalis toxicity.

Clinical features
The following features are seen:

- Rate is usually up to 130 beats/min.
- Gradual in onset and offset.
- ECG shows a narrow complex tachycardia, occasionally with retrogradely conducted P waves. It is difficult to distinguish from an AV nodal reentry tachycardia (AVNRT).

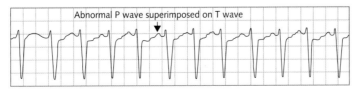

Fig. 14.8 Atrial tachycardia.

Management

Treatment is aimed at the underlying cause:

- Antiarrhythmic agents such as digoxin, β-blockers and calcium channel antagonists may be tried.
- Electrical cardioversion may be successful.

Atrioventricular nodal reentrant tachycardia

These tachycardias involve a reentry circuit in or close to the AV node that allows impulses to travel round and round, triggering the ventricles and the atria (in a retrograde manner) as they go.

Clinical features

These tachycardias display the following features:

- Rate is 150 to 260 beats/min.
- Usually sudden onset and offset.
- Narrow QRS complexes unless there is aberrant conduction. P waves are not always easy to see and may occur before, after, or within the QRS (Fig. 14.9).

Diagnosis

Differentiating a reentrant tachycardia from atrial flutter or fibrillation can be difficult in some cases. The irregularly irregular rhythm of atrial fibrillation is often noticeable, but this is not always the case with very fast heart rates. Diagnosis can be aided by:

- Performing Valsalva manoeuvre or carotid sinus massage.
- Giving IV adenosine.

These procedures block the AV node and, therefore, may show underlying P waves of atrial flutter or the baseline fibrillation of AF. In most cases, blocking the AV node breaks the reentry circuit and terminates the tachycardia. A ventricular ectopic beat can also terminate reentry tachycardia.

Management

These tachycardias often terminate spontaneously.

Vagal manoeuvres, such as carotid sinus massage and the Valsalva manoeuvre, are often effective in terminating the tachycardia and patients can be taught to do these themselves.

In the hospital, the following treatments can be effective:

- Vagal manoeuvres.
- IV adenosine.

- AV node blocking agents (e.g., β-blockers, digoxin and calcium channel blockers).
- Synchronized direct current (DC) cardioversion if less invasive methods are unsuccessful or if patient is haemodynamically unstable.

In a patient with recurrent troublesome AVNRT, electrophysiological testing can locate the site of the abnormal circuit, which can then be ablated. This is a curative procedure. The main risk is AV node ablation resulting in complete heart block and requiring a PPM.

Wolff-Parkinson-White syndrome

In this condition, there is an abnormal connection between the atrium and the ventricle along which an impulse can travel, known as an accessory pathway. In Wolff–Parkinson–White syndrome the accessory pathway is known as the bundle of Kent.

The bundle of Kent

The bundle of Kent is capable of:

- Both anterograde (atria to ventricle) and retrograde (ventricle to atria) conduction.
- Conducting impulses faster than the normal His conductive tissue. If the impulse is conducted down the bundle of Kent, the ventricle is activated sooner than normal, resulting in a short PR interval. This may be referred to as 'preexcitation'.

If, however, the impulse does not travel down the bundle of Kent, the P wave and QRS complex are normal. Therefore, it can be seen that the impulse can travel via two different routes from the atrium to the ventricle.

The impulse often travels both routes simultaneously; this results in a short PR interval and a slurred upstroke to the R wave (known as the delta wave of 'preexcitation'; Fig. 14.10).

Tachycardias associated with Wolff–Parkinson–White syndrome

Several different tachycardias may occur:

- AVNRT – the impulse is conducted from atrium to ventricle via the AV node and then back to the atrium via the accessory pathway, causing a narrow complex tachycardia.
- Similar tachycardia with conduction in the opposite direction (i.e., atrium to ventricle via accessory pathway),

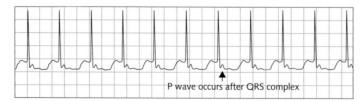

P wave occurs after QRS complex

Fig. 14.9 Atrioventricular nodal reentry tachycardia.

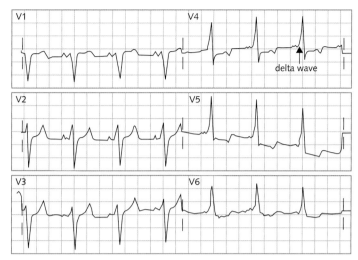

Fig. 14.10 Wolff–Parkinson–White syndrome. Note the short PR interval (0.08 s) and the slurred upstroke of the QRS complex (the delta wave). This is caused by part of the impulse travelling down the accessory pathway and causing ventricular preexcitation (early excitation), represented by the delta wave. The rest of the impulse travels via the atrioventricular node and is represented by the main QRS complex.

resulting in a broad complex tachycardia due to ventricular depolarization initiating at a point away from the bundle of His.

- AF/atrial flutter – can present a risk, as atrial impulses can be conducted very rapidly via the accessory pathway, giving ventricular rates of potentially 300 beats/min or greater (due to bypassing the AV node, which usually limits conduction rate). This rapid ventricular rate can lead to ventricular fibrillation (VF).

Clinical features
Wolff–Parkinson–White syndrome is a congenital condition. Patients present with recurrent palpitations or syncope. Sudden death is a risk due to ventricular tachyarrhythmias. The accessory pathway may cease to conduct as patients grow older, but other patients continue to have problems.

Management
Treatment of Wolff–Parkinson–White syndrome is indicated only in patients with tachyarrhythmias. Some patients have ECG evidence of accessory pathways (short PR and delta waves) but no tachyarrhythmia, and these do not require treatment. There are several treatment options, including pharmacological treatments and ablation (use of radiofrequency energy to cauterize an area of myocardium).

Pharmacological treatments
Drug therapy aims to slow conduction in the accessory pathway as well as to slow AV nodal conduction. Drugs that do both are Vaughan Williams classification IA, IC and III drugs.

Drugs such as digoxin and verapamil block the AV node but do not affect the accessory pathway, increasing the risk of rapid conduction of AF and flutter via the accessory pathway. This can sometimes result in loss of cardiac output and death; therefore, digoxin and verapamil **should not be used** as single agents to treat tachycardias in Wolff–Parkinson–White syndrome.

Ablation therapy
This is the preferred (and hopefully curative) treatment to abolish accessory pathways. It may be electrical or surgical:

- Electrical ablation (or radiofrequency catheter ablation) is performed after the accessory pathway has been located by electrophysiological testing.
- Surgical ablation is rare but may be useful if electrical ablation is not successful.

Atrial flutter

Atrial flutter has the following characteristics:

- Atrial contraction rate is regular and is 250 to 350 beats/min (usually 300 beats/min).
- Ventricular response is rarely 1:1 (300 beats/min) but more commonly 2:1 (150 beats/min), 3:1 (100 beats/min), etc.
- Severity of symptoms depends on the ventricular response rate (i.e., a rapid ventricular response is likely to cause palpitations, angina and cardiac failure).

Causes include:

- Structural heart disease (e.g., valve disease, cardiomyopathy).

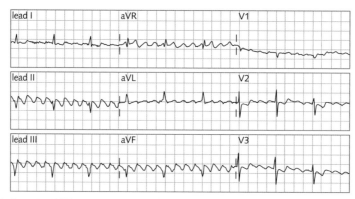

Fig. 14.11 Atrial flutter. Note 'saw-tooth' P waves at a rate of just over 300 beats/min and the ventricular response of 4:1 (around 75 beats/min).

- Pulmonary disease (e.g., pulmonary embolus, pneumothorax, infection).
- Toxins (including alcohol and caffeine).

Investigations and diagnosis

ECG (Fig. 14.11) may demonstrate:

- Regular 'saw-tooth' atrial flutter waves (P waves).
- Narrow QRS complexes (unless there is coexisting bundle branch block).

HINTS AND TIPS

ECG leads II and V1 often show P waves (and therefore flutter waves) best.

If diagnosis is unclear, then AV nodal blocking manoeuvres (adenosine administration or vagal manoeuvres) may help to slow ventricular response and reveal underlying saw-tooth P waves.

Management

Cardioversion is the best treatment, but if not possible, slowing ventricular rate will provide symptomatic relief and protect against cardiac failure. In some cases, direct current cardioversion using a **synchronized** shock will rapidly and safely restore sinus rhythm.

COMMON PITFALLS

Electrical cardioversion must be synchronized with the R or S wave of the QRS complex in patients with organized electrical activity. If the electrical discharge is delivered during the T wave, this can result in ventricular fibrillation.

Class IA, IC or III drugs may be useful for chemical cardioversion if DC cardioversion is unsuccessful or to maintain sinus rhythm after successful DC cardioversion.

Where cardioversion is not possible or not sustained, AV nodal blocking agents are used to slow the ventricular response rate (class II, class IV or digoxin). Some drugs (e.g., flecainide) may slow the flutter rate, leading to 1:1 conduction of flutter beats (rather than 2:1 or 3:1) with resultant *increase* in ventricular rate.

As with AF, there is increased risk of thrombus formation in atrial flutter, so anticoagulation is recommended before DC cardioversion.

If cardioversion is unsuccessful or flutter is recurrent, then ablation of the flutter circuit may be carried out. This is a relatively straightforward procedure and should be curative.

Atrial fibrillation

Atrial fibrillation is the most common sustained arrhythmia (over 5% of the population over 70 years of age) and has the following features:

- Disorganized random electrical activity in the atria results in ineffective atrial contraction (and varying ventricular response).
- Stasis of blood in the atria predisposes to thrombus formation and embolic episodes.

The rhythm disturbance may be paroxysmal (transient), persistent (lasting longer than 1 week), or permanent.

Causes

Common causes include:

- Ischaemic heart disease.
- Valvular heart disease (especially mitral valve disease).
- Hypertensive heart disease.
- Pulmonary disease (e.g., embolus, infection, pneumothorax).

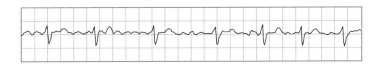

Fig. 14.12 Atrial fibrillation. Note the irregular baseline and absent P waves. The rhythm is irregularly irregular.

- Sepsis/underlying infection.
- Thyrotoxicosis.
- Alcohol excess.

Investigations and diagnosis

The ECG shows absent P waves and irregular baseline with a variable ventricular response rate (hence the irregularly irregular pulse; Fig. 14.12). Ventricular response ranges from 90 to 170 beats/min but can be faster or slower. The actual atrial rate may be from 300 to 600 beats/min. Absence of effective atrial contraction means there are no a waves in the jugular venous pressure waveform and there cannot be a fourth heart sound.

HINTS AND TIPS

It is more correct to refer to atrial fibrillation (AF) with tachycardia or bradycardia as 'AF with slow/fast ventricular response' than 'slow AF' or 'fast AF'. The atrial activity is always fast in AF. 'AF with slow/fast ventricular response' makes it clear that it is the ventricular rate (and therefore heart rate) that is either fast or slow.

Management

In AF, management generally involves either a rhythm control strategy (aiming to restore and maintain sinus rhythm) or rate control (controlling the ventricular response) alone (Table 14.3). The likelihood of successful cardioversion depends upon:

- Persistence of underlying cause (e.g., the patient with untreated mitral stenosis is unlikely to cardiovert successfully, unlike the patient with AF secondary to sepsis who is successfully treated with antibiotics).

Table 14.3 Factors to consider when deciding on rate vs. rhythm control to treat atrial fibrillation (AF)

Rhythm control	Younger patients First episode of AF AF secondary to treatable cause Medications used tend to have more side effects
Rate control	Older patients Preexisting coronary disease Contraindications to cardioversion Previous failed attempts to control rhythm

- Duration of the AF (i.e., the longer the duration, the smaller the chance of cardioversion – due to atrial remodelling).

Treatment options are similar to those in atrial flutter:

- Rate control alone if unlikely to be able to successfully cardiovert or maintain sinus rhythm – usually with an AV node blocking agent to slow the electrical response. This could be with a β-blocker or a rate-slowing calcium channel antagonist, e.g., verapamil or digoxin (especially in patients with heart failure).
- Synchronized DC cardioversion (often requiring higher energy than for atrial flutter) may cardiovert the patient into sinus rhythm.
- Pharmacological agents from group IC (e.g., flecainide, propafenone) (if there is no structural heart disease) or group III (e.g., amiodarone, sotalol) can be used to cardiovert or to maintain sinus rhythm after electrical cardioversion.
- Occasionally ablation can be considered – this is usually carried out by isolation of the pulmonary veins by burning around each pulmonary vein.

Anticoagulation in atrial fibrillation

AF carries an increased risk of thromboembolism due to stasis of blood in the atria leading to thrombus formation and subsequent cerebrovascular/peripheral embolization. Benefits of anticoagulation must be balanced against the risk of haemorrhage. The CHA_2DS_2-VASc scoring system is often used to risk-stratify patients' stroke risk prior to treatment (Table 14.4).

Each additional point on the CHA_2DS_2-VASc scoring system confers increased risk of thromboembolic stroke. This scoring system supersedes the older $CHADS_2$ score.

Table 14.4 The CHA_2DS_2-VASc scoring system for assessing risk of stroke in atrial fibrillation

Congestive heart failure history	+1 point
Hypertension history	+1 point
Age ≥75	+2 points
Diabetes history	+1 point
Stroke/TIA/thromboembolism history	+2 points
Vascular disease history	+1 point
Age 65–74	+1 point
Sex **c**ategory (female)	+1 point

TIA, transient ischemic attack.

Table 14.5 Treatment recommendations for CHA_2DS_2-VASc scores

Score	Risk	Recommendation
0 (male) or 1 (female)	Low	No anticoagulation therapy recommended.
1 (male)	Moderate	Oral anticoagulation should be considered.
2 or greater	High	Oral anticoagulation recommended.

Current guidelines recommend anticoagulant therapy in individuals with a CHA_2DS_2-VASc score of 2 or greater (Table 14.5). This scoring system means that females require a single additional point on the scoring system before anticoagulation would be recommended, whereas males would require 2 additional points for the same to apply.

However, in males with only a single risk factor for stroke (CHA_2DS_2-VASc score = 1), anticoagulation should be *considered* but is not mandated. Oral anticoagulation has been shown in this instance to provide net benefit for prevention of stroke when compared to no anticoagulation therapy (or aspirin).

Anticoagulation in AF was traditionally with warfarin (a vitamin K antagonist) but AF without coexisting valvular disease is increasingly treated with direct oral anticoagulants (DOACs). These medications were previously referred to as novel oral anticoagulants (NOACs) and include apixaban, rivaroxaban, dabigatran and edoxaban.

DOACs can easily provide adequate and predictable levels of anticoagulation without requiring monitoring therapeutic levels. However, their main disadvantages are that they need to be taken consistently (half-life is shorter than with warfarin) and some DOACs have no reversal agent in the case of major bleeding (unlike warfarin).

COMMON PITFALLS

Aspirin is no longer recommended for prevention of stroke in atrial fibrillation. Patients are either treated with oral anticoagulant therapy or not. Antiplatelet agents are not in current guidelines.

The National Institute for Health and Care Excellence (NICE) recommends bleeding risk on anticoagulation is assessed using the ORBIT tool (Table 14.6). Previously, the HAS-BLED scoring system was used for this purpose (and may still be used in some departments).

Bleeding risk:

- ORBIT score 0–2 = Low risk (2.4 bleeds per 100 patient-years)
- ORBIT score 3 = Medium risk (4.7 bleeds per 100 patient-years)
- ORBIT score 4–7 = High risk (8.1 bleeds per 100 patient-years)

Table 14.6 The ORBIT scoring system assesses risk of major bleeding for patients on anticoagulation. Scores range from 0 to 7.

Males with haemoglobin <130 g/L or a haematocrit <40%	+2 points
Females with haemoglobin <120 g/L or haematocrit <36%	+2 points
Patients with history of bleeding (e.g., gastrointestinal or intracranial bleeding)	+2 points
Age over 74 years	+1 point
Estimated glomerular filtration rate of less than 60 mL/min/1.73 m²	+1 point
On antiplatelet treatment	+1 point

Please note that a high ORBIT score is not necessarily a reason to withhold anticoagulation. In some patients, however, the risk of bleeding may be deemed greater than anticoagulation's benefits.

Anticoagulation and cardioversion of atrial fibrillation

There is an increased risk of thromboembolism for a few weeks after cardioversion of AF to sinus rhythm. This is thought to be due to the formation of atrial thrombus before cardioversion and the persistence of inefficient contraction in certain parts of the atrium (e.g., left atrial appendage) for a few weeks after apparently successful cardioversion. Note that:

- If AF onset is within 48 hours, it is reasonable to anticoagulate with IV heparin and cardiovert immediately.
- If the patient has a longer history, then full anticoagulation should be given (warfarin with an international normalized ratio (INR) 2–3 or DOAC treatment) for at least 4 weeks before cardioversion and continued for at least 6 months after cardioversion.
- In patients where emergency cardioversion is required (i.e., patients with severe heart failure secondary to AF), cardioversion should be performed with heparin cover immediately.
- Transoesophageal echocardiography (TOE) is sometimes used to assess safety to proceed to cardioversion immediately in a patient who is not anticoagulated. However, TOE cannot completely exclude the presence of any thrombus and, as indicated earlier, thrombus can form after successful cardioversion.

HINTS AND TIPS

Supraventricular tachyarrhythmias often concern patients but are not generally life-threatening; the main risk is stroke, which is reduced effectively with the treatment

---

strategies discussed. The only life-threatening supraventricular tachyarrhythmia is preexcited AF in patients with accessory pathways, as this may degenerate into ventricular fibrillation. These patients are usually treated as inpatients with radiofrequency ablation.

Investigation of supraventricular tachyarrhythmias

The following investigations are appropriate for patients presenting with a supraventricular tachyarrhythmia.

Blood tests
Relevant blood tests include:

- Full blood count and inflammatory markers – anaemia may precipitate ischaemia. Certain arrhythmias (such as sinus tachycardia, AF) may be predisposed to by infection.
- Electrolytes – derangement of sodium, potassium or calcium may predispose to arrhythmia. Hypokalaemia predisposes to digoxin toxicity.
- Thyroid function tests – hyperthyroidism may lead to atrial tachyarrhythmias, whereas hypothyroidism can predispose to bradyarrhythmia and sometimes ventricular tachyarrhythmias.
- Liver function tests – may be abnormal in patients with a history of alcohol excess (particularly γ-glutamyltransferase (GGT)).

Electrocardiography
12-lead ECG may demonstrate:

- The arrhythmia itself.
- Ischaemic changes – usually as the result of (or contributed to by) increased cardiac oxygen demand as the result of tachycardia.
- Hypertensive changes.
- Evidence of preexcitation (short PR interval, delta wave).

Measurement over a longer period (e.g., 24 hours, 48 hours or longer) may be useful in demonstrating paroxysmal tachyarrhythmias.

Chest radiography
Notable features may include in some cases:

- Signs of heart failure – such as cardiomegaly or pulmonary oedema.
- Valve calcification.

Echocardiography
May identify valve lesions or dilated cardiac chambers.

Electrophysiological studies
These studies involve inserting multiple electrodes into the heart via the great veins and positioning them at various intracardiac sites. Electrical activity can then be recorded from the atria, ventricles, bundle of His and so on to provide information on the conduction defect or rhythm disturbance.

These are useful for arrhythmias when it is difficult to identify the mechanism and also to help identify any possible focus or accessory pathway suitable for ablation. Ablation can be attempted during the investigation if the possible focus or an accessory pathway is identified.

Atrioventricular nodal blocking manoeuvres
These are used:

- Diagnostically – they slow ventricular response and enable P wave morphology to be seen.
- Therapeutically – they are used to terminate arrhythmias with reentry circuits involving the AV node.

The following may be appropriate:

- Valsalva manoeuvre – straining against a closed glottis (see Chapter 8).
- Carotid sinus massage.
- Adenosine administration (rapid IV injection).

Carotid sinus massage
This increases vagal tone and so prolongs AV node conduction time. The patient should be lying comfortably with the neck extended. Carotid bruits must be excluded (carotid artery massage may cause a stroke if thrombus or plaque is dislodged).

The patient should preferably be connected to a 12-lead ECG, running all leads simultaneously. The P waves might not be seen if only a few leads are running.

Initial gentle and then firm pressure is applied to the carotid pulse just below the angle of the jaw for a maximum of 5 to 10 seconds. Never do this on both sides simultaneously.

Adenosine administration
Again, the patient should be supine and connected to a 12-lead ECG continuous trace. Warn the patient that they may experience chest pain, flushing and dyspnoea for a few seconds after administration. Adenosine should not be administered to patients maintained on dipyridamole, as it prolongs dipyridamole's action and causes prolonged complete heart block.

Establish IV access in a good-sized vein (antecubital fossa is ideal). Start with a 6 mg rapid IV injection; follow with a rapid normal saline flush of 20 mL. If there is no response, this may be followed by a 12 mg bolus, followed by another 18 mg bolus if necessary.

Adenosine activates potassium channels and hyperpolarizes the cell membrane. It causes a reduction in AV nodal conduction velocity and transient AV block as a result.

The half-life of adenosine is very short (6 s) and it can be safely used in broad complex tachycardia to differentiate ventricular tachycardia (VT) from supraventricular tachycardia (SVT) with aberrant conduction. After adenosine administration, flutter waves may be revealed or the SVT may be terminated. **Do not use verapamil for this purpose**, as there is a risk of fatal myocardial depression in patients with VT.

VENTRICULAR ARRHYTHMIAS

Ventricular arrhythmias are arrhythmias generally characterized by broad QRS complexes. The arrhythmogenic focus is within the ventricles.

Differential diagnoses of ventricular arrhythmia are:

- Ventricular ectopic beats.
- Ventricular tachycardia (VT).
- Polymorphic VT (e.g., torsades de pointes).
- Ventricular fibrillation (VF).

Except for ventricular ectopic beats, all of these may be life-threatening.

Ventricular ectopic beats

These are also known as premature ventricular complexes and have certain ECG characteristics (Fig. 14.13), including:

- They occur before the next normal beat would be due.
- They are not preceded by a P wave.
- The QRS complex is abnormal in shape and has a duration of greater than 120 ms.
- They are followed by a compensatory pause so that the RR interval between the normal beats immediately preceding and immediately following the ectopic beat is exactly twice the normal RR interval (in premature atrial complexes the RR interval is less than this).

Clinical features

It is thought that ventricular ectopics occur in over half the normal population. This prevalence increases with age. These extra beats do not in themselves imply underlying heart disease.

Most people are asymptomatic; others may complain of missed or extra beats. Alternatively, others may experience thumping or heavy beats because the beat immediately following the ectopic does so after a compensatory pause during which there is a prolonged filling time, resulting in an increased stroke volume.

Several precipitating causes are recognized, including:

- Hypokalaemia.
- Excess caffeine consumption.
- Fever.
- Underlying cardiac abnormality (e.g., myocardial ischaemia, cardiomyopathy, mitral or aortic valve disease).

Management

No treatment is needed in patients with no underlying cardiac abnormality unless symptoms are severe. In this situation, a small dose of a β-blocker should suppress ectopic activity.

In the post-MI situation, there is controversy about the significance of ventricular ectopic beats. Treatment with certain antiarrhythmic agents increases mortality in these patients: in the CAST trial, encainide/flecainide increased the risk of death 3.6-fold.

Check serum electrolytes (especially potassium and magnesium) and prescribe a β-blocker unless contraindicated.

Definition of ventricular tachyarrhythmias

A ventricular tachyarrhythmia is an abnormal rapid rhythm originating in the ventricular myocardium or the His-Purkinje system. Ventricular tachyarrhythmias are broad complex – the QRS complex is longer than 120 ms in duration (three small squares on a standard ECG trace). Ventricular tachyarrhythmias include:

- Monomorphic VT.
- Polymorphic VT, including torsades de pointes.
- VF.

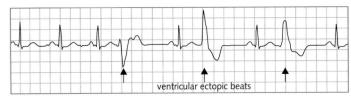
ventricular ectopic beats

Fig. 14.13 Ventricular ectopic beats, which are indicated by arrows.

Ventricular tachycardia

VT is defined as three or more consecutive ventricular beats occurring at a rate greater than 120 beats/min (Fig. 14.14).

Clinical features

VT is often a life-threatening arrhythmia. The reduction in cardiac output caused by this arrhythmia often causes dizziness or syncope. Common precipitants include acute MI, cardiomyopathy or inherited conduction disorders. Very occasionally, patients may tolerate this rhythm well and experience only palpitations.

Diagnosis

VT may be monomorphic (complexes on the surface ECG have the same shape) or polymorphic (beat-to-beat variations in morphology). The main differential diagnosis for VT is SVT with aberrant conduction (or bundle branch block) (Table 14.7). These arrhythmias can be difficult to differentiate. It helps if you remember the following points:

- VT is potentially fatal. If in doubt, treat as VT.
- Carotid sinus massage or adenosine may briefly block the AV node and slow the ventricular response in SVT (it will have no effect on VT).
- **Never** use verapamil to slow the ventricular response in this situation: the negative inotropic and vasodilatory effect of this drug could have disastrous effects if the rhythm is, in fact, VT, causing rapid development of cardiogenic shock or cardiac failure.

Management

VT is very dangerous and will result in cardiac failure or death if allowed to continue. Treatment must be prompt and depends upon the clinical scenario:

- A conscious patient with VT and no haemodynamic compromise – treatment should be with drugs (discussed later in the chapter).
- A conscious patient with VT and haemodynamic compromise – triggered (synchronized) DC cardioversion under general anaesthetic (fast bleep the anaesthetist).
- An unconscious patient with ongoing VT and no cardiac output ('pulseless VT') – unsynchronized DC cardioversion (defibrillation) as per ALS protocol (discussed later).

HINTS AND TIPS

Correct hypokalaemia promptly in all patients with ventricular arrhythmias. Potassium can be given orally or in a dilute form via a peripheral vein. Potassium can be given more rapidly via a central line with careful monitoring of cardiac rhythm and serum potassium levels. Warning: intravenous potassium can cause ventricular fibrillation.

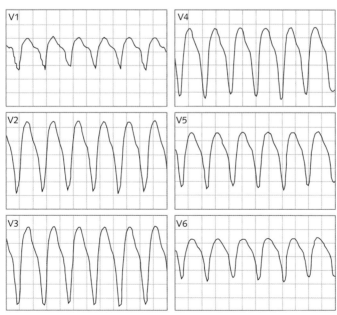

Fig. 14.14 ECG illustrating ventricular tachycardia. Note the concordance shown in the chest leads. No fusion or capture beats are visible in this example.

Table 14.7 Differences between ventricular tachycardia (VT) and supraventricular tachycardia (SVT) with bundle branch block (BBB)

Arrhythmia	VT	SVT with BBB
AV association	AV dissociation (no relationship between P waves and QRS)	P waves, if seen, are associated with the QRS
Variety of complexes	Capture beats (where a normal QRS complex occurs); fusion beats (a normal sinus beat coincides with a ventricular beat, producing a complex that is a hybrid of the two)	No capture or fusion beats
ECG pattern	May be RBBB or LBBB	Usually RBBB
Concordance	Present (the QRS complexes retain the same axis throughout the chest leads)	Absent (some QRS complexes will be positive, others will be negative)
QRS waveform	May vary from beat to beat	Constant

AV, atrioventricular; LBBB, left bundle branch block; RBBB, right bundle branch block.

Polymorphic ventricular tachycardia – torsades de pointes

Polymorphic VT occurs if there are multiple ventricular arrhythmogenic foci present. This results in a broad complex tachycardia with QRS complexes varying in amplitude, axis and duration. Torsades de pointes (twisting of the points) is a specific form of polymorphic VT that occurs in the context of prolonged QT interval – the name refers to the fact that QRS complexes seem to 'twist' around the isoelectric line (Fig. 14.15).

HINTS AND TIPS

The QT interval corresponds to the time from ventricular depolarization to repolarization (beginning of the Q wave to end of T wave, i.e., action potential duration) and varies according to the heart rate. Therefore, a long QT interval is approximated by a corrected QT interval (QTc) greater than 0.44 s in men or 0.46 s in women. QTc = QT/square root of RR interval.

Instead of correcting for heart rate, the QT interval can be plotted against heart rate on a QT nomogram (Fig. 14.16). This is often used to assess drug-induced QT prolongation in toxicology. The patient is considered to be at risk of torsades de pointes if their QT interval–heart rate pair is plotted above the line.

Clinical features

The patient usually feels faint or loses consciousness due to reduced cardiac output. Attacks may occur during periods of adrenergic stimulation (e.g., fear) or in some cases, in the context of bradycardia or during a compensatory pause following an ectopic beat. There are many causes, all of which act through a prolonged QT interval (Table 14.8).

Management

Treatment of torsades de pointes is different to treatment of other ventricular arrhythmias:

- Identify and treat any precipitating factors (e.g., stop offending drugs, correct electrolyte imbalance).
- IV magnesium – effective even in patients with normal serum magnesium levels.
- Atrial or ventricular pacing to maintain a heart rate of no less than 90 beats/min to prevent lengthening of the QT interval – IV isoprenaline may also be used to reduce the QT interval.
- In congenital long QT syndromes, high-dose β-blockers (β-adrenoceptor antagonists) or high left thoracic sympathectomy may be used. PPMs are increasingly used in

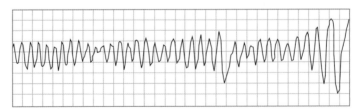

Fig. 14.15 Torsades de pointes. Note the irregular rhythm and twisting axis.

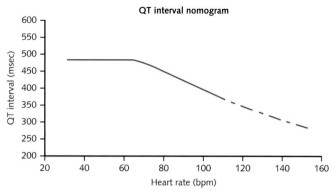

Fig. 14.16 QT interval nomogram.

Table 14.8 Causes of a long QT interval

Cause	Examples
Congenital	Jervell and Lange-Nielsen syndrome (autosomal recessive, sensorineural deafness) Romano-Ward syndrome (autosomal dominant, no deafness)
Drugs (a long list!)	Class IA, IC, III antiarrhythmic agents (e.g., quinidine, flecainide, amiodarone) Tricyclic antidepressants (e.g., amitriptyline) Other antidepressants (including citalopram, venlafaxine) Antipsychotics (e.g., chlorpromazine, haloperidol, olanzapine) Antihistamines (e.g., loratadine, diphenhydramine) Macrolides (e.g., erythromycin, clarithromycin) Methadone
Electrolyte abnormalities	Hypokalaemia Hypomagnesaemia Hypocalcaemia
Others	Acute myocardial infarction Central nervous system disease Mitral valve prolapse Organophosphate pesticides

individuals who remain symptomatic despite maximally tolerated β-blocker dosage. ICDs are sometimes useful if episodes of torsades continue despite drug therapy.

- Torsades may degenerate into VF, requiring defibrillation. Avoid DC cardioversion in otherwise stable patients, as torsades de pointes is generally paroxysmal and often recurs following cardioversion.
- Do not use antiarrhythmic drugs.

Ventricular fibrillation

VF is irregular rapid ventricular depolarization (Fig. 14.17). There is no organized ventricular contraction; therefore, the patient has no pulse, rapidly causing loss of consciousness and cardiorespiratory arrest.

Clinical features

The most common cause of VF is acute MI. However, VF is also seen as the end-stage of many disease processes and signifies the presence of severe myocardial damage (sometimes referred to as secondary VF and usually results in death despite resuscitation attempts). VF may be precipitated by:

- VT, including torsades de pointes.
- Ventricular ectopic beats.
- Supraventricular arrhythmias.
- **Unsynchronized** DC cardioversion during ventricular repolarization ('R on T' phenomenon), e.g., in an unstable patient with SVT (make sure cardioversion in these cases is **synchronized**).

Management

VF must be treated promptly with simple (nonsynchronized) DC cardioversion (see resuscitation protocol later). It is vital to start effective chest compressions as soon as possible while the defibrillator is charging. For secondary prevention, an ICD is indicated.

CLINICAL NOTES

Use of precordial thump is no longer recommended routinely, as there is a very low success rate for cardioversion of a shockable rhythm. It should only be considered in monitored VF (or pulseless VT) arrest if used without delay while awaiting the arrival of a defibrillator.

Following defibrillation, management can be divided into pharmacological and nonpharmacological therapies. Pharmacological treatments are discussed later in this chapter (see Antiarrhythmic drugs).

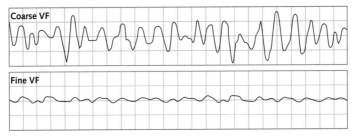

Fig. 14.17 Ventricular fibrillation (VF) can have a coarse or fine pattern.

Nonpharmacological treatments of ventricular tachyarrhythmias

Nonpharmacological treatments are used in patients with recurrent VT or VF because:

- If successful, complete cure is achieved without the need for drugs.
- Localization of the arrhythmogenic focus is becoming possible in more cases due to increased understanding of the mechanisms of these arrhythmias.

Common methods of treatment involve electrophysiological studies and radiofrequency ablation or ICD insertion.

Electrophysiological studies

These studies are used mostly:

- To elucidate the mechanism of tachyarrhythmias.
- Diagnostically to evaluate the risk of sudden cardiac death in patients with possible ventricular tachyarrhythmias.
- Diagnostically to determine conduction defects in patients with recurrent syncope.
- Therapeutically to terminate a tachyarrhythmia by overdrive pacing or shock.
- Therapeutically to ablate potential source of recurrent tachyarrhythmia. This is intended to be curative, with the patient no longer needing antiarrhythmic agents. Note that even though these ventricular arrhythmias can sometimes be prevented, this does not in itself reduce the incidence of sudden death.

Patients who have survived a cardiac arrest will often be treated with an implantable cardioverter-defibrillator (ICD) without an electrophysiological study beforehand.

Implantable cardioverter-defibrillators

ICDs are regularly used in the management of sustained or life-threatening ventricular arrhythmias. These devices are slightly larger than a PPM but implanted in the same way. The device can sense VT and VF, antitachycardia pacing of the ventricle can attempt to cardiovert VT and prevent a painful shock, or DC shock can be delivered when required.

Indications for ICDs are detailed in Table 14.9.

Devices may also be recommended in patients with:

- Left ventricular systolic dysfunction with ejection fraction ≤35%.
- Coexisting broadening of the QRS interval or presence of left bundle branch block.

These patients may sometimes be treated with ICD, cardiac resynchronization therapy with pacing (CRT-P) or cardiac resynchronization therapy with defibrillator (CRT-D).

The impact of an ICD on a patient's occupation and ability to drive needs to be made clear to the patient. Following ICD implantation:

- Patients are **permanently** barred from driving buses or lorries.
- If implanted due to an arrhythmia associated with incapacity, the patient must not drive cars or motorcycles for 6 months. If not implanted for this reason, the patient is

Table 14.9 Indications for implantable cardioverter-defibrillators

Primary prevention	Secondary prevention
• Familial cardiac condition with increased risk of sudden death – long QT syndrome, hypertrophic cardiomyopathy, Brugada syndrome or arrhythmogenic ventricular dysplasia • Previous surgical repair of congenital heart disease	• Survivors of cardiac arrest caused by either ventricular tachycardia (VT) or ventricular fibrillation (VF) • Spontaneous sustained VT causing significant haemodynamic compromise or syncope • Sustained VT without syncope or cardiac arrest and left ventricular ejection fraction ≤35% but symptoms no worse than New York Heart Association class III

barred for 1 month. The patient may then return to driving assuming there are no other contraindications.

- If the device delivers a shock, this has further implications upon driving cars and motorcycles. The period a patient must not drive for varies based on the context of the shock, whether there was any incapacity at the time and whether steps are taken to prevent recurrence.

ANTIARRHYTHMIC DRUGS

Drugs used to treat tachyarrhythmias

The older Vaughan Williams classification is still sometimes used:

- Class I – Sodium channel blockers.
- Class II – Beta blockers.
- Class III – Potassium channel blockers (which inhibit repolarization, thereby prolonging the action potential and refractory period).
- Class IV – Calcium channel blockers.
- Other – Other or unknown mechanisms such as digoxin, adenosine and magnesium.

A summary of the electrophysiological actions of antiarrhythmic drugs is given in Table 14.10. The Vaughan Williams classification of antiarrhythmic drugs allows agents to be grouped according to mode of action on the myocardium and may make selecting appropriate treatment agents more straightforward.

A summary of pharmacokinetics and side effects of the antiarrhythmic agents is shown in Table 14.11. These medications have a large number of interactions with other medications, particularly other antiarrhythmic agents. It is important to fully check the other medications a patient takes prior to administering an antiarrhythmic agent.

HINTS AND TIPS

Antiarrhythmic agents can cause bradyarrhythmias as well as being arrhythmogenic. This can be serious and extreme caution with close monitoring is important when using antiarrhythmic agents, especially when used in combination.

Pharmacological treatments of supraventricular tachyarrhythmias

Class IA, IC and III drugs and adenosine affect conduction in atrial and ventricular tissue and are useful for cardioverting many rhythms to sinus by breaking reentry circuits or reducing the excitability of ectopic foci. Class III drugs have the added advantage of slowing AV conduction and also therefore ventricular response.

Table 14.10 Electrophysiological actions of antiarrhythmic drugs

Vaughan Williams class	Examples	Site of action	Sinus node rate	Atrial conduction rate	AV node refractory period	Ventricular contraction rate
IA	Quinidine, procainamide, disopyramide	Blocks fast sodium channels	No effect	Decreased	Increased	Decreased
IB	Lidocaine, mexiletine, tocainimide	Blocks fast sodium channels	No effect	No effect	Little effect	Decreased
IC	Flecainide, propafenone	Blocks fast sodium channels	Reduced	Decreased	Increased	Decreased
II	Bisoprolol, atenolol, metoprolol, sotalol	Blocks β–adrenergic receptors	Reduced	No effect	Increased	No effect
III	Amiodarone, sotalol, bretylium	Blocks potassium channels; mechanism not entirely understood	Reduced	Decreased	Increased	Decreased
IV	Verapamil, diltiazem	Blocks slow calcium channels	Small reduction	Small reduction	Increased	No effect
Digoxin		Blocks Na^+/K^+ ATPase	No effect	Increased	Increased	Slows AV conduction
Adenosine		Slows conduction through the AV node	Reduced	Decreased	Increased	Temporarily pauses AV conduction

ATPase, Adenosine triphosphatase; AV, atrioventricular.

Table 14.11 Pharmacokinetics and adverse effects of antiarrhythmic drugs

Medication	Route of administration	Half-life	Mode of excretion	Adverse effects
Procainamide	Oral, IV or IM	3–5 h	Renal	Skin rashes, Raynaud syndrome, hallucinations; toxicity – cardiac failure, long QT, ventricular tachyarrhythmias
Lidocaine	IV	1–2 h	Hepatic	Myocardial depression, cardiac failure, long QT; toxicity – dizziness, confusion, paraesthesia
Flecainide	Oral, IV	20 h	Renal (partly hepatic)	Myocardial depression, ventricular arrhythmias (a major problem, especially in patients with ischaemic heart disease)
Atenolol	Oral, IV	6–7 h	Renal	Myocardial depression, bronchospasm, peripheral vasoconstriction
Sotalol	Oral, IV	10–15 h	Renal	Myocardial depression, long QT, ventricular tachyarrhythmias
Amiodarone	Oral, IV	3–6 weeks	Hepatic	Pulmonary fibrosis, liver damage, peripheral neuropathy, hyper- or hypothyroidism, corneal microdeposits, photosensitivity, myocardial depression (but safe in cardiac failure), long QT
Verapamil	Oral, IV	3–7 h	Renal	Myocardial depression, constipation
Digoxin	Oral, IV	36–48 h	Renal	Toxicity – heart block, atrial tachycardia, ventricular arrhythmia, xanthopsia
Adenosine	IV	<10 s	Rapidly broken down by enzymes in the circulatory system	Light-headedness, sweating, nausea, 'sense of impending doom', metallic taste

Pharmacological treatments of ventricular tachyarrhythmias

In the acute situation, if the patient is unconscious or has no cardiac output, give prompt DC cardioversion (see Cardiac arrest and resuscitation section of this chapter).

Antiarrhythmic agents may be given after sinus rhythm has been established in an effort to stabilize the myocardium. Medications used to treat ventricular tachyarrhythmias other than torsades de pointes are mainly either class I or class III.

Amiodarone is commonly used, but alternative agents include flecainide and lidocaine:

- Amiodarone is useful in cardiac failure because it has little negative inotropic effect. If given IV, after the initial bolus dose, amiodarone should ideally be given centrally because it is damaging to peripheral veins. Amiodarone has a very long half-life (25 days) and oral loading takes at least 1 month. IV loading is faster.
- If there is no contraindication to β-blockers, sotalol may be considered, as it has none of the long-term side effects of amiodarone. It must be used in high doses to gain the class III effect but should be uptitrated gradually, measuring the QT interval before each dose increase.
- Flecainide is effective but avoided in patients with suspected ischaemic heart disease because this may increase its proarrhythmic side effects.

Drug treatment alone for the secondary prevention of ventricular arrhythmia is ineffective, although β-blockers should be used where possible in patients post-MI or with heart failure. Drugs are a useful adjunct to reduce the frequency of arrhythmic events in conjunction with ICD therapy.

ALGORITHMS FOR MANAGEMENT OF ARRHYTHMIAS

Perform a comprehensive A–E assessment on all patients presenting with arrhythmia.

Many patients with arrhythmias will be stable but if patients demonstrate any of the following life-threatening (or 'adverse') features, then urgent action is required:

- Shock (usually defined as SBP <90 mmHg, symptoms of increased sympathetic activity and decreased cerebral perfusion).
- Syncope – due to reduced cerebral perfusion.
- Myocardial ischaemia – either as anginal chest pain, finding on 12-lead ECG or from biochemical markers (e.g., elevation of troponin).
- Severe heart failure – pulmonary oedema (left ventricular failure) +/– raised JVP (right ventricular failure).

Adult bradycardia algorithm

See Fig. 14.18 for an algorithm for treatment of bradycardia in adults.

Adult tachycardia algorithm

See Fig. 14.19 for an algorithm for management of tachycardia in adults.

CARDIAC ARREST AND RESUSCITATION

Cardiac arrest occurs when there is an absence of cardiac output. Cardiopulmonary resuscitation (CPR) is the term used to describe attempts to maintain adequate breathing and circulation in a patient who cannot do so for themself. CPR aims to restore respiration and adequate cardiac output as soon as possible to prevent death or permanent disability. CPR involves two types of protocol:

1. Basic life support (BLS).
2. Advanced life support (ALS).

In ALS and BLS, these three areas must be assessed and supported in order of priority:

- Airway.
- Breathing.
- Circulation.

Basic life support

BLS refers to the maintenance and support of the airway, breathing and circulation without specialized equipment (Fig. 14.20). This should be commenced immediately upon recognizing cardiac arrest. BLS aims to maintain adequate ventilation and cardiac output until the underlying problem can be reversed. There are several points to note:

- Open the airway if necessary, and assess if the patient is breathing (with look, listen and feel) for no more than 10 seconds. If trauma to the cervical spine is possible, the airway should be maintained without tilting the head.
- If there are two rescuers, one should seek help as soon as possible. If there is only one, the rescuer should shout for help and, if necessary, very quickly (i.e., taking seconds) go to obtain help after establishing that the patient is not breathing. If, however, the patient is a child and there is no phone available, give five rescue breaths and 1 min of CPR before going to get help – in these situations, the collapse is likely due to respiratory arrest and rescue breaths, if given early, will improve prognosis.
- Chest compressions are performed by placing the heel of the hand over the sternum's lower half. Enough pressure should be applied to depress the sternum 5 to 6 cm and no more.
- The rescuer should be vertically above the patient's chest, and the arms should be kept straight. The rate of compressions should be 100–120/min. After each compression, the pressure should be released and the chest wall allowed to rise back up. The sequence is 30 compressions followed by 2 rescue breaths. If the rescuer is not trained or not willing to give rescue breaths, continuous compressions are recommended.
- Each rescue breath is given by mouth-to-mouth inflation, ensuring a good seal and the nose is occluded. The rescuer should watch the patient's chest wall to ensure that it rises and falls with each breath. It is essential to allow the chest wall to fall back completely before taking the next breath.

Use of automated external defibrillators

Automated external defibrillators (AEDs) are increasingly prevalent in public places and can be used with minimal or no training. They allow for early defibrillation, often long before professional help arrives. AEDs provide full instructions to the user throughout the defibrillation process. AEDs are useful in areas with high densities of people (e.g., airports, railway stations, stadiums, etc.) but also in remote areas where the response would be significantly delayed if an arrest occurred.

Recovery position

This position should be adopted if an unresponsive patient is breathing and has a pulse whilst the rescuer seeks help. It has several important functions (Fig. 14.21), including keeping the patient's airway straight, allowing the tongue to fall forward and not obstruct the airway, and minimizing aspiration risk.

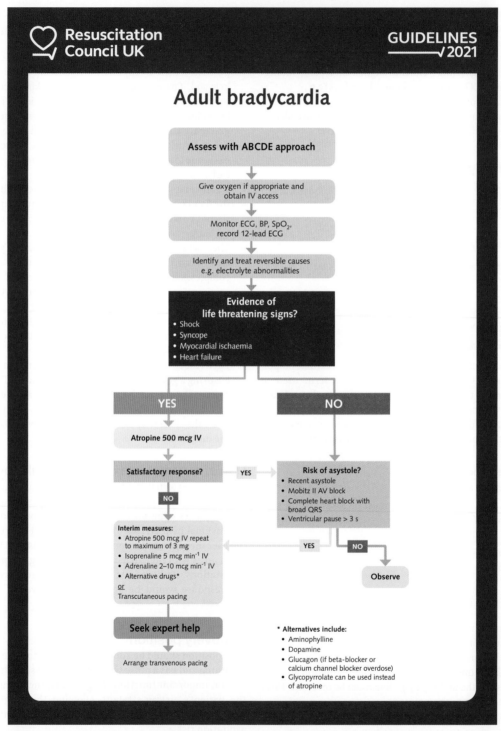

Fig. 14.18 Adult bradycardia (with pulse) algorithm (Reproduced with the kind permission of Resuscitation Council UK, https://www.resus.org.uk/sites/default/files/2021-04/Bradycardia%20Algorithm%202021.pdf. Linked to from this page: https://www.resus.org.uk/library/2021-resuscitation-guidelines/adult-advanced-life-support-guidelines).

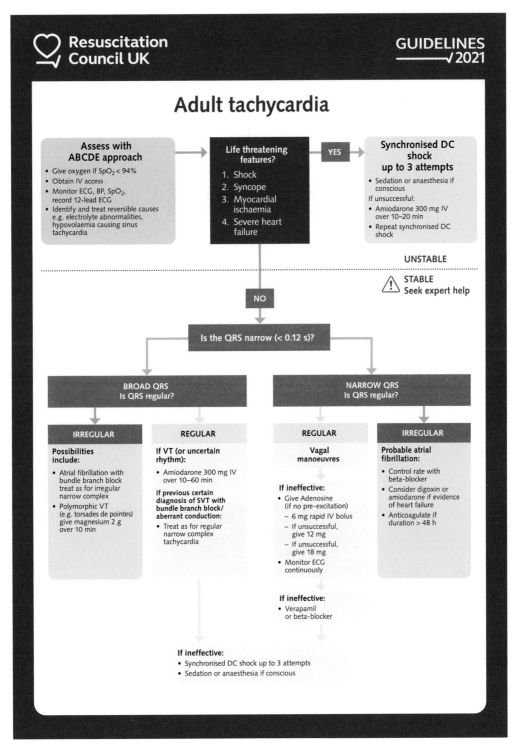

Fig. 14.19 Adult tachycardia (with pulse) algorithm (Reproduced with the kind permission of Resuscitation Council UK, https://www.resus.org.uk/sites/default/files/2021-04/Tachycardia%20Algorithm%202021.pdf).

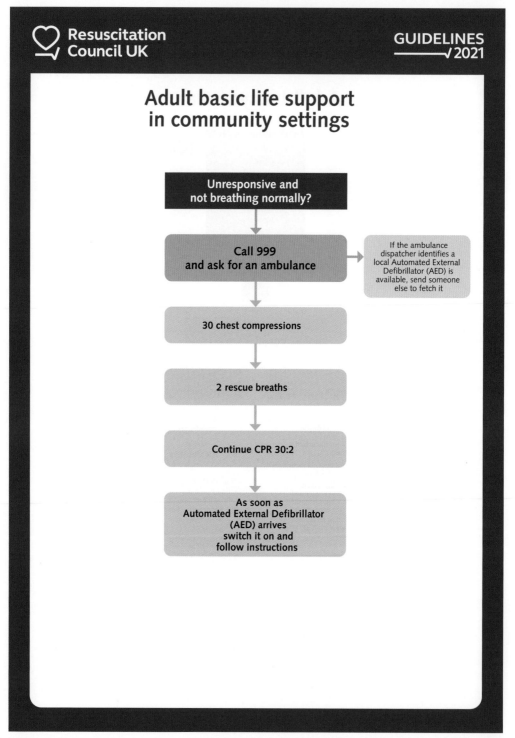

Fig. 14.20 Adult basic life support algorithm (Reproduced with the kind permission of Resuscitation Council UK, https://www.resus. org.uk/sites/default/files/2021-04/Adult%20Basic%20Life%20Support%20Algorithm%202021.pdf). *CPR*, cardiopulmonary resuscitation.

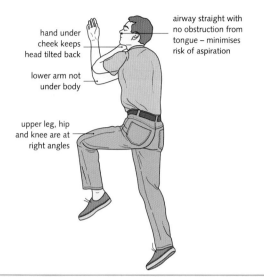

airway straight with no obstruction from tongue – minimises risk of aspiration

hand under cheek keeps head tilted back

lower arm not under body

upper leg, hip and knee are at right angles

Manoeuvres

Remove patient's glasses (if worn).

Kneel beside patient and make sure their legs are straight.

Place patient's near-side arm at right angles to their body, elbow bent with palm up.

Bring patient's far-side arm across the chest and hold back of their hand against the cheek on near-side.

With other hand, grasp far-side leg above the knee and pull it up, keeping the foot on the ground.

Keeping their hand against the cheek, pull on the far-side leg to roll the patient towards you.

Adjust the upper leg so the hip and knee are both at right angles.

Tilt the head back to ensure airway remains open.

If necessary, adjust hand under the cheek to keep head tilted.

Reassess breathing regularly.

Fig. 14.21 The recovery position.

Advanced life support

The Resuscitation Council's current adult ALS guidelines were most recently updated in 2021 (Fig. 14.22). This guideline divides cardiac arrest patients into two main groups, those with:

1. Shockable rhythms – VF/pulseless VT (pVT).
2. Nonshockable rhythms – asystole/pulseless electrical activity (PEA).

Points to note

For optimum efficacy of ALS:

- Ensure BLS is commenced immediately and, once a cardiac monitor is available, that defibrillation is administered immediately if shockable rhythm is present. Minimize interruptions to CPR.
- Ensure the airway is protected throughout – the gold standard is with insertion of a cuffed endotracheal (ET) tube, preferably by an anaesthetist. This minimizes aspiration risk and can increase the efficacy of ventilation. If there is not a trained person highly competent at intubating with an ET tube or there is any delay with difficult intubation, an i-gel (supraglottic airway device) usually provides a good seal and can be inserted quickly with minimal training, therefore minimizing any gaps in chest compressions. Once an advanced airway is in place, ventilate the patient at a constant rate of 10 breaths/min and continue chest compressions at a rate of 100–120 compressions/min without pauses for ventilation.
- The defibrillator pads should be placed to allow optimum energy delivery to the myocardium – the right pad should be below the clavicle in the mid-clavicular line and the left pad should be on the lower rib cage on the anterior axillary line.

'Shockable rhythms' arm of the advanced life support algorithm

In the event of pVT or VF, one DC shock should be administered as soon as the rhythm is identified and it is safe to deliver the shock. Generally, an energy setting of at least 150 J should be used in the first instance when using a biphasic defibrillator. Following delivery of the shock, CPR should be resumed immediately. Rhythm and pulse is assessed following a further 2-minute cycle of CPR. A further shock may be delivered at this time if indicated. 1 mg IV adrenaline is given after the third shock and then every 3 to 5 minutes (generally every two rhythm checks). Amiodarone (300 mg IV) should also be given after the third shock. Look for reversible causes of cardiopulmonary arrest.

'Nonshockable rhythms' arm of the advanced life support algorithm

Prognosis in asystole, PEA and profound bradyarrhythmias is generally poorer than for patients with shockable rhythms. Defibrillation is not indicated unless the rhythm check changes to VF/pVT. 1 mg IV adrenaline should be given as soon as IV access is achieved. This may be repeated every 3 to 5 minutes. Look for reversible causes of cardiac arrest.

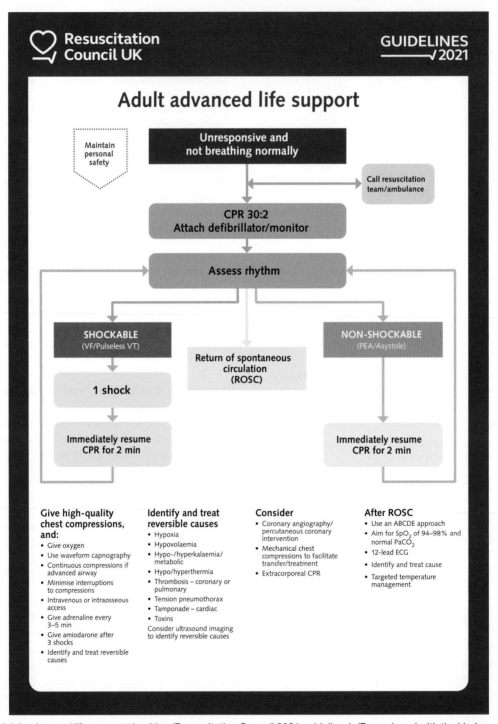

Fig. 14.22 Adult advanced life support algorithm (Resuscitation Council 2021 guidelines). (Reproduced with the kind permission of Resuscitation Council UK, https://www.resus.org.uk/sites/default/files/2021-04/Adult%20Advanced%20Life%20Support%20Algorithm%202021.pdf). *CPR*, cardiopulmonary resuscitation; *PEA*, pulseless electrical activity; *VF*, ventricular fibrillation; *VT*, ventricular tachycardia.

Reversible causes – '4 Hs and 4 Ts'

Several reversible causes of cardiac arrest have been identified and are sometimes referred to as the *4 Hs and 4 Ts*. Attempts should be made to rule these out or treat as appropriate during all cardiac arrests:

- **H**ypoxia – ensure maximal possible inspired oxygen is delivered during CPR and that ventilation is adequate. Ensure the chest is rising and falling and that there are bilateral breath sounds.
- **H**ypovolaemia – attempt to stop any obvious haemorrhage and restore circulating volume with fluids and/or blood products.
- **H**ypo-/hyperkalaemia, hypoglycaemia or other metabolic disorders – patient history may suggest a metabolic abnormality; ABG and blood glucose may allow for rapid diagnosis/treatment.
- **H**ypo-/hyperthermia – may be suggested by the history, e.g., cardiac arrest associated with drowning.
- **T**hrombosis (coronary or pulmonary) – if pulmonary embolus is suspected, consider giving thrombolysis if there are no contraindications. Consider performing CPR for at least 60–90 minutes if thrombolysis is given before resuscitation efforts are terminated.
- **T**ension pneumothorax – suspect in trauma cases or after insertion of a central line; it is also seen spontaneously in fit young men and patients with asthma or COPD. Look for unilateral absence of chest movements and breath sounds. Treat it with a large-bore cannula into the pleural space at the second intercostal space in the mid-clavicular line, followed by the insertion of a chest drain.
- **T**oxins – may be suggested by the history; may occur due to prescribed medications, over-the-counter medications or recreational drugs. Use a toxicology database (e.g., Toxbase) for specific guidelines.
- **T**amponade (cardiac) – suspect in trauma cases and postthoracotomy patients. Tamponade can be confirmed by ultrasound imaging. It needs rapid insertion of a pericardial drain.

In-hospital cardiac arrest

When a cardiac arrest occurs in the hospital, a call is made to the arrest team. Most hospitals in the UK have a standard number (2222), which is a direct line to the switchboard operator. The caller should state in a clear voice, 'Cardiac arrest, ward X'. The switchboard operator will then repeat the information to the caller before alerting the arrest team. Generally, the arrest team comprises at least an anaesthetist, a medical registrar, a senior house officer and an FY1, as well as a porter who can take urgent blood samples to the laboratory. The anaesthetist or registrar usually leads the resuscitation effort.

Many hospitals now use audit forms to analyze the response to each cardiac arrest call. These forms collect information on the patient's condition on arrival, events during the arrest and whether resuscitation was successful. The results of audit sheets are used as part of ongoing quality improvement and to direct further training of the arrest team.

ETHICS

'Do Not Attempt Cardiopulmonary Resuscitation' or 'DNACPR' orders are written by senior staff members when it is thought that death is expected, resuscitation under the circumstances would be futile or the patient's quality of life would subsequently be very poor. These are difficult decisions, and a sound knowledge of ethical principles and medical law is essential. The principles of beneficence and nonmaleficence are particularly important here; CPR should not be carried out if felt not in the patient's best interests. Even if CPR is a valid treatment option, patients may exert their autonomy and refuse resuscitation in advance.

Chapter Summary

- The term 'arrhythmia' describes irregularity in the normal heartbeat. Many patients with arrhythmia may be asymptomatic, whereas others can be critically unwell.
- Certain patients with bradycardia (e.g., patients with complete heart block) warrant pacemaker insertion.
- Patients with atrial fibrillation are at increased risk of stroke – it is important to balance stroke risk against the increased bleeding risk of anticoagulation.
- Familiarity with antiarrhythmic agents' indications (and contraindications) is vital – some can cause profound instability if given inappropriately.
- Arrhythmia and the presence of myocardial ischaemia (either in the form of chest pain, on the ECG or from elevated troponin), syncope, shock (systolic blood pressure <90 mmHg, increased sympathetic activity and decreased cerebral perfusion), or signs of severe heart failure indicate the arrhythmia is 'unstable' – urgent intervention is required.
- If the patient has a pulse but warrants a shock, remember to use synchronized DC cardioversion. In ventricular fibrillation or pulseless ventricular tachycardia, proceed with unsynchronized defibrillation immediately.
- For cardiac arrest and resuscitation, follow the BLS and ALS algorithms.
- Rapid recognition of arrest with early CPR, early defibrillation and prompt postresuscitation care improve arrest outcomes.

UKMLA Conditions
Arrhythmias
Cardiac arrest
Vasovagal syncope

UKMLA Presentations
Blackouts and faints
Cardiorespiratory arrest
Dizziness
Driving advice
Palpitations

Valvular disease can manifest as either stenosis or regurgitation, or sometimes both simultaneously. Stenosis is a narrowing or obstruction to normal flow through the valve. In regurgitation, the valve fails in its function to prevent backflow of blood and is 'leaky'. This can also be described as an incompetent or insufficient valve.

Valvular disease can be caused by:

1. Direct damage to valve leaflets (usually the case in stenosis).
2. Damage to the valve ring (the annulus).
3. Damage to supporting structures (papillary muscles, chordae tendineae).

The most commonly affected valves are the aortic and mitral valves due to the high pressures to which they are exposed (compared to those in the right side of the heart). Multiple valves may be diseased. Any valvular abnormality will predispose to infective endocarditis (IE).

See Chapter 10 for a summary of causes of valvular disease (and other murmurs) and clinical findings on examination.

> **HINTS AND TIPS**
>
> Valve lesions are a common short-case question both in finals and in membership examinations. Be sure you have a good understanding of the common valvular pathologies.

RHEUMATIC HEART DISEASE

Rheumatic fever is now rare in the developed world due to improved sanitation, reduced overcrowding, effective antibiotic therapy and a reduction in virulence of β-haemolytic streptococcus. It is still a major problem in the developing world, where it is the most common cause of acquired valvular disease. Acute rheumatic fever most frequently affects children aged 5 to 15 years.

Acute rheumatic fever is an inflammatory disease caused by an autoimmune reaction initiated by infection with group A β-haemolytic streptococcal pharyngitis 2 to 3 weeks earlier. Antibodies directed against bacterial cell membrane antigens cross-react with the patient's own proteins (a type II hypersensitivity reaction). It may cause multiorgan disease, affecting the heart, skin, joints and central nervous system.

Rheumatic heart disease is a consequence of rheumatic fever that may have occurred many years previously. The acute process can leave the valves scarred and deformed, and progressive fibrosis can occur, causing chronic rheumatic heart disease. It is more common in females.

Clinical features

The patient may not recall a preceding sore throat. Diagnosis of rheumatic fever is based on the revised Jones criteria.

Major criteria:

1. Carditis – involves all three layers (pancarditis).
2. Arthritis – a migrating polyarthritis affecting the large joints.
3. Sydenham chorea – occurs months after the initial disease and is characterized by rapid, involuntary purposeless movements of the face and limbs due to inflammation of the caudate nucleus, also known as *St Vitus' dance*.
4. Erythema marginatum – seen mainly on the trunk; the shape of the lesions change with time and the asymptomatic rash spreads outwards with raised red circular edges and a centre that clears.
5. Subcutaneous nodules – pea-sized, firm, painless, subcutaneous nodules on the extensor surfaces (overlying joints, on the scalp and over vertebrae).

Minor criteria are:

1. Fever.
2. Raised erythrocyte sedimentation rate (ESR) or C-reactive protein (CRP).
3. Prolonged PR interval (only if carditis is not a major criteria).
4. Arthralgia.
5. Previous rheumatic fever.

Diagnosis requires two major criteria, or one major and two minor criteria, plus evidence of preceding streptococcal infection (e.g., increased antistreptolysin O (ASO) titres). Evidence of streptococcal infection is not required if there is isolated pancarditis or chorea and if all other causes of these are excluded. If diagnosing recurrent rheumatic fever, only evidence of previous streptococcal infection and two minor criteria are required.

Carditis predominantly affects the valves (valvulitis) but can affect the endocardium, myocardium and pericardium concomitantly (pancarditis). It is usually asymptomatic even though a murmur or echocardiographic evidence may be found. The patient may present with breathlessness, chest pain or palpitations. Signs may include a new murmur, features of pericarditis or heart failure.

Commonly, rheumatic fever affects the mitral valve (65%) or the mitral and aortic valves (25%). In the long-term, progression can lead to commissural fusion (fusing of valve leaflets), shortening/thickening of the chordae and cusp fibrosis. The most common chronic sequelae are mitral stenosis (MS) with or without regurgitation, although other valves may be affected.

Aschoff nodules (granulomatous lesions with a central necrotic area) are pathognomonic of rheumatic fever and initially have an inflammatory infiltrate that is eventually replaced by fibrous tissue.

Investigations

Blood tests usually show raised inflammatory markers (ESR and CRP) and leucocytosis.

Evidence of streptococcal infection should be looked for. A throat swab should be taken for culture (although often too late for positive results when rheumatic fever presents) and may be used for the rapid streptococcal antigen detection test (RADT) if available. Blood tests 2 weeks apart may demonstrate rising antibodies, e.g., ASO titres.

First-degree atrioventricular (AV) block may be seen on the ECG, although this is not a specific finding despite being a minor criterion. Features of pericarditis or other nonspecific ST or T wave changes may be seen.

A chest X-ray may demonstrate cardiomegaly or evidence of heart failure.

An echocardiogram may demonstrate valvular abnormalities, cardiac enlargement and pericardial effusion in acute rheumatic fever. The so-called fish-mouth or button-hole mitral valve deformity can be seen on an echocardiogram in MS secondary to chronic rheumatic heart disease.

Management

Treatment with high-dose penicillin (benzylpenicillin, single intramuscular injection or phenoxymethylpenicillin, 10-day oral course) is started immediately to eradicate the causative organism.

Antiinflammatory agents are given to suppress the autoimmune response and to relieve arthritis. Aspirin is effective, and although in children there is a small risk of Reye syndrome, it is still sometimes used in preference to nonsteroidal antiinflammatory drugs at small doses. Corticosteroids are used if there is carditis.

Bed rest reduces cardiac workload and reduces joint pain. Cardiac failure is treated with supportive therapy, although sometimes rheumatic fever causes severe mitral regurgitation (MR), which does not respond to medical treatment and requires valve replacement.

Long-term antibiotics (usually penicillin) are recommended for a minimum of 5 years (or until the patient is 21) to prevent recurrent rheumatic fever. Long-term follow-up is needed to identify any valve disease.

HINTS AND TIPS

Acute rheumatic fever is not common in the developed world, but there are still many elderly people suffering the after-effects of childhood infection.

AORTIC STENOSIS

Aortic stenosis (AS) is the commonest valvular disease in the developed world and is usually due to degenerative valvular calcification. However, AS may also occur at the sub- or supravalvular level in congenital disease (Table 15.1).

CLINICAL NOTES

Congenitally bicuspid valves are one of the most common congenital cardiac abnormalities; however, most do not cause problems until later in life. On average, patients with bicuspid valves develop aortic stenosis 10 years earlier than those with normal valves. It is also associated with aortic aneurysm and dissection.

Table 15.1 Causes of aortic stenosis

Site of aortic stenosis (AS)	Causes
Valvular AS	Degenerative calcification of normal tricuspid valve or congenitally abnormal valve (tends to occur at a younger age) Rheumatic fever Congenital, males > females (malformed valve can be uni-, bi- or tricuspid)
Subvalvular AS	Fibromuscular ring Hypertrophic cardiomyopathy
Supravalvular AS	Associated with hypercalcaemia in Williams syndrome (elfin facies, intellectual disability, affable 'cocktail party' personality, strabismus, hypervitaminosis D and hypercalcaemia; autosomal dominant inheritance although mostly arises de novo)

Pathophysiology

In adults, left ventricular outflow obstruction usually develops over a number of years. The stenosis increases afterload on the left ventricle (LV), increasing the force required to eject blood into the aorta. This causes left ventricular hypertrophy (LVH) and an increase in myocardial oxygen demand. More vigorous and prolonged contraction aims to overcome the obstruction and maintain an adequate cardiac output, but as systole is prolonged, diastole is shortened. Coronary artery flow occurs during diastole; therefore, myocardial blood supply from the coronary arteries is reduced. If myocardial perfusion is outstripped by demand, angina occurs even with normal coronary arteries. Inadequate tissue perfusion (e.g., of the brain) may cause syncope. Reduced cardiac output and pulmonary oedema may cause breathlessness.

Clinical features

Although patients are often asymptomatic, there is a classic triad of symptoms:

1. Angina – see earlier.
2. Dizziness and syncope – especially on exertion.
3. Dyspnoea – initially exertional due to the inability to increase cardiac output adequately. May lead to orthopnoea and paroxysmal nocturnal dyspnoea as the LV fails.

Sudden death and systemic emboli may occur but these are rare.

HINTS AND TIPS

Patients who have aortic stenosis may present with angina, but an exercise test is usually contraindicated in patients with severe aortic stenosis, as exertion can cause syncope or sudden death. It is therefore crucial to examine every patient carefully before recommending an exercise ECG.

Examination

The following findings are common in valvular AS (Fig. 15.1):

1. Slow rising, low volume pulse – best felt at the carotid pulse.
2. Narrow pulse pressure.
3. Heaving apex beat – rarely displaced.
4. Ejection systolic murmur heard loudest over the aortic area, may radiate to the carotids and be accompanied by a palpable thrill.
5. Quiet or absent aortic component of the second heart sound (A_2).
6. Signs of left ventricular failure (LVF).

Investigations

Electrocardiography

This usually shows sinus rhythm and LVH with strain – a tall R wave in lead V5–V6, with a deep S wave in lead V1 and T wave inversion in the lateral leads.

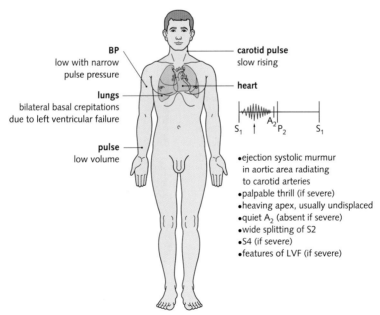

Fig. 15.1 Possible clinical findings in aortic stenosis. A_2, aortic component of second heart sound; *LVF*, left ventricular failure; P_2, pulmonary component of second heart sound; S_1, first heart sound; S_2, second heart sound.

Chest radiography

The heart is often normal size in LVH but can be enlarged if there is coexistent aortic regurgitation (AR) or LVF. The aorta is often enlarged due to turbulent blood flow. There may also be evidence of pulmonary oedema in LVF.

Echocardiography

This is the standard method to assess and follow up AS. It will show the valve in great detail, including the number of cusps and their mobility and the presence of calcification. Doppler echocardiography allows blood flow velocity to be measured and the calculation of the effective orifice area and aortic valve gradient, which are all measures of AS severity. It will also demonstrate resultant LVH or LVF. Aortic size can be measured, and coexistent AR or mitral valve disease may be seen.

Computed tomography

This may show thickened, calcified valve leaflets or evidence of bicuspid valve. Noncontrast calcium scoring of the valve can be used in part of the assessment of severity of AS. CT may also show sequelae of AS, including evidence of LVF or LVH as well as evidence of other pathology (e.g., aortic, coronary or pulmonary disease).

Cardiac catheterization

This may provide information on the valve gradient and LV function, although echocardiography is sufficient in the vast majority. The main indication is assessment of coronary arteries prior to surgical valve replacement to identify patients who may benefit from concurrent bypass grafting.

Management

Medical management

Prognosis is good if the patient is asymptomatic. Patients with asymptomatic severe AS may be followed up with intermittent echocardiography as the patient may attribute gradual decrease in exercise tolerance to age. Patients should be educated to look out for warning symptoms, such as chest pain, syncope and breathlessness. As soon as mild symptoms are present, survival becomes poor unless left ventricular outflow tract obstruction is promptly relieved either surgically or percutaneously. The average time between symptom onset and death is 5 years with angina, 3 years with syncope and 2 years with heart failure. Valve replacement may prevent LVF or sudden death.

Medication use is limited. Diuretics can be helpful to remove abnormal fluid accumulation in heart failure, but use cautiously – hypovolaemia will overcome the compensatory raised end-diastolic LV pressure and reduce cardiac output. The positive inotropic effects of digoxin also have some theoretical benefits and can be used in patients with AS and heart failure. Many antianginal

drugs and angiotensin-converting enzyme (ACE) inhibitors are avoided in AS because they theoretically might:

1. Have a negative inotropic effect and result in acute pulmonary oedema (if LV function is impaired).
2. Cause vasodilatation, resulting in worsening of the gradient across the aortic valve, and inability to produce a compensatory increase in cardiac output.

However, there is interest in the potential protective effects of ACE inhibitor therapy, especially longer-acting agents that do not cause such acute falls in blood pressure.

Endovascular management

Endovascular management includes:

- Transcatheter aortic valve implantation (TAVI) – balloon or self-expandable valves that can be deployed either through percutaneous catheters or using a trocar through the apex of the heart (Fig. 15.2). This is a valuable treatment in patients at high surgical risk due to comorbidities and is increasingly being used in elderly patients (>75–80 years old).
- Balloon aortic valvuloplasty (BAV) – this procedure stretches the stenotic valve with a balloon inserted via a percutaneous catheter. It is not a long-term solution and is associated with significant risks; therefore, it is only used as a palliative measure or bridge to surgery.

Surgical management

Aortic valve replacement (AVR) is still the treatment of choice and should be considered without delay in all patients with

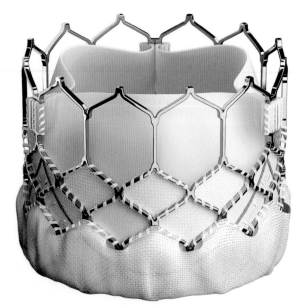

Fig. 15.2 Example of a transcatheter heart valve (Sapien 3). (Courtesy Prof. D Newby.)

symptomatic severe AS. Most centres have experience operating on elderly patients with improved quality of life and survival. AVR is usually performed via median sternotomy and requires cardiopulmonary bypass. Aortic valvotomy is performed to repair congenital AS in children.

AORTIC REGURGITATION

Aortic regurgitation may be due to an abnormality of the valve cusps themselves and/or dilatation of the aortic root and therefore the valve ring (Table 15.2).

Pathophysiology

Regurgitation of blood into the LV after each systole results in increase in end-diastolic volume and stroke volume. The LV works harder, becoming hypertrophied and dilated. The aorta may also dilate with increased stroke volumes, worsening AR. As AR progresses, the LV may no longer be able to compensate, resulting in LVF and pulmonary congestion. LV backpressure may also cause pulmonary hypertension and right ventricular failure (RVF) but this is uncommon.

If onset is acute (e.g., ruptured valve with IE), compensatory structural changes cannot take place and increased LV pressure causes premature closure of the mitral valve, preventing diastolic filling.

Table 15.2 Causes of aortic regurgitation

Site of disease	Cause
Valve disease	Infective endocarditis Rheumatic fever Congenital – e.g., prolapse with ventricular septal defect Rheumatoid arthritis Systemic lupus erythematosus
Aortic root disease	Osteogenesis imperfecta Type A aortic dissection Aortic root aneurysm Trauma Takayasu arteritis Reiter syndrome Psoriatic arthritis Syphilis
Both	Degenerative Hypertension Connective tissue disease (e.g., Marfan syndrome) Bicuspid aortic valve Ankylosing spondylitis

Clinical features

Moderate and mild AR is usually asymptomatic. Patients often have an increased awareness of their heartbeat due to increased stroke volume years before any other symptom. Dyspnoea is the main presenting symptom and develops insidiously in chronic severe AR with accompanying features of LVF, such as orthopnoea and paroxysmal nocturnal dyspnoea. Angina can develop as hypertrophy increases demand and abnormally low diastolic blood pressure decreases coronary flow.

Acute severe AR may present with profound hypotension (due to cardiogenic shock), weakness and breathlessness.

Examination

Characteristic findings in chronic AR (Fig. 15.3) are:

1. Collapsing high-volume pulse.
2. Wide pulse pressure.
3. Downward and laterally displaced apex, which has a thrusting nature.
4. Murmur best heard with the diaphragm at the lower left sternal edge with the patient sitting forward and in full expiration. It is a soft, high-pitched, early diastolic murmur, sometimes difficult to hear – be sure to listen closely with the stethoscope diaphragm.
5. Increased flow across the aortic valve in significant AR frequently produces an ejection systolic murmur even without AS, which is often louder than the early diastolic murmur.
6. Third heart sound due to rapid ventricular filling.
7. A number of eponymous signs (see Chapter 10).
8. Austin Flint murmur – heard when the regurgitant jet causes vibration of the anterior mitral valve leaflet. The murmur is similar to that of MS but with no opening snap.
9. May include signs of LVF.

> **CLINICAL NOTES**
>
> A collapsing pulse (or *water hammer pulse*) is due to increased stroke volume and rapid run-off of blood back into the left ventricle after systole. It is accentuated at the radial pulse by lifting the arm rapidly – use the base of your fingers across the patient's radial artery at the wrist to best appreciate the tapping quality of the collapsing pulse. Remember to check whether the patient has any shoulder pain first! The abrupt expansion and collapse can be better felt at the carotid pulse (Corrigan sign).

In acute AR, the patient may appear very unwell, with cyanosis, hypotension and pulmonary congestion. Tachycardia occurs to compensate for the inability of the heart to dilate and

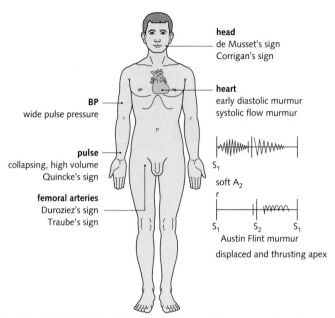

head
de Musset's sign
Corrigan's sign

heart
early diastolic murmur
systolic flow murmur

S_1

soft A_2

r

S_1 S_2 S_1

Austin Flint murmur

displaced and thrusting apex

BP
wide pulse pressure

pulse
collapsing, high volume
Quincke's sign

femoral arteries
Duroziez's sign
Traube's sign

Fig. 15.3 Possible clinical findings in aortic regurgitation. A_2, aortic component of second heart sound; S_1, first heart sound; S_2, second heart sound.

hypertrophy quickly. This usually leads to shortening of the murmur, and most of the other peripheral signs are also less evident.

Investigations

Electrocardiography
Normal in early AR. As AR progresses, there may be left axis deviation, then LVH with strain pattern.

Chest radiography
The LV does not have time to enlarge in acute AR but may be markedly enlarged in chronic AR. Aortic root enlargement may also be the cause of AR. There may be features of LVF.

Echocardiography
Aortic valve structure can be evaluated and fluttering of the anterior mitral valve leaflet is frequently seen as the regurgitant jet hits the leaflet from above. Size and velocity of the regurgitant jet is a measure of severity. Left ventricular size and function can be assessed. Aortic root size can sometimes be assessed. Transthoracic echo is usually sufficient, although sometimes transoesophageal echo may provide more detailed information.

Cardiac catheterization
Enables assessment of aortic root size, severity of AR, left ventricular function and coexistent coronary artery disease.

Cardiac MRI
Allows accurate assessment of AR severity, aortic flow reversal, LV volume and mass. MRI is helpful when echocardiography has not provided optimal views.

Management

Medical management
Treatment of underlying cause (e.g., IE) may be required. Isolated systolic hypertension can increase regurgitant volume and therefore should be treated – vasodilators (e.g., ACE inhibitors, nifedipine) are preferred. Diuretics and ACE inhibitors are used to treat cardiac failure.

Prognosis for asymptomatic patients is generally good in chronic AR. Once symptoms develop, prognosis is poor without valve replacement (average time from symptom onset to death is 4 years with angina, 2 years with LVF). Irreversible dilatation and significant LV systolic impairment can occur in some patients before symptoms occur; therefore, follow-up is valuable. It is important to diagnose and surgically treat before the LV dilatation and failure becomes irreversible. Patients with severe AR should be educated to look out for symptoms and are followed up with echocardiography.

Surgical management
AVR is considered promptly in chronic AR if the patient is symptomatic, if there is significant progressive LVF or if there are signs

of progressive LV dilatation (end systolic diameter >55 mm). The aortic root may also need to be replaced if grossly dilated. Concurrent coronary artery bypass graft may also be required. Rarely, aortic valve repair rather than replacement may be possible.

In acute AR, urgent AVR is recommended – in the case of IE in haemodynamically stable patients, this may be deferred for 5 to 7 days for intensive antibiotic treatment.

MITRAL STENOSIS

MS is almost always caused by rheumatic fever. Other causes are rare:

1. Calcification of the mitral valve annulus in old age.
2. Congenital.
3. Malignant – lung carcinoid (systemic carcinoid causes right-sided valve disease).
4. Systemic lupus erythematosus.
5. Rheumatoid arthritis.

Other conditions may mimic MS by causing obstruction of inflow to the LV. These include left atrial (LA) myxoma, LA thrombus, large vegetations (IE) and hypertrophic cardiomyopathy.

Pathophysiology

Rheumatic fever causes thickening of the cusps and fusion of the cusps and commissures, which then become immobile and stenosed in a fish-mouth configuration. An immobile valve cannot open properly and is often regurgitant as well.

The stenosis limits passive diastolic filling of the LV, increasing the contribution of atrial systole. It also increases LA pressure, producing atrial distension, often causing atrial fibrillation (AF) and increasing pulmonary venous pressure. In turn, this can cause pulmonary hypertension and right heart failure (Fig. 15.4). This may occur over decades.

Tachycardia shortens diastole (LV filling time) and increases LA pressure. In AF, loss of coordinated LA contraction (upon which the heart has become dependent) reduces cardiac output by ~20%. Both tachycardia and AF are poorly tolerated and may precipitate the onset of pulmonary oedema in previously asymptomatic patients.

Clinical features

The main presenting features of MS are exertional dyspnoea and fatigue:

1. Dyspnoea – may be due to pulmonary oedema or pulmonary hypertension. Patients with MS are more susceptible to chest infections, which may cause dyspnoea.
2. Fatigue – due to reduced cardiac output.
3. Ankle swelling – if right heart failure develops.
4. Palpitations – AF is common in MS (due to LA enlargement) and may cause palpitations, often accompanied by a sudden deterioration in dyspnoea.
5. Haemoptysis – either frank blood (bronchial vein or alveolar capillary rupture) or frothy pink sputum (pulmonary oedema).

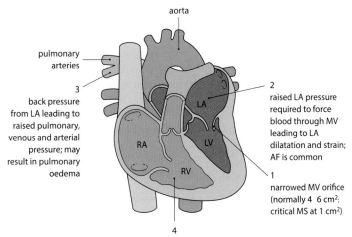

aorta

pulmonary arteries

3
back pressure from LA leading to raised pulmonary, venous and arterial pressure; may result in pulmonary oedema

2
raised LA pressure required to force blood through MV leading to LA dilatation and strain; AF is common

1
narrowed MV orifice (normally 4 6 cm^2; critical MS at 1 cm^2)

4
back pressure from pulmonary artery causes RV strain, hypertrophy and eventually RV failure with raised JVP, ascites, hepatomegaly and peripheral oedema; dilatation of RV may lead to dilatation of tricuspid valve ring and TR

Fig. 15.4 Pathophysiology of mitral stenosis. *AF*, atrial fibrillation; *LA*, left atrium; *LV*, left ventricle; *JVP*, jugular venous pressure; *MV*, mitral valve; *RA*, right atrium; *RV*, right ventricle; *TR*, tricuspid regurgitation.

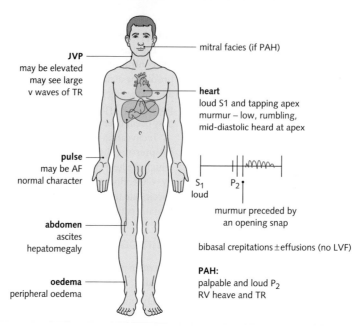

Fig. 15.5 Possible clinical findings in mitral stenosis. *AF*, atrial fibrillation; *JVP*, jugular venous pressure; *LVF*, left ventricular failure; *P₂*, pulmonary component of second heart sound; *PAH*, pulmonary arterial hypertension; *RV*, right ventricular; *RVF*, right ventricular failure; *S₁*, first heart sound; *SR*, sinus rhythm; *TR*, tricuspid regurgitation.

6. Chest pain – thought to be due to severe pulmonary hypertension.
7. Systemic emboli (higher risk with AF) – a dilated LA predisposes to thrombus formation and thromboembolism, e.g., stroke, acute limb ischaemia, renal emboli causing hypertension.

Rare symptoms secondary to LA enlargement include:

1. Hoarseness due to stretching of the recurrent laryngeal nerve.
2. Dysphagia due to oesophageal compression.
3. Left lung collapse due to compression of the left main bronchus.

Examination

Clinical findings (Fig. 15.5) include:

1. Loud first heart sound (S₁) due to slow diastolic filling.
2. Tapping apex beat (palpable S₁) that is not displaced.
3. Opening snap after the second heart sound (S₂). Both the opening snap and loud S₁ may be absent if the valve is heavily calcified.
4. Low rumbling mid-diastolic murmur following the opening snap – heard loudest with the bell at the apex with the patient lying on their left side and in full expiration. Presystolic accentuation of the murmur if the patient is in sinus rhythm (absent in AF). Severity is related to the duration, not the intensity, of the murmur.

5. Irregularly irregular pulse in AF (common as the disease progresses and with older age).
6. Signs of pulmonary oedema (bibasal crepitations, possible effusions).
7. As the pulmonary vascular resistance rises, if the patient is still in sinus rhythm, prominent a waves in the jugular venous pressure (JVP) are seen. Pulmonary hypertension in MS can cause mitral facies (malar flush), a loud palpable pulmonary component of the second heart sound (P₂), a Graham Steell murmur (pulmonary regurgitation (PR) early diastolic murmur), and a parasternal heave due to right ventricular hypertrophy. Right ventricular dilatation can cause tricuspid regurgitation (TR) with a pansystolic murmur and giant v waves in the JVP.
8. If RVF develops, signs include a raised JVP, peripheral oedema, ascites and hepatomegaly.

HINTS AND TIPS

The murmur of mitral stenosis is difficult to identify, and it is vital to listen where it is best heard: with the bell of the stethoscope at the apex with the patient lying on his or her left side and in full expiration. Without undertaking this accentuation manoeuvre, the murmur of MS cannot be excluded. The murmur is also louder after exercise.

Investigations

Electrocardiography

AF may be seen. P mitrale may be shown in LA enlargement (only in sinus rhythm) – the P wave in lead II is abnormally long (>0.12 s) and may have a bifid 'M' shape. There may also be evidence of right ventricular hypertrophy (right axis deviation, tall R wave in V1 or deep S wave in V6 >7 mm).

Chest radiography

This may show evidence of an enlarged LA (the normal concave upper left heart border can be straightened or convex, the left atrium can indent the right lung to cause the double density sign at the right heart border and the carina can be splayed with a horizontal left main bronchus). The mitral valve or valve annulus may be calcified and visible. There may be prominent pulmonary vessels or frank pulmonary oedema.

Echocardiography

This is the most accurate investigation to assess MS (Fig. 15.6). The mitral valve structure and mobility can be visualized and the cross-sectional area measured. Velocity of blood flow through the valve can be measured using Doppler (as a marker of severity). Left ventricular function, LA size, pulmonary hypertension and right ventricular complications can be evaluated. Transoesophageal echocardiography (TOE) can be helpful sometimes to identify LA thrombus.

Cardiac catheterization

This is performed on most patients before valve replacement to exclude coexistent coronary artery disease and evaluate any MR or pulmonary hypertension that may be present.

Management

Medical management

Medical treatment of MS may consist of antibiotic prophylaxis, management of AF and heart failure and follow-up.

If MS is due to rheumatic heart disease, antibiotics are given to prevent worsening of MS from recurrent rheumatic fever.

AF management is similar to that of any other cause of AF (see Chapter 14):

1. Digoxin, small dose of β-blocker or rate-limiting calcium channel antagonist – helpful for ventricular rate control in AF, as prolonging diastole allows the LV more time to fill. A β-blocker may be lifesaving in pregnancy (MS is often previously undiagnosed).
2. Direct current (DC) cardioversion – may be successful in AF of recent onset, although rhythm control can be difficult to achieve in MS. Only attempt it if confident that onset was within 48 hours or the patient has been fully anticoagulated for at least 4 weeks to reduce the risk of embolization.
3. Anticoagulation – recommended in all patients with AF or previous embolic complications; aim for international normalized ratio (INR) between 2 and 3.

Diuretics are useful to treat pulmonary and peripheral oedema.

Prognosis is good in asymptomatic MS; follow-up is helpful to determine optimal timing of intervention. Consider valve intervention in patients with symptomatic severe MS (poor outcomes if stenosis is not relieved) or pulmonary hypertension.

Endovascular management

Mitral balloon valvuloplasty is the intervention of choice if suitable. A balloon is passed across the mitral valve and inflated, separating the commissures of the stenosed valve. This procedure

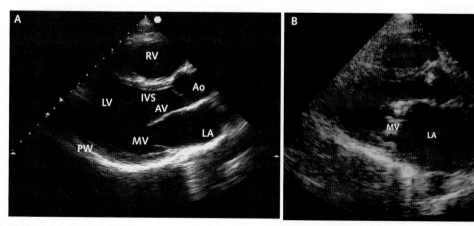

Fig. 15.6 (A) Normal echocardiogram of the parasternal long axis view (diastolic frame) (*Ao*, aorta; *AV*, aortic valve; *IVS*, intraventricular septum; *LA*, left atrium; *LV*, left ventricle; *MV*, mitral valve; *PW*, posterior LV wall; *RV*, right ventricle). (B) Echocardiogram of mitral stenosis (long axis). The mitral valve (MV) leaflets are densely thickened and the left atrium (LA) is severely dilated. (Courtesy Dr A Timmis and Dr S Brecker.)

is carried out percutaneously and only requires a local anaesthetic and light sedation. The following features make a patient unsuitable for this procedure:

1. Severe MR.
2. LA thrombus (must have TOE to exclude) or history of systemic emboli.
3. Calcified or thickened rigid mitral valve leaflets or subvalvular apparatus.

Complications include embolization, cardiac perforation and MR requiring valve replacement.

Surgical management

This is indicated in patients who have severe MS (mitral valve area ≤ 1 cm^2) with significant symptoms (New York Heart Association class III or IV), severe pulmonary hypertension (pulmonary artery systolic pressure >60 mmHg), or persistent LA thrombus. Note that restenosis may occur after percutaneous valvuloplasty or surgical valvotomy and patients should be followed up. In some patients, this does not occur for many years, whereas early restenosis within 5 years may occur in those with thickened or rigid valves.

Open mitral valvotomy

Open mitral valvotomy is performed under general anaesthetic using a median sternotomy incision and requires cardiopulmonary bypass. Any thrombus in the LA (or LA appendage) is removed, the mitral valve commissures are separated under direct vision and fused chordae tendineae can be split. It is used when balloon valvuloplasty is not suitable, e.g., in mitral valves that are too calcified or distorted, coexistent mild MR amenable to surgical repair, presence of LA thrombus, previous failed balloon valvuloplasty and coexistent disease of other heart valves.

Closed mitral valvotomy

This has been superseded by mitral valvuloplasty. It does not require cardiopulmonary bypass; access is gained through a submammary incision (curved, under the left breast) with a dilator passed into the LV apex to separate the valves. It is worth knowing this because patients in finals examinations may have this scar.

Mitral valve replacement

Mitral valve replacement (MVR) can be used for calcified or very rigid valves that cannot be split with valvuloplasty or valvotomy without causing significant regurgitation or if there is already significant coexistent MR not amenable to repair.

MITRAL REGURGITATION

MR can occur if any of the following components of the mitral valve apparatus are abnormal (Table 15.3):

Table 15.3 Causes of mitral regurgitation

Site of pathology	Cause
Mitral annulus	Senile calcification LV dilatation and annular enlargement – IHD, dilated cardiomyopathy IE (abscess formation)
Mitral valve leaflets	IE (vegetations preventing leaflet closure or causing perforation) Chronic rheumatic heart disease MVP Congenital malformation Connective tissue disorders – Marfan syndrome, Ehlers-Danlos syndrome, osteogenesis imperfecta, pseudoxanthoma elasticum Systemic lupus erythematosus (Libman-Sacks lesion)
Chordae tendineae	Idiopathic rupture Myxomatous degeneration (MVP, connective tissue disorders) Acute rheumatic fever IE
Papillary muscle	Myocardial infarction Infiltration – amyloidosis, sarcoidosis Myocarditis

IE, infective endocarditis; IHD, ischaemic heart disease; LV, left ventricular; MVP, mitral valve prolapse.

1. Mitral valve annulus.
2. Mitral valve leaflets.
3. Chordae tendineae.
4. Papillary muscles.

The most common causes are mitral valve prolapse (MVP), ventricular and annular dilatation, rheumatic heart disease, IE and ischaemic damage to the chordae tendineae or papillary muscles.

Pathophysiology

In chronic MR, to accommodate the increased volume of blood flowing back into the LA during systole, LA dilatation occurs over time, often causing AF. Regurgitant flow also increases pulmonary backpressure, leading to pulmonary hypertension, which may eventually cause RVF. The LV also gradually dilates as it compensates for chronic volume overload, which can then further worsen MR and lead to LVF. Therefore, untreated severe MR may result in biventricular failure. MS, on the other hand, does not cause LVF.

In acute MR, the left atrium does not have time to dilate to accommodate the increased volume, and the pressure increase is transmitted directly to the pulmonary veins, resulting in pulmonary oedema.

Clinical features

These vary depending upon whether the MR is chronic or acute:

1. Chronic MR develops slowly, allowing the heart to compensate, and usually presents with fatigue and reduced exercise tolerance (primarily decreased cardiac output); dyspnoea can be due to eventual LVF. Palpitations can occur due to increased stroke volume or AF. Peripheral oedema may occur with development of pulmonary hypertension.
2. Acute MR presents with severe dyspnoea due to acute pulmonary oedema or cardiogenic shock.

   Acute MR can be rapidly fatal. Look for this in patients following MI (papillary muscle rupture or dysfunction occurs in the first 7 days after MI) and in patients with IE.

Examination

Features that may be seen (Fig. 15.7) include:

1. Irregularly irregular pulse – AF is common, especially in chronic MR.
2. Displaced thrusting apex – downward and lateral displacement as the LV dilates – eventually LVF may result. Note that in MS, the apex is not displaced, as the LV is protected by the stenosed mitral valve.
3. Soft S_1 – quiet if mitral valve leaflets are malfunctioning.
4. Pansystolic murmur – best heard at the apex, may radiate to the axilla. May obliterate the second heart sound. Note that murmur intensity is not an indicator of MR severity.
5. May have a mid-systolic click and late systolic murmur in MVP.
6. Signs of LVF – i.e., bilateral basal inspiratory crepitations, basal dullness due to effusions. S_3 is less useful, as it is often present without LVF due to the increased flow volume and rapid LV filling in MR.
7. Signs of RVF (more common in acute MR or if pulmonary hypertension develops) – elevated JVP, peripheral oedema, ascites and congestive hepatomegaly.
8. Loud P_2 and right ventricular heave – may be present with pulmonary hypertension.

Investigations

Electrocardiography

There may be P mitrale or AF, and LVH. Evidence of right ventricular hypertrophy may be present in late stages.

Chest radiography

Cardiothoracic ratio may be increased due to LV enlargement. LA enlargement, pulmonary venous congestion or overt pulmonary oedema may be seen. The mitral valve or valve annulus may be visible if calcified.

Echocardiography

The mitral valve leaflets (including any vegetations) and supporting structures (e.g., ruptured chordae tendineae) can be clearly

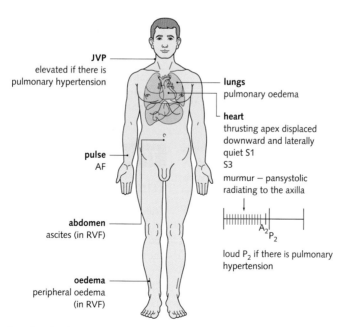

JVP
elevated if there is
pulmonary hypertension

lungs
pulmonary oedema

heart
thrusting apex displaced
downward and laterally
quiet S1
S3
murmur – pansystolic
radiating to the axilla

A_2 P_2

loud P_2 if there is pulmonary
hypertension

pulse
AF

abdomen
ascites (in RVF)

oedema
peripheral oedema
(in RVF)

Fig. 15.7 Possible clinical findings in mitral regurgitation. A_2, aortic component of second heart sound; *AF*, atrial fibrillation; P_2, pulmonary component of second heart sound; *RVF*, right ventricular failure; S_1, first heart sound; S_3, third heart sound.

visualized. The regurgitant jet is seen and severity quantified using colour Doppler. The LA and LV may be enlarged; LV dysfunction may be seen in severe MR. Pulmonary artery pressures can be estimated. Suitability for mitral valve repair is better evaluated with TOE.

Cardiac catheterization

This is performed to further assess the severity of the MR, to measure pulmonary hypertension and to exclude other valve lesions and coronary artery disease in the assessment for valve replacement. Most patients have minimal MR on echocardiography and do not require catheterization.

Management

Medical management

Vasodilators (e.g., ACE inhibitors) are valuable in hypertension or cardiac failure to prevent increased afterload worsening MR. If LV function is impaired, other standard management (e.g., β-blockers, diuretics) is helpful. Management of AF is important with rate-limiting medicines and anticoagulation.

Percutaneous mitral valve repair

In the last few years, percutaneous devices have been developed to reduce MR by drawing in the mitral valve ring or clipping together the centre of the two mitral valve leaflets: transcatheter edge-to-edge repair (TEER). This is considered in patients unsuitable for surgery and those with heart failure.

Cardiac resynchronization therapy

In functional MR (dilated annulus secondary to e.g., dilated or ischaemic cardiomyopathy), cardiac resynchronization therapy (CRT) with dual ventricular pacing is indicated in patients with significantly reduced LV ejection fraction and left bundle branch block. It may improve leaflet coaptation and reduce the severity of MR.

Surgical intervention

Patients are considered for surgery if there is symptomatic severe MR, progressive cardiac enlargement or deterioration of LV function. Surgery may be considered if AF or pulmonary hypertension has developed in asymptomatic patients, as these are associated with a worse prognosis. If possible, it is important to act before irreversible LV damage and severe pulmonary hypertension have occurred.

In acute MR, in addition to aggressive medical therapy, surgery is indicated if there is acute LVF; without it, the patient is unlikely to survive.

Mitral valve repair

This may take the form of mitral annuloplasty, repair of a ruptured chorda or repair of a mitral valve leaflet. These procedures are performed on patients with mobile noncalcified and nonthickened valves. Both repair and replacement of the mitral valve require a median sternotomy incision and cardiopulmonary bypass.

Mitral valve replacement

This is only performed if mitral valve repair is not possible and the higher operative risks are deemed necessary. Replacement may paradoxically worsen LV function by preventing reduction of afterload through MR or interrupting the continuity of the annulus with the chordae tendineae and the papillary muscles.

Mitral valve prolapse

MVP is also known as floppy mitral valve or click-murmur syndrome. Important points include:

1. This is common (2%–3% of the population), with a female preponderance.
2. The mitral valve may billow minimally into the LA with a click but no regurgitation, or it may cause varying degrees of MR.
3. Most cases are idiopathic, but it is seen more frequently in connective tissue disorders, e.g., Marfan syndrome.
4. Most patients are asymptomatic and are diagnosed incidentally on examination. Infrequently, some patients present with fatigue, atypical chest pain, palpitations, infective endocarditis or embolic phenomena.
5. Examination reveals a mid-systolic click at the apex. If there is regurgitation, this may be followed by a systolic murmur of MR. The murmur may be best heard at the left sternal edge or round the patient's back.
6. Most patients require no further treatment other than reassurance, as MVP generally follows a benign course. However, it is one of the commonest causes of MR, which can become severe as the chordae tendineae elongates. Rarely, rupture can cause acute severe MR. It is a common predisposing condition to IE.

TRICUSPID DISEASE

Tricuspid stenosis

Tricuspid stenosis (TS) is rare. It is almost always due to rheumatic fever but only affects a small subset of patients – the mitral and aortic valves are usually also affected. Infrequently, it can be due to carcinoid syndrome or congenital tricuspid atresia.

Clinical features

The most prominent symptoms are usually related to concurrent left-sided valvular disease. However, if TS is severe, this may prevent enough forward flow to cause breathlessness; conspicuously little orthopnoea or paroxysmal nocturnal dyspnoea should raise suspicion of severe TS. Fatigue may be present due to reduced cardiac output. Systemic congestion (hepatic congestion, ascites and peripheral oedema) may be pronounced; severe generalized oedema is known as anasarca.

The most obvious examination findings are those of venous congestion. The JVP is raised with large a waves (if the patient is in sinus rhythm) and slow y descent. There may be hepatomegaly, ascites and peripheral oedema. A soft mid-diastolic murmur at the lower left sternal edge may be heard, although this can be difficult to differentiate from the murmur of MS. Lack of the parasternal heave of RV hypertrophy may be helpful.

Management

The mainstay of management in severe TS is surgery; this may be either valve replacement or valvotomy. Concurrent operation on other valves might be necessary. Balloon valvuloplasty is very rarely used. Medical management with salt restriction and diuretics may help with systemic congestion.

Tricuspid regurgitation

Most cases of TR are due to dilatation of the tricuspid annulus resulting from RV dilatation. This may be due to any cause of RVF or pulmonary hypertension.

Occasionally, the tricuspid valve is affected by IE (usually in intravenous drug abusers). Rheumatic disease can cause TR uncommonly. Rarer causes include congenital malformations, including Ebstein anomaly and carcinoid syndrome.

> ### CLINICAL NOTES
>
> Ebstein anomaly is a congenital malformation where there is downward displacement of the tricuspid valve into the body of the RV. The valve is regurgitant and malformed. The condition is associated with other structural cardiac abnormalities and a high incidence of both supraventricular and ventricular tachyarrhythmias.

Clinical features

The symptoms and signs are due to the backpressure effects of the regurgitant jet into the RA.

The most common features are fatigue due to reduced cardiac output and symptoms of RVF, including discomfort secondary to hepatic congestion, ascites or peripheral oedema. Patients usually present with symptoms of the disease causing the underlying RVF; the TR is often an incidental finding.

Examination

The regurgitant jet is transmitted to the venous system, causing a 'giant' v wave in the jugular venous waveform (Fig. 15.8). There are signs of RVF with systemic venous congestion, and there may

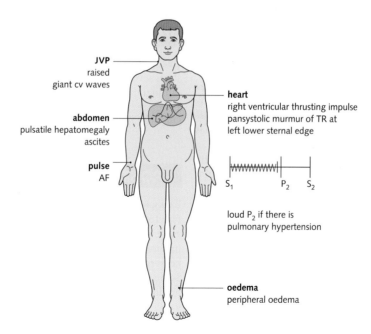

Fig. 15.8 Possible clinical findings in tricuspid regurgitation. Look out for signs of an underlying cause of right-heart failure such as mitral valve disease or pulmonary disease. *AF*, atrial fibrillation; *JVP*, jugular venous pressure; *P₂*, pulmonary component of second heart sound; *S₁*, first heart sound; *S₂*, second heart sound.

be pulsatile hepatomegaly. AF is common. There may be signs corresponding to the cause in functional TR.

Management

TR due to right ventricular overload can improve with treatment of the cause. The mainstay of management is medical, with diuretics and ACE inhibitors to treat the fluid overload (which is due to LVF in most cases). Isolated RVF is less common; in this case, use caution with diuretics, as they may adversely reduce left ventricular preload and consequently cardiac output. Instead, cautious fluid challenges may be helpful (see Chapter 13). Annuloplasty in functional dilatation or tricuspid valve replacement may be considered in very severe cases. In IE, the excision of the infected valve without immediate replacement is usually well tolerated if there is no concurrent pulmonary hypertension and avoids infection of the prosthetic valve; the valve is replaced when the infection is controlled.

PULMONARY DISEASE

Pulmonary stenosis

Pulmonary stenosis (PS) is usually congenital, e.g., tetralogy of Fallot, Noonan syndrome, congenital rubella syndrome, but rarely can be caused by carcinoid syndrome or rheumatic heart disease.

Clinical features

If mild, PS is asymptomatic. If severe, there may be features of RVF (systemic venous congestion). If PS occurs in a neonate, there may be cyanosis due to right-to-left shunting. In neonates and infants, PS may present with failure to thrive or as an incidental murmur at neonatal check. In older children and adults, there may be an RV equivalent of AS symptoms (exertional fatigue, exertional light-headedness and angina).

Possible signs on examination include an ejection systolic murmur in the pulmonary area, an ejection click preceding the murmur and wide splitting of second heart sound or quiet P2. In severe PS, there may be a prominent a wave in the JVP, RV heave and features of RVF.

Management

Balloon valvuloplasty is the mainstay of treatment, with surgical valvotomy less common.

Pulmonary regurgitation

PR is most frequently due to dilatation of the valve ring or pulmonary artery. This can be secondary to pulmonary hypertension due to left-sided heart disease, for instance, in MS (Graham Steell murmur), primary pulmonary hypertension or Eisenmenger syndrome. Marfan syndrome can also cause dilatation. The valves can be affected by disease, such as IE, rheumatic fever, carcinoid syndrome and tetralogy of Fallot (or previous surgical correction).

Clinical features

Frequently, the clinical features of the underlying disease causing PR are the main issue, and the murmur of PR is found incidentally without causing much problem. If isolated, PR is frequently asymptomatic, although in severe cases may cause RVF. In association with pulmonary hypertension, it can exacerbate RVF, and pulmonary septic emboli may be seen if PR is due to IE.

Possible signs include a low-pitched early diastolic murmur in the pulmonary and tricuspid area, which may also be accompanied by an ejection systolic flow murmur due to increased RV stroke volume. In severe PR, the murmur is high-pitched due to the forceful jet and best heard at the left parasternal edge (i.e., similar to that in AR but with signs of severe pulmonary hypertension, wide splitting of S_2, RV heave and RVF).

Management

Treat any underlying disease. PR is usually benign and mostly does not require treatment. Valve replacement may be considered in PR caused by surgical correction of tetralogy of Fallot.

ASSESSING THE SEVERITY OF A VALVE LESION

Once a valve lesion has been diagnosed, it is important to evaluate its severity. This is judged in most cases by clinical and echocardiographic means; angiography is occasionally also helpful. The more common left-sided valvular lesions are discussed here (Table 15.4).

PROSTHETIC HEART VALVES

Examples of mechanical and biological heart valves are shown in Fig. 15.9 and Table 15.5. Aim to be familiar with mechanical valve sounds, as they are common in exams. Mechanical valves impart a metallic quality to the first (mitral) or second (aortic) heart sound, and both opening and closing clicks can be heard. Some patients may have both types of valves. Biological valves produce normal heart sounds. All patients with prosthetic aortic valves (even tissue valves) will have a systolic flow murmur. Patients with mitral valves may have a quiet pansystolic murmur due to turbulent LV blood flow, but loud pansystolic murmurs require investigation. Diastolic murmurs are generally a worrying sign and require investigation for endocarditis, valve

Table 15.4 Severity markers for valve disease

Valve disease	Severity markers
AS	Presence of AS symptoms. Slow-rising pulse and narrow pulse pressure, obscured or absent A_2, paradoxical splitting of S_2, S_4, associated thrill, generally a louder/harsher or later peaking murmur (NB: if severe AS complicated by LVF, murmur may be very quiet or disappear; may only have signs of severe LVF and low CO). Severe AS (jet velocity >4 m/s, aortic valve area <1.0 cm^2, mean gradient >40 mmHg) and poor LV function on echo or cardiac catheterization.
AR	Symptoms and signs of LVF (may be one of the only signs in acute AR). Collapsing pulse and wide pulse pressure, eponymous signs, S_3, increased decrescendo murmur duration, Austin Flint murmur. Size of regurgitation jet and LV enlargement/dysfunction on echo or cardiac catheterization.
MS	Symptoms of pulmonary congestion or RVF. OS earlier and closer to S_2 (OS/loud S_1 may be lost in severe MS), soft S1, increased murmur duration (quieter if reduced CO), mitral facies, signs of pulmonary congestion, signs of pulmonary hypertension and RVF, Graham Steell murmur, signs of TR. Severe MS (valve area <1.0 cm^2, mean gradient >10 mmHg) or significant pulmonary HTN (pulmonary artery systolic pressure >50 mmHg) on echo or cardiac catheterization.
MR	Symptoms and signs of LVF, pulmonary HTN or RVF. Size of regurgitant jet, LA enlargement, LV enlargement/dysfunction or evidence of pulmonary HTN on echo and cardiac catheterization.

A_2, aortic second heart sound; AR, aortic regurgitation; AS, aortic stenosis; CO, cardiac output; echo, echocardiography; HTN, hypertension; LA, left atrial; LV, left ventricular; LVF, left ventricular failure; MR, mitral regurgitation; MS, mitral stenosis; OS, opening snap; RVF, right ventricular failure; S_1, first heart sound; S_2, second heart sound; S_3, third heart sound; S_4, fourth heart sound; TR, tricuspid regurgitation.

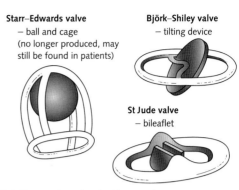

Fig. 15.9 Types of mechanical heart valve.

Table 15.5 Types of biological heart valve

Type of valve	Features
Xenograft	Manufactured from porcine valve or bovine pericardium and mounted on a frame (on chest X-ray, only the mounting ring can be seen).
Homograft	Cadaveric valve graft, does not require prosthetic mounting ring. A subtype is an autograft (from the same patient), e.g., a pulmonary valve transplanted into the aortic position.

thrombosis, paravalvular leak or valve failure. A short, quiet diastolic murmur in a mitral prosthesis may be innocent but it is better to investigate if there is any doubt.

RED FLAG

Remember to investigate urgently for valvular dysfunction if a patient with a prosthetic valve develops unexplained heart failure.

All patients must be anticoagulated for life with mechanical valves. The target INR varies between 2.5 and 3.5, depending on the type of valve, the position of the valve and other patient risk factors for thromboembolism. Lower target INRs are used when thromboembolic risk is lower, e.g., the St Jude valve is less thrombogenic than the Starr-Edwards valve, and aortic valves are less thrombogenic than mitral or tricuspid valves. Targets vary with local, national and international guidelines. Anticoagulation is not required with bioprosthetic valves, unless there is another indication, e.g., coexistent AF (common in mitral disease).

Bileaflet valves are currently the most widely used mechanical valve due to their superior haemodynamic characteristics and lower risk of thromboembolism.

Mechanical valves last longer than bioprosthetic valves. Bioprosthetic valves may last an average of 10 years, but failure may occur in as early as 4 to 5 years or as late as 20 years. Mechanical valves have been shown to usually last more than 25 years.

In general, older patients (e.g., over 65) are suitable for bioprosthetic valves, as the valves are likely to last the patient's lifetime. Younger patients should be considered for mechanical valves (even though this will entail the risks of lifelong anticoagulation), as the mortality for repeat valve replacement is much higher. However, some younger patients may choose bioprosthetic valves for lifestyle reasons, accepting the risk of tissue valve deterioration and the likely need for a future second valve replacement. Increasingly, patients with bioprosthetic valve failure are being treated with a 'valve-in-valve' procedure where a TAVI valve is inserted into the bioprosthetic valve.

In MS, mechanical valves are used frequently, as MS tends to present at a younger age and often the patient is in AF, for which they will already require long-term anticoagulation. Bioprosthetic valves are generally preferred in the tricuspid position, as mechanical valves in this position have a much higher risk of thromboembolism.

Although guidelines have changed to state that antibiotic prophylaxis against IE is not required in native valve disease, it should still be considered in those with prosthetic valves, especially during procedures with a high risk of bacteraemia, as the outcome of IE in prosthetic valves is much worse.

INFECTIVE ENDOCARDITIS

IE is an infection of the endocardium. This usually involves the heart valves (native or prosthetic), but it can affect the chordae tendineae, the surface of the cardiac chambers or blood vessels, and indwelling cardiac devices (e.g., pacemakers leads).

The development of IE depends on a number of factors:

1. Endocardial abnormalities.
2. Cardiac haemodynamic abnormalities.
3. Presence of bacteraemia.
4. Host immune response.
5. Organism virulence.

Transient bacteraemia is common, e.g., brushing teeth and chewing, as well as with both dental and nondental procedures. Despite this, IE is rare; therefore, the endothelium of a healthy individual with normal cardiac anatomy is well protected.

IE occurs more commonly at sites of endothelial injury, for example, on damaged or congenitally abnormal valves, or any area damaged by a high-pressure jet through a narrow orifice (e.g., ventricular septal defect). The resultant inflammation and platelet and fibrin aggregation at the site are easier for bacteria to adhere to; the infecting organism becomes incorporated into the site to form a vegetation. This causes further destruction of the valve(s), often leading to valvular regurgitation (either perforation of the valve leaflets or vegetations and adhesions impeding valve closure). These vegetations can also throw off emboli to other organs, causing ischaemia or infection.

There is mortality of up to 20% even with treatment, largely due to these potentially fatal complications:

1. Local destructive effects – valve regurgitation (occasionally stenosis with large vegetations), paravalvular abscess or fistulae, prosthetic valve dehiscence, arrhythmia, pericarditis and myocardial rupture. These can cause cardiac failure and cardiogenic shock, sometimes rapidly.
2. Embolization of infected or noninfected fragments (may be clinically silent) – left-sided IE can result in mycotic

(infected) aneurysm, stroke or cerebral abscesses, digital infarcts, renal/hepatic/splenic abscesses, renal/splenic infarcts (hepatic infarcts are rare because the liver is supplied by the hepatic artery and the hepatic portal system), MI from coronary emboli and ischaemic bowel. Right-sided IE can lead to septic pulmonary emboli.
3. Type III autoimmune reaction to the organism – resulting in the deposition of immune (antibody-antigen) complexes and a subsequent inflammatory response. A diffuse or focal glomerulonephritis or arthritis may occur.

HINTS AND TIPS

If you remember these three classes of complications, it is easy to fit symptoms and signs into each category. Classifying signs according to the pathophysiology shows that you have a full understanding of the disease process and will impress examiners.

Previously, endocarditis was classified by onset as acute or subacute; now it is classified according to the valves involved, whether native or prosthetic, whether community or healthcare-acquired and the causative organism.

Diagnostic criteria

The modified Duke criteria are used in the diagnosis of IE (Table 15.6).

COMMON PITFALLS

The modified Duke criteria do not require either major criteria to be met, as infective endocarditis can be culture-negative and vegetations are not always visualized. Conversely, not all endocarditis is infective (termed *marantic endocarditis*) and can occur with systemic lupus erythematosus, other connective tissue diseases and malignancy.

In injection drug users, microorganisms are introduced via the intravenous route or from injection-related soft tissue infections, increasing risk of developing IE (actually several times higher than in patients with predisposing heart conditions, such as rheumatic heart disease or prosthetic valves).

Epidemiology

Traditionally, the main predisposing condition was rheumatic heart disease; however, the incidence of rheumatic fever in developed countries has dropped significantly because of improved social conditions and antibiotic therapy. Now, incidence of

Table 15.6 Modified Duke criteria for the diagnosis of infective endocarditis (IE)

Criteria	Description
Major	
1	Positive **blood culture** – one of:
1	1 – Typical IE microorganism from two separate blood cultures: • Viridans streptococci, *Streptococcus gallolyticus (S. bovis)* or HACEK* group, or • *Staphylococcus aureus* or community-acquired enterococci, in the absence of a primary focus
1	2 – Persistently positive blood cultures with microorganism consistent with IE, defined as: • Two positive cultures drawn >12 h apart • All of three or majority of four separate cultures (first and last samples drawn >1 h apart)
	3 – Single positive blood culture for *Coxiella burnetii* or anti–phase I IgG antibody titre >1:800
2	Evidence of **endocardial involvement** – one of:
	1 – Positive echocardiogram: vegetation, abscess, pseudoaneurysm, intracardiac fistula, valvular perforation or aneurysm, or new partial dehiscence of a prosthetic valve
	2 – New valvular regurgitation (worsening or changing of preexisting murmur not sufficient)
Minor	
1	**Predisposition**: predisposing heart condition or injection drug use
2	**Fever** ≥38.0°C (100.4°F)
3	**Vascular phenomena**: major arterial emboli, septic pulmonary infarcts, mycotic aneurysm, intracranial haemorrhage, conjunctival haemorrhages, Janeway lesions
4	**Immunological phenomena**: glomerulonephritis, Osler nodes, Roth spots, rheumatoid factor
5	**Microbiological evidence**: positive blood culture but does not meet a major criterion as noted above, or serological evidence of active infection with an organism consistent with IE

Clinical diagnosis of infective endocarditis (IE) is based on:

Definite IE:
• Two major criteria, or
• One major and three minor criteria, or
• Five minor criteria

Possible IE:
• One major and one minor criteria, or
• Three minor criteria

* HACEK group: Haemophilus spp., Aggregatibacter spp. [previously known as Actinobacillus spp.], Cardiobacterium spp., Eikenella corrodens, Kingella spp.

infective endocarditis in the UK is increasing due to an increase in the following:

1. Number of prosthetic valve insertions, pacemakers and long lines.
2. Number of patients with congenital heart disease surviving to adulthood.
3. Elderly population.
4. Injection drug abuse.
5. Antibiotic resistance.

With this change in the population affected by IE, the organisms are also changing. Staphylococci have overtaken streptococci as the most common cause due to increased healthcare-associated infection and injection drug abuse. Coagulase-negative staphylococci, which used to be uncommon, are now the most common organisms seen on prosthetic valves (Table 15.7).

There are a number of conditions that put people at increased risk of IE (see clinical note box on the next page). Previously, such patients were routinely given antibiotic prophylaxis before procedures anticipated to cause bacteraemia. Since 2008, the National Institute for Health and Care Excellence (NICE) no longer recommends routine antibiotic prophylaxis and recommends that infections are treated promptly in those at risk (CG64). NICE recommends patients receive prophylactic antibiotics (chosen to cover common organisms that cause endocarditis) only when they undergo gastrointestinal or genitourinary procedures where there is already suspected infection. This change was made due to lack of evidence of benefit (there is no association between these procedures and the development of IE) and a known risk of harm (including anaphylaxis and the development of antibiotic resistance). This has caused controversy, and antibiotics should still be considered in patients at the highest risk.

Table 15.7 Common causative organisms in infective endocarditis

Organism	Comments
Staphylococcus aureus	Acute; highly invasive, can cause rapid destruction of previously normal valves, abscesses, septic emboli and high mortality; common in patients with indwelling lines, skin and soft tissue infections, postoperatively and in injection drug users; has overtaken streptococci to become the most common cause.
Viridans streptococci [α-haemolytic] (e.g., *S. mutans*, *S. mitis*, *S. sanguinis*, *S. anginosus* group, *S. gallolyticus*)	Subacute; common with brushing teeth, poor dentition and after dental procedures, tonsillectomy or bronchoscopy, as they are upper respiratory commensals; predominantly found on rheumatic heart valves or congenitally abnormal valves, although can be found in other situations. *S. gallolyticus* (formerly *S. bovis*) and *Streptococcus anginosus* group (formerly *S. milleri*) are found in the gastrointestinal tract and are associated with colorectal malignancies, and patients should be considered for colonoscopy.
Coagulase-negative staphylococci (e.g., *S. epidermidis*, *S. lugdunensis*)	*S. epidermidis* (a skin commensal) is the most common cause within 2 months of prosthetic valve replacement (the high-risk period), may be introduced from a wound infection; after the early period, the risk is much lower and the above organisms are more common. *S. epidermidis* can also be found on native valves. *S. lugdunensis* is more invasive. May be mistaken for a contaminant.
Enterococci (*E. faecalis*, *E. faecium*)	May be acute but more often subacute; third most common cause after staphylococci and streptococci; usually in patients with gastrointestinal or urinary tract infections or surgery; can cause endocarditis in any situation.
HACEK group (fastidious gram-negative bacteria)	These fastidious, slow-growing organisms are commensals of the upper respiratory tract and require prolonged culture to be detected. May be resistant to penicillin.
Coxiella burnetii (Q fever)	Subacute; usually a history of contact with farm animals; can be associated with a purpuric rash, pneumonia or hepatitis.
Other gram-negative bacteria (e.g., *Chlamydia*, *Brucella*, *Bartonella*), diphtheroids	These are less common causes of endocarditis. Brucellosis is associated with contact with farm animals. *Bartonella* may be from cats (cat scratch fever) or infected lice (trench fever). Diphtheroids (*Corynebacterium spp.*) are gram-positive bacilli and an important cause in prosthetic valves.
Fungi (*Candida*, *Aspergillus*, *Histoplasma*)	More common in immunocompromised patients, injection drug users (*Candida* from contaminated lemon juice used to dissolve heroin) and in those with indwelling catheters or prosthetic valves; invasive and can affect normal valves; associated with abscesses, emboli and high mortality. There may be concurrent bacterial infection.

Note that infective endocarditis may be polymicrobial (involve multiple organisms), and a significant number of cases are culture negative (grow no organism).

CLINICAL NOTES

Conditions predisposing to infective endocarditis (**Bold denotes highest risk group**):

- Acquired valvular heart disease.
- **Prosthetic valve.**
- Congenital heart disease (**especially cyanotic heart disease with residual defect, within 6 months of complete repair with prosthetic material, or residual defect at the site of repair with prosthetic material**).
- Hypertrophic cardiomyopathy.
- **Previous infective endocarditis.**

Clinical features

History

The duration of the symptoms is variable, from a few days to several months. This tends to reflect the virulence of the organism – *Staphylococcus aureus* causes rapid valvular destruction and presents early, whereas a *Staphylococcus epidermidis* infection of a prosthetic valve may take a few months to present. Previous antibiotics (partially treated endocarditis) also cause a subacute picture, and symptoms and signs vary by site of infection. Common symptoms are:

1. Fever
2. Sweats
3. Anorexia and weight loss
4. General malaise

Other symptoms may relate to cardiac complications, embolic events and vasculitic phenomena:

1. Valve dysfunction and heart failure in severe cases.
2. Stroke (may be the presenting complaint).
3. Other systemic emboli (symptoms depending on site) – bear in mind IE if the source of emboli is unknown.
4. Septic pulmonary emboli from tricuspid IE (pleuritic chest pain, breathlessness, cough and haemoptysis).
5. Myalgia and arthralgia (relatively common).

COMMON PITFALLS

Given symptoms are frequently nonspecific, the diagnosis of IE can be easily missed unless there is a high index of suspicion. Early treatment reduces the risk of severe complications, such as stroke and rapid valve destruction (with heart failure or cardiogenic shock), and therefore lowers mortality. Until proven otherwise, any patient with a fever and a new murmur should be investigated and potentially treated for endocarditis.

For clues about the causative organism, enquire about:

1. History of rheumatic fever, other valvular disease, valve replacement or indwelling cardiac devices/lines.
2. History of any dental work, operations or infections.
3. History of intravenous drug abuse.
4. Occupation and any pets or environmental contacts.

It is also important to find out about any drug allergies – this may affect the choice of long-term intravenous antibiotics. Ensure you clarify the nature of drug allergies, as ruling out penicillins unnecessarily may result in prolonged drug combinations particularly toxic to the kidneys, e.g., vancomycin and gentamicin.

Examination

A thorough examination of all systems is vital (Fig. 15.10). Aim to identify the multiple components of the modified Duke criteria and cardiac complications not included in the criteria (e.g., heart failure); also look for other possible sources of infection or fever.

COMMON PITFALLS

Some findings (e.g., finger clubbing, splenomegaly) take a few weeks to develop and do not occur with a short history of illness (i.e., acute endocarditis). Although some of these signs (e.g., Osler nodes, Roth spots) are famously associated with IE, they are rare, and none of the characteristic findings in IE are pathognomonic. However, the diagnosis is suggested by the constellation of signs and symptoms.

The following signs are characteristic of IE:

1. Finger clubbing – seen with chronic subacute endocarditis. Other causes include cyanotic congenital heart disease, suppurative lung disease, lung cancer and inflammatory bowel disease.

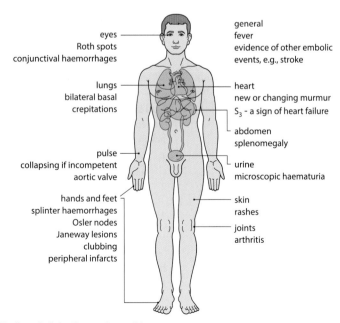

eyes
Roth spots
conjunctival haemorrhages

lungs
bilateral basal
crepitations

pulse
collapsing if incompetent
aortic valve

hands and feet
splinter haemorrhages
Osler nodes
Janeway lesions
clubbing
peripheral infarcts

general
fever
evidence of other embolic
events, e.g., stroke

heart
new or changing murmur
S_3 - a sign of heart failure

abdomen
splenomegaly

urine
microscopic haematuria

skin
rashes

joints
arthritis

Fig. 15.10 Possible clinical findings in infective endocarditis.

2. Splinter haemorrhages – infrequent in IE (~10%); in most patients, these relate to trauma.
3. Osler nodes – painful raised papules on the pulps of digits (infrequent) due to immune complex deposition with vasculitic changes.
4. Janeway lesions – nontender erythematous flat lesions on the palms or soles (rare). They represent peripheral microabscesses from emboli.
5. Pulse – collapsing pulse may be found in AR with IE. Occasionally, bradycardia (due to complete heart block) may be present if there is an aortic root abscess complicating aortic valve endocarditis.
6. Murmur – usually that of a regurgitant valve, although large vegetations may cause stenosis and, of course, a flow murmur is possible in sepsis of any origin. It is important to perform regular cardiac auscultation because the murmur may change due to progressive valve damage; this may signify imminent valve failure, and a repeat echocardiogram may be necessary to evaluate any progression.
7. Congestive cardiac failure – remember to look for this complication. In IE, this is most commonly due to valve disruption or rupture of chordae tendineae.
8. Splenomegaly – common in subacute endocarditis.
9. Rash – a vasculitic (purpuric) rash may be found.
10. Roth spots (retinal haemorrhages with a pale centre) and subconjunctival or buccal haemorrhages.
11. Examine for neurological features carefully – there may be a cerebral infarct from emboli, a haemorrhagic stroke from a mycotic aneurysm or multiple cerebral abscesses. Confusion is common.
12. There may be evidence of other peripheral emboli, such as digital or nailfold infarcts, or abdominal tenderness from splenic or mesenteric infarcts.
13. Inflamed joints – although joint pain is common, a truly swollen hot joint is uncommon; if it occurs, it should be considered as a possible septic arthritis and source of IE until excluded.
14. Look for poor dentition, which may be the source of bacteraemia.

> **HINTS AND TIPS**
>
> Remember to listen for prosthetic valve sounds – this is a risk factor for endocarditis, an infection that is notoriously difficult to eradicate; patients will often require cardiac surgery to remove infected material, and prosthetic valve infective endocarditis has a higher mortality rate than that in native valves. Working closely with microbiologists and cardiothoracic surgeons is crucial.

Investigations

As expected with the modified Duke criteria, blood cultures and echocardiography are central to the diagnosis and management of IE.

Blood tests
Blood cultures

These are the most important of all the investigations, as it is crucial to identify the causative organism and its sensitivities to guide the prolonged antibiotic therapy required. Positive blood cultures are usually obtained in around 95% of cases of bacterial endocarditis if taken before antibiotic therapy.

In contrast to most other infections, *three to six sets* of (aerobic and anaerobic) cultures should be performed to increase the chances of isolating the cause. If possible, at least three sets should be taken with the first and last at least 1 hour apart *before* commencing antibiotic therapy. If the patient is very ill and there is a high index of suspicion of IE, it is appropriate to start antibiotics after one or two sets have been obtained; otherwise, it is preferable to establish the microbial cause first.

> **HINTS AND TIPS**
>
> When taking blood cultures, strict aseptic technique, multiple venepuncture sites and avoiding indwelling lines are crucial to reduce risk of contamination. Clean the skin thoroughly with a 2% chlorhexidine swab and allow to dry, and do not re-palpate. Take the blood and then inject it into the culture bottles using new needles, or if available, use direct attachments between the needle and swabbed culture bottles. Maintain aseptic technique throughout.

Full blood count

Anaemia of chronic disease is common (~90%) in patients who have a subacute presentation. Other findings can include:

1. Leucocytosis – a sign of inflammation (usually a neutrophilia).
2. Thrombocytosis – may be seen as part of the acute phase response.
3. Thrombocytopenia – may occasionally be an indication of disseminated intravascular coagulopathy, a severe disorder with a high mortality rate.

Inflammatory markers

ESR and CRP are raised (>90%). CRP is particularly valuable as an acute marker of disease activity, and repeated measurements every few days provide information on the patient's response to treatment.

Renal function

This may be impaired due to infarction or immune complex-mediated glomerulonephritis, or due to reduced renal perfusion in cardiac failure. This should be monitored during treatment, as aminoglycoside (gentamicin) and glycopeptide (vancomycin) antibiotics and disease progression may all cause renal impairment.

Liver function tests

These may be deranged due to septic microemboli.

Serological tests

These may be considered for *Coxiella*, *Brucella*, *Bartonella*, *Legionella* and *Chlamydia* if there is possible exposure and blood cultures remain negative.

Urinalysis

Microscopic haematuria is common in ~90% of patients with IE; therefore, if you suspect this diagnosis, always perform a bedside urine dipstick (quick, easy and cheap). Formal urine microscopy may also reveal casts in associated immune-complex glomerulonephritis.

Electrocardiography

In aortic abscess formation, development of AV block may be seen – regular ECGs are helpful in patients with IE at the aortic valve due to this risk. Embolization to the coronary arteries may cause MI with ECG changes.

Chest radiography

This may show signs of pulmonary oedema or evidence of pulmonary abscesses from septic emboli in right-sided IE.

Echocardiography

Echocardiography (echo) may demonstrate vegetations and their size, valvular regurgitation and its severity, para-valvular leak with prosthetic valves, and complications such as abscesses or systolic dysfunction. Repeat echo is helpful to assess progression or development of complications. Transthoracic echo is not as sensitive for IE as transoesophageal echo (which is over 90% sensitive).

Echo may help confirm the diagnosis, but even if vegetations are not detected, IE cannot be excluded if the clinical picture is suggestive, as echo is not 100% sensitive. It is also not 100% specific – oscillating masses thought to be vegetations may be noninfective in origin.

Management

There are two main aims in the management of IE:

1. To treat the infection effectively with the minimum of antimicrobial-related complications, surgery if required and source control.

2. To diagnose and treat complications (e.g., congestive cardiac failure, severe valvular regurgitation, peripheral abscesses, renal failure).

Treatment of infection

If IE is suspected and the patient is unwell, empirical intravenous antibiotic therapy is started as soon as the blood cultures have been taken. The choice of agent can then be modified once the organism is known. Most commonly, therapy will consist of antibiotics, although antifungals may be required. Surgery may be required. Any identifiable source of infection should be controlled to prevent recurrent bacteraemia. The patient requires a thorough dental examination and, for example, a tooth with an apical abscess should be extracted.

Choice of antibiotic regimen

Antibiotics not only treat infection but also reduce risk of complications, such as embolization of vegetations. Always discuss the choice of antibiotic regimen with the microbiologist as soon as possible. Choice of empirical therapy depends on whether the valve affected is native or prosthetic, most likely organisms (likely route of infection), local epidemiology (including resistance), any prior antibiotic therapy and patient allergies.

Penicillin-based antibiotics are effective against gram-positive cocci (usually benzylpenicillin for streptococci, flucloxacillin for staphylococci, and ampicillin or amoxicillin for enterococci, as they are resistant to benzylpenicillin). Bactericidal regimens are more effective to eradicate infection, as bacteriostatic therapy inhibits microbial growth but allows resurgence of infection once antibiotics are stopped. Aminoglycosides (e.g., gentamicin) are typically combined with the above penicillins for synergistic activity to achieve bactericidal action. A reasonable first-line regimen may be amoxicillin, flucloxacillin and gentamicin in native valve infections before the organism is known.

In empirical treatment for prosthetic valves or if methicillin-resistant *Staphylococcus aureus* is found, vancomycin is generally used instead of penicillin and rifampicin may be added.

When the organism and its sensitivity is known, discuss the most suitable ongoing agents and duration with the microbiologist. Sensitivity of the organisms to antibiotics may be reported with the minimum inhibitory concentration; if it is not satisfactory, an antimicrobial may be added or switched.

Duration of antibiotic therapy

The avascular nature of the valves protects the microorganism from host defences, and formation of a biofilm on prosthetic material can further prevent clearance using antimicrobials. Antibiotic tolerance (bacteriostatic rather than bactericidal action) is another problem. This is why prolonged antibiotic courses are required to fully eradicate infection and prevent serious complications.

Required duration of therapy depends on the:

- Presence of a prosthetic valve (always at least 6 weeks).
- Causative organism and its sensitivity to the antibiotics used.
- Size of the vegetation(s).
- Presence of complications.
- Clinical response to therapy.

Most bacterial infections require 4 to 6 weeks of intravenous therapy. As little as 2 weeks may be sufficient if response is swift with small vegetations on native valves without any complications and if the organism is suitable. In some situations, it may be possible to switch to oral antibiotics. Remember, the patient must be closely monitored after changing to oral or finishing therapy. If there is any evidence of recurrent disease activity, intravenous therapy should be recommenced.

Surgery

Although operative intervention in active IE carries a significant morbidity and mortality rate, in some high-risk cases, surgery is required to control infection or prevent worsening heart failure or embolism. This is especially the case in endocarditis associated with prosthetic valves or those caused by *Staphylococcus aureus* or fungi. The difficult decision regarding whether to undertake surgery and the timing of surgery is made in collaboration with cardiothoracic surgeons after consideration of high-risk IE features and comorbidities.

Surgery may involve drainage of abscesses or debridement of infected material, repair or valve replacement; indications are listed in the box below. The patient should complete a full course of intravenous antibiotic treatment postoperatively.

CLINICAL NOTES

Indications for surgery in infective endocarditis:
- Heart failure.
- Uncontrolled infection (or abscess/fistula).
- Large left-sided vegetations with systemic embolization or high embolic risk.

Management of complications

There are numerous complications, as listed earlier. Treatment of these may require input from other teams, e.g., stroke, renal, etc.

Cardiac failure should be treated appropriately – if this continues to be severe despite medical treatment, valve repair or replacement may be required.

Conduction defects are uncommon and may be temporary (related to inflammation); therefore, pacemakers for high-grade AV block are not always required.

The use of antithrombotic therapy can be controversial, as there is limited evidence, and it may theoretically prevent thromboembolic complications but increase the risk of haemorrhage from mycotic aneurysms. Indications in IE patients are the same as in other patients. If there are thromboembolic complications, such as pulmonary embolus or deep vein thrombosis, anticoagulation is used as it is normally. Patients with metal prosthetic valves should remain on anticoagulation, although it is often preferable to change from warfarin to heparin, as this is more easily reversed. Patients with ischaemic stroke are not anticoagulated because of the risk of haemorrhage into the infarct, which can worsen the outcome.

Monitoring of patients who have infective endocarditis

To follow the course of infection and identify new complications early, this should include:

1. Daily history and examination – this is the most important. Look for signs of worsening valvular incompetence, cardiac failure, new splinter haemorrhages, Roth spots, Osler nodes and so on, all of which are suggestive of active disease.
2. Temperature chart – an increase in temperature after the patient has been apyrexial for some time can represent reactivation of infection. Blood cultures (as well as other samples of possible infection) should be sent immediately, with reconsideration of possible sources (e.g., endocarditis, abscess formation, embolism of vegetation, other infections, reaction to drugs, etc.).
3. Blood tests – monitor full blood count and CRP. Renal function and liver function may deteriorate due to disease activity or as a side effect of medications. Closely monitor antibiotic levels (e.g., gentamicin, vancomycin) and adjust doses for renal function.
4. ECG – in some cases, this may be required daily to look for PR interval prolongation; the highest risk is in left-sided IE. If an aortic root or septal abscess develops, this can affect the AV node and lead to complete heart block.
5. Echocardiography – used as frequently as weekly to monitor response or urgently if there is clinical deterioration. This will assess vegetation size, abscess formation, severity of valvular regurgitation and left ventricular function.

HINTS AND TIPS

Close monitoring is crucial in patients with IE to identify and treat new complications early. Indications for surgery may develop, and deterioration may lead to severe morbidity and mortality.

● **Chapter Summary**

- Echocardiography is key to the diagnosis and management of all valvular diseases.
- Rheumatic fever is an important cause of valvular disease in the developing world, although there are still numerous affected patients in the developed world. It is caused by an autoimmune reaction to group A β-haemolytic streptococci.
- Diagnosis of rheumatic fever is made according to the revised Jones criteria. Treatment is with antibiotics and antiinflammatory drugs.
- Left-sided valvular diseases and tricuspid regurgitation are the most common valvular abnormalities; knowing the causes, clinical signs, severity markers, complications and management is essential for exams.
- Patients with valvular disease may benefit from follow-up, as the timing for possible valve replacement or repair is critical.
- Development of heart failure in valvular disease is usually a sign of decompensation and the need to consider further intervention in addition to medical management.
- Prosthetic valves can be metallic or bioprosthetic; metallic valves require lifelong anticoagulation.
- Infective endocarditis is a serious infection with a high mortality rate. Diagnosis is made using the modified Duke criteria; multiple minor criteria may be fulfilled with careful examination of the patient. Taking multiple blood cultures at an early stage is crucial to the subsequent management of infective endocarditis.
- Remember to conduct urinalysis in suspected infective endocarditis, as microscopic haematuria is found commonly due to immune-complex glomerulonephritis and may provide an early part of the puzzle in a frequently nonspecific presentation (but bear in mind other causes). Haematuria is much more common than the famous but rare signs, e.g., Osler nodes and Janeway lesions.
- Treatment of infective endocarditis involves prolonged antibiotics with infectious diseases input, source control (if identified), surgery (if any of the three indications are met), and multidisciplinary management of any complications.

UKMLA Conditions
Aortic valve disease
Infective endocarditis
Mitral valve disease
Right heart valve disease

UKMLA Presentations
Fever
Heart murmurs

Diseases of the myocardium and pericardium | 16

DISEASES OF THE MYOCARDIUM

Myocardial damage can be caused by a number of processes. Ischaemia/infarction, arrhythmia, valvular disease and hypertension have all been discussed elsewhere. There are also a number of conditions that cause intrinsic damage to the myocardium, including myocarditis and cardiomyopathy.

Myocarditis

Myocarditis is inflammation of the myocardium and may be either acute or chronic. It can present in a similar way to myocardial infarction (MI). Substantial damage to the myocardium may result in dilated cardiomyopathy (DCM). Table 16.1 lists the numerous causes of myocarditis.

Clinical features

The clinical course is very variable. Many patients present with chest pain with features that often overlap with pericarditis. Patients with evidence of myocarditis may be asymptomatic and only recognized following identification of electrocardiography (ECG) changes. Other patients may present with severe heart failure, arrhythmia or even sudden cardiac death.

Table 16.1 Causes of myocarditis

Aetiology	Examples/comment
Idiopathic	No specific cause found in many cases.
Viral infections	Numerous – including coxsackie virus, echovirus, human immunodeficiency virus (HIV).
Bacterial infections	Numerous – including *Staphylococcus*, tuberculosis, diphtheria.
Other infections	Various fungal, parasitic, protozoal causes.
Immunological	Including systemic lupus erythematosus, sarcoidosis, rheumatoid arthritis, Kawasaki disease, scleroderma.
Toxins	Numerous – including ethanol, cocaine, doxorubicin, cyclophosphamide, heavy metal poisoning (e.g., lead, iron, cadmium), arsenic, various insect bites/stings.
Other	Radiotherapy, electric shock.

Symptomatic patients may complain of:

- Lethargy/malaise.
- Chest pain – either from pericarditis or myocardial damage.
- Fever.
- Breathlessness.
- Palpitations.
- Ankle swelling.

Examination may be unremarkable. There may be clinical evidence of heart failure or arrhythmia.

Investigation

The following investigations may be appropriate:

- Blood tests – inflammatory markers such as erythrocyte sedimentation rate (ESR) and C-reactive protein (CRP) may be raised. Full blood count, urea and electrolytes, and liver function tests may be helpful. Troponin is often elevated – the magnitude and pattern of troponin release is very important.
- ECG – may show nonspecific ST segment changes, T wave changes or conduction abnormalities (e.g., bundle branch block).
- Chest X-ray – may be normal. There may be signs of cardiac failure or coexisting pericarditis (e.g., pericardial effusion).
- Echocardiogram – may identify left ventricular dysfunction, ventricular wall motion abnormalities or altered myocardial image texture. Useful for serial monitoring of cardiac function.
- Cardiac magnetic resonance imaging (MRI) – is particularly helpful to differentiate between myocarditis and MI. Certain sequences are used to look for oedema of the myocardium. Areas of myocarditis often demonstrate late enhancement following gadolinium (MRI contrast) administration.
- Myocardial biopsy – rarely performed. Histological analysis may identify inflammatory infiltrates with significant numbers of lymphocytes and macrophages.

Management

Management is focused on treatment of the underlying cause if possible. Patients who develop florid myocarditis and marked impairment of left ventricular function may require cardiovascular support in an intensive care or high dependency setting. Treatments are generally supportive (administration of oxygen, intravenous fluids, etc.) but management may also include:

- Treatment of heart failure or arrhythmia if present.
- Restriction of physical activity – sometimes for months, to reduce strain on the heart.

- β-Blocker therapy ± angiotensin-converting enzyme (ACE) inhibitor therapy.

Cardiomyopathy

Cardiomyopathy is heart muscle disease, often of unknown cause. Ischaemic cardiomyopathy is heart failure due to underlying coronary artery disease (discussed elsewhere). There are several other types (Fig. 16.1):

- DCM.
- Hypertrophic cardiomyopathy (HCM).
- Restrictive cardiomyopathy.
- Arrhythmogenic ventricular dysplasia.
- Others, including Takotsubo cardiomyopathy.

Dilated cardiomyopathy

DCM is the most common type of cardiomyopathy and results in dilated ventricles and poor systolic function. The coronary arteries are often normal. Often DCM is a result of a combination of different factors, with causes including:

- Idiopathic – in many cases, no obvious cause is identified.
- Genetics (familial DCM) – usually autosomal dominant but not exclusively.
- Alcohol excess.
- Thyrotoxicosis.
- Autoimmune disease – including rheumatoid arthritis and systemic lupus erythematosus.
- Viral infection – numerous infective agents including adenovirus, parvovirus, echovirus, coxsackievirus and human immunodeficiency virus (HIV).
- Drugs and toxins – including cocaine, doxorubicin, cyclophosphamide, trastuzumab (Herceptin), and lead.
- Infiltrative conditions – haemochromatosis, amyloidosis, sarcoidosis, etc.
- Untreated hypertension.
- Tachycardia cardiomyopathy – chronic tachyarrhythmia causing heart failure.

Clinical features

Progressive biventricular cardiac failure leads to fatigue, dyspnoea, peripheral oedema and ascites.

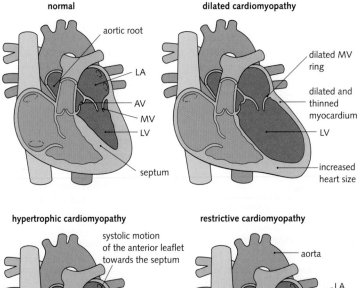

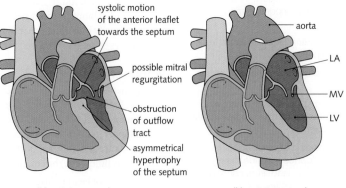

Fig. 16.1 Different types of cardiomyopathy. *AV*, aortic valve; *LA*, left atrium; *LV*, left ventricle; *MV*, mitral valve.

Other complications secondary to the progressive dilatation of the ventricles include:

- Mural thrombus with systemic or pulmonary embolization.
- Dilatation of the tricuspid and mitral valve rings leading to functional valve regurgitation.
- Atrial fibrillation (AF).
- Ventricular tachyarrhythmias and sudden death.

Investigation

Investigations to aid diagnosis include:

- Blood tests – thyroid function tests, calcium (sarcoidosis), ferritin and iron binding studies (haemachromatosis), creatine kinase (to look for primary muscle diseases), a full blood count (anaemia), and autoimmune screen. Viral titres may be useful.
- Chest radiography – may show cardiomegaly, signs of pulmonary oedema (upper lobe blood diversion or interstitial shadowing), or pulmonary effusions.
- ECG – may show tachycardia, poor R wave progression across chest leads, and aberrancy of conduction (e.g., bundle branch block).
- Echocardiography – may identify dilated ventricles or regurgitant valves. Occasionally, intracardiac thrombus may be seen (easier to identify on transoesophageal echocardiography than transthoracic echocardiography).
- Cardiac catheterization – it is important to exclude coronary artery disease (the most common cause of ventricular dysfunction).
- MRI – an excellent noninvasive tool for assessment of patients with cardiomyopathy, and late enhancement with gadolinium can provide useful information about the aetiology and prognosis.

Management

Management of DCM follows four basic steps (the same applies for any other case of cardiac failure):

1. Search for and treat any underlying cause (e.g., abstinence from alcohol).
2. Treat cardiac failure (diuretics, ACE inhibitors and β-blockers).
3. Treat any arrhythmias (β-blockers, digoxin or amiodarone for AF, or amiodarone for ventricular arrhythmias).
4. Consider anticoagulation to prevent mural thrombi.

After optimization of medical therapy, device therapy should be considered. Cardiac transplantation may also be a treatment option.

Hypertrophic cardiomyopathy

HCM is characterized by ventricular hypertrophy. The pattern of hypertrophy is variable but tends to preferentially affect the interventricular septum.

HCM may be diagnosed following detection of left ventricular wall thickness of ≥15 mm, or ≥13 mm if the patient is a known gene carrier or has a first-degree relative with known HCM.

The majority of mutations resulting in HCM are autosomal dominant and affect genes encoding sarcomere proteins.

The myocytes of the left ventricle (LV) are abnormally thick when examined microscopically and their layout is disorganized ('myocardial disarray'). This makes left ventricular filling more difficult than normal and grossly disordered.

This condition was previously known as hypertrophic obstructive cardiomyopathy (HOCM). Dynamic left ventricular outflow tract (LVOT) obstruction occurs in around 25% of cases at rest but up to 70% of patients with provocation, most commonly due to systolic anterior motion of the mitral valve into the thickened septum, but sometimes the cavity can become occluded. The term HOCM is only used if there is evidence of obstruction (and HCM otherwise).

> **HINTS AND TIPS**
>
> The management of HCM involves alleviation of symptoms in some patients, but risk assessment for sudden death is vital in everyone. Certain mutations are particularly associated with sudden death, so genetic testing can sometimes help.

Clinical features

There are four main symptoms:

1. Angina (even in the absence of coronary artery disease) – due to increased oxygen demand of the hypertrophied muscle.
2. Palpitations – there is an increased incidence of AF and ventricular arrhythmias in this condition.
3. Syncope and sudden death – may be due to LVOT obstruction by the hypertrophied septum or due to a ventricular arrhythmia. Syncope may result from inappropriate vasodilatation on exercise.
4. Dyspnoea – due to the stiff LV, which leads to reduced cardiac output and pulmonary venous congestion.

Signs (Fig. 16.2) on examination include:

- Jerky peripheral pulse – the second rise palpable in the pulse is due to the rise in left ventricular pressure as the LV attempts to overcome the LVOT obstruction.
- Double apical beat – the stiff LV causes raised left ventricular end-diastolic pressure. The atrial contraction is, therefore, very forceful to fill the LV. It is this atrial impulse that can be felt in addition to the LV contraction that gives this classical sign.

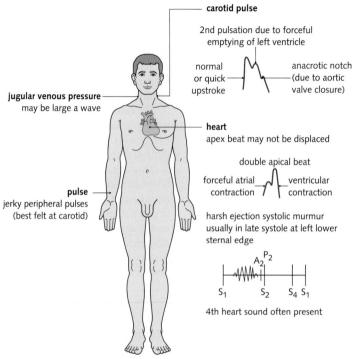

carotid pulse

2nd pulsation due to forceful emptying of left ventricle

normal or quick upstroke

anacrotic notch (due to aortic valve closure)

jugular venous pressure
may be large a wave

heart
apex beat may not be displaced

double apical beat

forceful atrial contraction ventricular contraction

pulse
jerky peripheral pulses
(best felt at carotid)

harsh ejection systolic murmur usually in late systole at left lower sternal edge

A_2 P_2

S_1 S_2 S_4 S_1

4th heart sound often present

Fig. 16.2 Important clinical signs in hypertrophic cardiomyopathy.

- Systolic thrill – felt at the left lower sternal edge.
- Systolic murmur – crescendo-decrescendo in nature, best heard between the apex and the left lower sternal edge.

It can be difficult to differentiate between HCM and aortic stenosis (AS) on examination. Use the following features to help:

- Pulse character – slow rising in severe AS, jerky or with a normal upstroke in HCM.
- Second heart sound – reduced in intensity in significant AS.
- Thrill and murmur – found in the second right intercostal space in AS and at the left lower sternal edge in HCM.
- Variation of the murmur with Valsalva manoeuvre or with standing from squatting – the murmur of HCM (but not AS) is increased because LV volume is reduced by these manoeuvres and, therefore, the outflow gradient worsens.

HINTS AND TIPS

Remember that the outflow obstruction of aortic stenosis is fixed and is present throughout systole, whereas the obstruction of HCM is often absent at the start of systole and worsens as the ventricle empties.

Investigation

Investigation of HCM involves:

- ECG – usually abnormal (most common abnormalities are T wave and ST segment abnormalities). Signs of left ventricular hypertrophy may also be present. Q waves due to the hypertrophied septum may mimic old MI.
- Continuous ambulatory ECG – presence of nonsustained ventricular tachycardia (VT) is common and is a risk factor for sudden death. Sustained VT is relatively uncommon.
- Echocardiography – may be used to confirm the diagnosis and assess the degree of LVOT obstruction. There may be evidence of unexplained hypertrophy or abnormal systolic anterior motion of the anterior leaflet of the mitral valve.
- Exercise testing – lack of the normal rise (or a fall) in blood pressure on exercise is a risk factor for sudden death in HCM. All patients with HCM should have an exercise test to look for this, and it should be repeated periodically.
- MRI – fibrosis is associated with a worse prognosis.

Prognosis

For the majority of patients, HCM carries a relatively benign prognosis. Approximately 90% will be asymptomatic at diagnosis and most remain so long term.

Patients who present with symptoms generally experience slow progression over time.

Children diagnosed when under 14 years of age have a poor prognosis and a high incidence of sudden death. Adults have a better prognosis, but they also have a higher sudden cardiac death rate than the general population.

Another outcome is progressive cardiac failure with cardiac dilatation, which carries a poor prognosis and a high mortality rate after symptoms develop. Risk factors for cardiac failure in HCM patients include young age at diagnosis, severe symptoms, large left ventricular cavity and family history of advanced cardiac failure.

AF is common (seen in roughly 20% of adult patients) and often tolerated poorly. The presence of AF is a poor prognostic marker due to the increased risk of death from heart failure.

Pharmacological treatments

As with AS, vasodilators should be avoided because they worsen the gradient across the obstruction. Therefore, patients with HCM should not receive nitrates.

β-Blockers (β-adrenoceptor antagonists) are used because their negative inotropic effect acts to decrease the contractility of the hypertrophied septum and reduces the outflow tract obstruction. Disopyramide may be used in combination or alone to treat obstruction – it is a negative inotrope that reduces myocardial contractility and, as a result, reduces resting pressure gradients and improves symptoms. Verapamil or diltiazem may be given in symptomatic HCM in the absence of obstruction. Antiarrhythmic agents are important in patients with documented arrhythmias. Amiodarone or sotalol may be used for AF (along with anticoagulation).

A novel cardiac myosin inhibitor, mavacemten, appears to provide symptomatic benefit in patients with HOCM.

Nonpharmacological treatments

These include:

- Device therapy – dual chamber pacing to reduce the outflow gradient may be considered in selected patients. An implantable cardioverter defibrillator (ICD) should be considered in patients at high risk of sudden cardiac death.
- Percutaneous treatment (alcohol septal ablation) – alcohol can be injected down the septal branch of the left anterior descending coronary artery, causing necrosis of the myocardial tissue that gives rise to the obstruction.
- Surgery – a myomectomy is performed on the abnormal septum. This is the treatment of choice if other cardiac structural abnormalities need surgical correction.
- Cardiac transplant – may be necessary in patients with advanced heart failure.

Restrictive cardiomyopathy

Restrictive cardiomyopathy is an uncommon cause of cardio-myopathy in developed countries where most cases of restrictive cardiomyopathy are a variant of HCM – first-degree relatives may have classical HCM.

In this condition, the ventricular walls are excessively stiff and impede ventricular filling; therefore, end-diastolic pressure is increased. Ventricular systolic function is often normal.

Presentation is identical to that of constrictive pericarditis, but the two must be differentiated because pericardial constriction can be treated with surgery.

Possible causes of restrictive cardiomyopathy include:

- Idiopathic – no particular cause identified.
- Infiltrative diseases – such as amyloidosis (most common cause), sarcoidosis and haemochromatosis.
- Numerous other rare conditions including scleroderma, glycogen storage diseases, endomyocardial fibrosis, hypereosinophilic syndrome, etc.

Clinical features

The main features are:

- Dyspnoea and fatigue due to poor cardiac output.
- Peripheral oedema and ascites.
- Elevated jugular venous pressure (JVP) with a positive Kussmaul sign (increase in JVP during inspiration).

Management

In most cases, there is no specific treatment and the condition usually progresses towards death relatively quickly; most patients do not survive beyond 10 years after diagnosis. Treatment focuses on management of causative conditions (if identified) and heart failure treatments.

For transthyretin amyloidosis (a subtype of amyloidosis), disease-modifying drugs (including tafamidis and diflunisal) have recently shown promise in a hereditary form of this condition. Although these medications do not remove amyloid deposits, they have been shown to slow progression.

Arrhythmogenic ventricular dysplasia

Arrhythmogenic ventricular dysplasia, or arrhythmogenic cardiomyopathy, is a rare condition characterized by fibrofatty replacement of the myocardium, particularly in the right ventricular free wall. It was previously known as arrhythmogenic right ventricular cardiomyopathy (ARVC), as it was previously thought to only affect the right ventricle but more recently, it has been shown to affect either the right or left ventricle (or in some cases both). The main problem that this causes is heart rhythm disturbance, ranging from ectopic beats to sustained ventricular arrhythmias, and even sudden cardiac death. There may also be impairment of right ventricular function.

Patients present with palpitation, syncope, heart failure or sudden death. Characteristic features are often seen on cardiac MRI.

There is no curative treatment, so management is aimed at preventing complications. This includes the use of ACE inhibitors and diuretics for the treatment of heart failure, antiarrhythmic agents and consideration of ICD implantation in patients at high risk of sudden cardiac death.

Takotsubo cardiomyopathy

'Takotsubo' cardiomyopathy is named after a type of Japanese octopus pot, which resembles the characteristic shape of the LV in this condition (see Figs. 16.3 and 16.4). Typically, the apex dilates ('ballooning'), with the rest of the ventricle spared, though mid- and basal versions have been described.

The cardiomyopathy frequently presents after a stressful event, most commonly in postmenopausal women, and patients may complain of chest pain or shortness of breath, with ischaemic ECG changes, often initially being mistaken for MI. After the

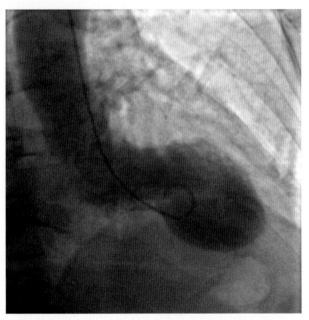

Fig. 16.4 Takotsubo cardiomyopathy seen during angiography, with the catheter tip in the left ventricle. Note how the contrast demonstrates the unusual shape of the left ventricle.

initial presentation (which may be life-threatening), the prognosis is usually good, with full resolution of the cardiomyopathy in weeks or months. A small proportion die acutely of arrhythmia (generally torsades de pointes due to QT prolongation) or cardiogenic shock. The disease often recurs and is associated with long-term major adverse cardiovascular events.

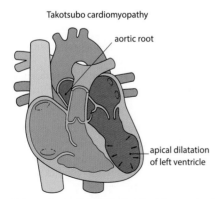

Takotsubo cardiomyopathy

aortic root

apical dilatation of left ventricle

Fig. 16.3 Takotsubo cardiomyopathy. Sudden weakening of the myocardium results in ballooning of the left ventricular apex to take on a shape resembling a Japanese octopus pot.

DISEASES OF THE PERICARDIUM

The pericardium forms a strong protective sac around the heart. It is composed of an outer fibrous and an inner serosal layer with approximately 50 mL of pericardial fluid between these in the healthy state. The main clinical conditions affecting the pericardium and the pericardial space are:

- Pericarditis – inflammation of the pericardium.
- Pericardial effusion – increased fluid in the pericardial space.

Pericarditis

Acute pericarditis is more common (history of less than 6 weeks) but pericarditis can, in some cases, be chronic and have a clinical course that runs over many months. There is a wide differential for patients presenting with pericarditis (Table 16.2).

Table 16.2 Causes of pericarditis

Aetiology	Examples/comment
Idiopathic	No specific cause found in many cases.
Viral infections	Numerous – including coxsackie virus, echovirus, Epstein-Barr virus, human immunodeficiency virus (HIV).
Bacterial infection	Numerous – including *Staphylococcus*, tuberculosis.
Fungal infections	Especially in immunosuppressed patients – including aspergillosis, histoplasmosis.
Rheumatological	Including systemic lupus erythematosus, sarcoidosis, rheumatoid arthritis.
Neoplastic	Both primary (e.g., sarcoma) and metastatic.
Pharmacological	Numerous – including hydralazine, procainamide.
Other	Numerous – including uraemia, mediastinal radiotherapy, myocardial infarction (acutely), postmyocardial infarction or pericardiotomy (weeks later, i.e., Dressler syndrome).

Table 16.3 ECG changes in pericarditis

First few hours to 2 weeks	Widespread concave ST segment elevation (often in all leads except aVR and V1). PR segment depression is more specific for acute pericarditis.
1 to 3 weeks	Subsequently, the ST segments return to normal and T wave flattening occurs.
3 to several weeks	T waves later may become inverted.
Several weeks to months	Finally, all of the changes resolve and the ECG trace returns to normal.

Not all changes may be seen in every patient and time course may vary.

- Antibodies for HIV, coxsackie virus, and Epstein-Barr virus.
- Autoantibody titres (e.g., antinuclear antibodies and rheumatoid factor).
- Antistreptolysin titres.

Electrocardiography

Superficial myocardial injury caused by pericarditis characteristically results in four stages of ECG changes (Table 16.3), although all four are only present in approximately 50% of patients. Some patients may be left with permanent ECG changes.

Other investigations

Other investigations may be appropriate:

- Chest X-ray – may demonstrate an enlarged, globular or 'flask-shaped' cardiac shadow which may be a sign of large volume pericardial effusion. Pleural effusions can sometimes be seen.
- Echocardiography – useful if suspicion of pericardial effusion. May be normal in acute uncomplicated pericarditis.
- Computed tomography (CT)/MRI – can be useful if diagnosis is unclear. These may show pericardial thickening >5 mm or pericardial effusion.
- Pericardial fluid analysis – if large effusion present and pericardiocentesis carried out. Fluid can be sent for biochemical, microbiological and pathological analysis.
- Pericardial biopsy – rarely done but may be useful in recurrent or chronic pericarditis.

Clinical features

History

The chest pain of acute pericarditis is usually central or left-sided, sharp in nature and classically relieved by sitting forwards. Aggravating factors include lying supine, coughing or swallowing.

Dyspnoea may be caused by the pain of deep inspiration or the haemodynamic effects of an associated pericardial effusion.

Examination

The patient may have a fever and tachycardia.

A pericardial friction rub may be heard on auscultation of the heart. This is a high-pitched scratching sound (heard best with the diaphragm). It characteristically varies with time and may appear and disappear from one examination to the next. It occurs in both systole and diastole.

Investigation

Blood tests

A number of blood tests may be helpful:

- Full blood count, ESR and CRP – may provide evidence of active inflammation and also clues as to the underlying cause.
- Urea, creatinine and electrolytes.
- Cardiac biomarkers (e.g., troponin) – may be elevated, suggesting that the inflammatory process involves the myocardium (myopericarditis).
- Blood cultures.

HINTS AND TIPS

Aortic dissection may occasionally present as acute pericarditis or a pericardial effusion. Therefore, be careful to look for a widened mediastinum on the chest radiograph and, if clinically suspicious, a CT scan of the aorta should be performed to avoid missing this diagnosis.

Management

Treat any identifiable underlying cause. Most cases of pericarditis are viral or idiopathic. The main aims of management are, therefore, analgesia and bed rest. Nonsteroidal antiinflammatory agents are the most effective for this condition. Colchicine may be useful and occasionally, a short course of oral corticosteroids is required.

A pericardial effusion may be present. If large or causing tamponade, this can be drained. Analysis of the effusion may provide clues about the underlying cause of the pericarditis. Recurrence is rare but, if it does recur, colchicine or steroids will generally abort the episode.

Dressler syndrome

Dressler syndrome is a syndrome of fever, pericarditis and pleurisy occurring generally 2 to 8 weeks (although can occur as late as 3 months) after a cardiac operation or MI. It can occur only if the pericardium has been exposed to blood. Antibodies form against the pericardial antigens and then attack the pericardium in a type III autoimmune reaction.

Patients present with fever, malaise and chest pain. They exhibit the classic signs of acute pericarditis; they may also have arthritis. Pericardial effusions are common, but cardiac tamponade is not.

Chest radiography may show pleural effusions. Echocardiography may reveal a pericardial effusion.

Initial management consists of aspirin or nonsteroidal antiinflammatory agents; corticosteroids may be added if the symptoms persist.

Chronic pericarditis

Any cause of acute pericarditis can persist and lead to chronic pericarditis. Some diseases, however, may result in chronic pericarditis more commonly, including:

- Viral infection.
- Tuberculosis.
- Mediastinal radiotherapy.
- Mediastinal malignancy.
- Cardiac surgery.
- Autoimmune disease.

There are two main types of chronic pericarditis:

- Constrictive pericarditis.
- Effusive-constrictive pericarditis.

Constrictive pericarditis

Constrictive pericarditis occurs when the pericardium becomes fibrosed and thickened and eventually restricts the filling of the heart during diastole. Restricted filling of all four cardiac chambers results in low-output failure. Initially, the right-sided component is more marked, resulting in a high venous pressure and hepatic congestion. Later, left ventricular failure becomes apparent with dyspnoea and orthopnoea.

On examination, the signs of right and left ventricular failure are evident, but the ventricles are not enlarged. The most important feature in the examination of such a patient is the JVP, which is elevated. Kussmaul sign – an increase in the JVP during inspiration – may be evident. Another important feature of the JVP is a rapid x and y descent (quite difficult sign), the presence of which excludes cardiac tamponade. The heart sounds are often soft. AF is common.

Investigation of constrictive pericarditis is as follows:

- Blood tests – as for acute pericarditis.
- Chest radiography – heart size may be normal. There may be signs of a neoplasm or tuberculosis. Pleural effusions are not uncommon. Tuberculous pericarditis may be associated with visible calcification.
- Chest CT often raises the diagnosis with extensive pericardial calcification or thickening (see Fig. 16.5).
- Echocardiography usually shows good left ventricular function.
- Cardiac catheterization – usually diagnostic, showing the classic pattern of raised and equal left and right end-diastolic pressures with normal left ventricular function on the ventriculogram.

The only definitive management is with pericardiectomy (surgical removal of part or the whole of the pericardium). Antituberculous therapy may be required if the underlying cause is tuberculosis and should be continued for 1 year.

Effusive-constrictive pericarditis

This is a rare variant of chronic pericarditis characterized by the presence of both pericardial effusion and pericardial constriction. It is not uncommon for these patients to present with evidence of cardiac tamponade or increased ventricular filling pressures.

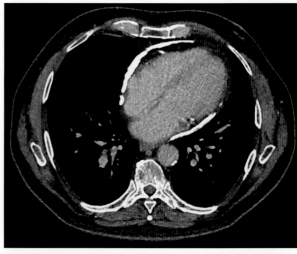

Fig. 16.5 CT scan showing thick pericardial calcification in a patient with constrictive pericarditis.

Patients may present with a variety of symptoms, including dyspnoea on exertion, chest pain (or discomfort), syncope, light-headedness, palpitations, cough, lethargy, etc. Many patients will be asymptomatic until pericardial effusion is very large.

Patients may require treatment with repeated pericardiocentesis or pericardiectomy.

Pericardial effusions

A pericardial effusion is an accumulation of fluid in the pericardial space.

Causes

Pericardial effusion can be caused by a number of different pathologies. Any cause of acute pericarditis may cause an effusion. Pericardial effusions may be classified based on the nature of the fluid in the pericardial space (Table 16.4).

Clinical features

Clinical features depend on the rate and volume of fluid accumulation.

A pericardial effusion may remain asymptomatic, even if very large, if it accumulates gradually (due to the pericardium having time to stretch). As much as 2 L of fluid can be accommodated without increased intrapericardial pressure if it accumulates slowly.

Cardiac tamponade describes the condition where a pericardial effusion increases the intrapericardial pressure such that it leads to haemodynamic compromise.

As little as 100 mL of fluid (or blood) can cause tamponade if it accumulates suddenly.

History

The only symptoms produced by a large chronic effusion may be a dull ache in the chest or dysphagia from compression of the oesophagus.

If cardiac tamponade is present, however, the patient may complain of dyspnoea, light-headedness, abdominal swelling (due to ascites), and peripheral oedema.

Examination

The classic signs of cardiac tamponade (Beck triad) include:

- Hypotension – due to low end-diastolic volume (and therefore stroke volume). If severe, then shock may be present.
- Muffled heart sounds.
- Raised JVP.

Other signs to examine for include:

- Pulse – tachycardia with low volume pulse.
- Pulsus paradoxus – exaggerated reduction of the blood pressure of >10 mmHg during inspiration. This in combination with a pericardial effusion is diagnostic of cardiac tamponade. This occurs due to increased venous return during inspiration filling the right heart and restricting left-ventricular filling (because the pericardium forms a rigid sac with limited space within). This results in reduced stroke volume during inspiration and, consequently, a drop in blood pressure.
- Kussmaul sign – a paradoxical rise in JVP during inspiration (raised intrapericardial pressure impairs right ventricular filling and results in impaired venous return to the heart).

Investigation

Investigation of pericardial effusions include:

- ECG – small voltage complexes with variable axis may be seen (electrical alternans is caused by the movement of the heart within the fluid).
- Chest radiography – the heart may appear large and globular.
- Echocardiography – reveals the pericardial effusion. Right ventricular diastolic collapse is a classical sign of tamponade.

Management

The pericardial effusion should be drained if it is causing haemodynamic compromise or it may be drained to aid diagnosis. If the patient is in cardiogenic shock due to tamponade, then emergency needle aspiration (pericardiocentesis) should be performed, followed by formal drainage once the patient has been resuscitated. Aspirated fluid should be sent for biochemical, microbiological and pathological analysis.

Long-term treatment depends upon the underlying cause; a surgical pericardial 'window' may be required if effusion is recurrent.

Table 16.4 Causes of pericardial effusions

Type of effusion	Examples
Transudate (<30 g/L protein)	Congestive cardiac failure, hypoalbuminaemia.
Exudate (>30 g/L protein)	Infection (viral, bacterial or fungal), immediately postmyocardial infarction and Dressler syndrome, malignancy, systemic lupus erythematosus.
Haemorrhagic (known as haemopericardium)	Malignancy, uraemia, aortic dissection, chest trauma, ventricular wall rupture, following cardiac surgery.

COMMUNICATION

Following drainage of pericardial effusion and prior to discharge from the hospital, patients should be made aware of the symptoms they may experience should the effusion reaccumulate; patients should seek medical help should these symptoms occur.

Chapter Summary

- Cardiomyopathies are rare and presentation can be very variable – some patients may be symptomatic while others present with sudden cardiac death.
- Risk of sudden cardiac death is important to assess in patients with cardiomyopathy – some patients may warrant insertion of implantable cardioverter defibrillators (ICDs) if there is a high risk of arrhythmia.
- Genetic testing/counselling is important with inherited forms of cardiomyopathy.
- Myocarditis and pericarditis have numerous causes; treatment generally consists of supportive measures and attempting to treat the underlying cause.
- Pericardial effusion can be acute or chronic – small volumes of pericardial fluid can cause tamponade if accumulation is rapid, whereas large volumes (up to 2 L) may be relatively asymptomatic if accumulation is slow.
- The classic signs of cardiac tamponade are described by Beck triad: hypotension, muffled heart sounds and raised jugular venous pressure.
- Cardiac tamponade is an emergency and warrants urgent needle aspiration (pericardiocentesis), followed by formal drainage of effusion.

UKMLA Conditions

Cardiac failure
Myocarditis
Pericardial disease

UKMLA Presentations

Breathlessness
Cardiorespiratory arrest
Chest pain
Palpitations

Congenital heart disease

Congenital heart disease refers to cardiac lesions present from birth.

The embryological development of the heart is complex and involves many coordinated steps. Defects arise if the process does not occur correctly. Congenital heart defects have an incidence of 6 to 8 per 1000 live-born infants. They may present in the first year of life or during childhood, or a person may remain asymptomatic for life.

CLINICAL NOTES

The following conditions are not counted in the traditional incidence statistics for congenital heart disease, but are more common:

- Patent foramen ovale (PFO) – seen in 25% to 30% of adults; clinical significance in many patients is unclear.
- Bicuspid aortic valve (two of the aortic valve leaflets fuse during development, which results in an aortic valve with two leaflets rather than three) – present in 1% to 2% of the population and often asymptomatic. Aortic stenosis may develop around 10 years earlier than in the general population. Patients are also at slightly higher risk of aortic root/ascending aorta aneurysm/dissection.

There are a number of different congenital abnormalities; they are listed below in descending order of incidence:

- Ventricular septal defect (VSD).
- Atrial septal defect (ASD).
- Patent ductus arteriosus (PDA).
- Pulmonary stenosis.
- Coarctation of the aorta.
- Aortic stenosis.
- Tetralogy of Fallot.
- Transposition of the great arteries.
- Other – e.g., pulmonary atresia, hypoplastic left heart, Ebstein anomaly.

CAUSES OF CONGENITAL HEART DISEASE

There are many different genetic and environmental factors affecting foetal cardiac development. Genetic associations include:

- Trisomy 21 – atrioventricular septal defect, ASD, VSD, PDA and tetralogy of Fallot.
- Turner syndrome (XO) – coarctation of the aorta, bicuspid aortic valve, partial anomalous pulmonary venous drainage and aortic dilatation.
- Other chromosomal abnormalities, such as Patau syndrome (trisomy 13) and Edwards syndrome (trisomy 18).
- A number of rare single gene mutations have been associated with specific defects, e.g., mutations in a gene coding for alpha-myosin heavy chain (a cardiac muscle protein) are associated with ASDs.

Maternal infection or exposure of the foetus to drugs or toxins may result in a number of congenital defects:

- Maternal rubella – in addition to cataracts, deafness and microcephaly, this can cause PDA, ASD and pulmonary valvular and/or arterial stenosis.
- Maternal alcohol use – may result in foetal alcohol syndrome, which can cause a number of cardiac defects (especially septal defects) as well as microcephaly, micrognathia, microphthalmia and growth retardation.
- Maternal systemic lupus erythematosus – associated with foetal complete heart block (due to transplacental passage of anti-Ro and anti-La antibodies).
- Numerous other toxins/medications – e.g., thalidomide, lithium, etc.

COMPLICATIONS OF CONGENITAL HEART DISEASE

Before discussing individual lesions, it is important to have a grasp of the significance of congenital heart disease. A lesion's effects vary depending on its size/severity and location.

Many (but not all) of the complications of congenital heart disease are due to shunting of blood within the heart or great vessels. It is important to visualize the pressure changes that occur in the cardiac cycle to work out which shunting mechanism and murmur occurs with each defect; this will, for the most part, allow you to understand the symptoms and signs that arise. Shunts may be described as:

- Left to right – results in oxygenated blood going from the left side of the heart to the right side of the heart and therefore will not cause cyanosis at birth.
- Right to left – results in deoxygenated blood going from the right side of the heart to the left side of the heart. This commonly results in cyanosis early in life.

Clinical presentations that occur as the result of congenital heart disease include:

- Central cyanosis – defined as the presence of more than 5 g/dL of deoxyhaemoglobin in arterial blood. Central cyanosis can be caused by congenital heart disease due to shunting of venous blood straight into the arterial circulation, bypassing the lungs.
- Congestive cardiac failure – this occurs due to the inability of the heart to maintain sufficient tissue perfusion as a result of the cardiac lesion. This may occur in infancy (e.g., due to a large VSD or transposition of the great arteries) or in adulthood in less severe conditions.
- Pulmonary hypertension and Eisenmenger syndrome – discussed later.
- Infective endocarditis – congenital heart disease may result in lesions prone to bacterial colonization. Appropriate

antibiotic prophylaxis is occasionally considered where appropriate to prevent this – it is not needed with some lesions, e.g., ASD.

- Paradoxical emboli – venous emboli entering the systemic arterial circulation via a right-to-left shunt leading to stroke or other arterial thrombosis.
- Aortic dilatation/dissection – certain defects, such as bicuspid aortic valves or coarctation of the aorta, may put patients at increased risk of aneurysm or dissection of the aortic root or ascending aorta.
- Sudden death – this may be due to arrhythmias (more common in these disorders) or outflow tract obstruction as seen in aortic stenosis.

Pulmonary hypertension and Eisenmenger syndrome

In left-to-right shunts (e.g., VSD), the higher pressure in the left ventricle results in blood flowing from the left to the right, increasing right heart and pulmonary pressures. Over time, the increased pulmonary blood flow results in changes to the pulmonary vessels, with smooth muscle hypertrophy and obliterative changes. The pulmonary vascular resistance increases causing pulmonary hypertension. The patient becomes increasingly dyspnoeic with the progression of pulmonary hypertension.

Echocardiography allows assessment of the pulmonary pressures. This is vital because the shunt should be corrected before significant pulmonary hypertension develops. Eventually, as pulmonary hypertension progresses, pulmonary pressure exceeds systemic pressure causing reversal of the left-to-right shunt, resulting in a syndrome of cyanotic heart disease called Eisenmenger syndrome (Fig. 17.1).

In Eisenmenger syndrome, dyspnoea is usually relatively mild considering the profound hypoxia these patients have (oxygen saturations of 50% are not uncommon). There is no definitive

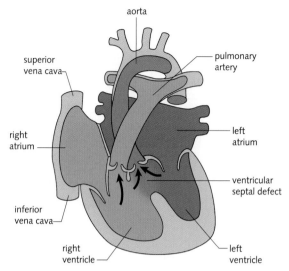

aorta

superior
vena cava

pulmonary
artery

right
atrium

left
atrium

ventricular
septal defect

inferior
vena cava

right
ventricle

left
ventricle

Fig. 17.1 Eisenmenger syndrome with ventricular septal defect. Patients initially will have a left-to-right shunt with ventricular septal defect; this has reversed due to pulmonary hypertension (and now flows from right to left). Less blood now passes through the pulmonary circulation and the patient becomes cyanosed. (Courtesy Lissauer T, Clayden G. *Illustrated textbook of paediatrics,* 2nd edn. London: Mosby, 2001.)

treatment at this late stage, save for combined heart and lung transplantation; therefore it is important to intervene early, before pulmonary hypertension and Eisenmenger syndrome develop.

HINTS AND TIPS

Cyanosis caused by pulmonary disease or cardiac failure improves on increasing inspired oxygen. Cyanosis caused by a right-to-left shunt bypassing the lungs does not improve on increasing inspired oxygen.

Complications of Eisenmenger syndrome include:
- Clubbing – develops in the fingers and toes (can be just in toes when Eisenmenger syndrome occurs with a PDA).
- Polycythaemia and hyperviscosity – with resulting complications of stroke and venous thrombosis. Regular venesection or anticoagulation may be necessary.
- Cerebral abscesses – especially in children.
- Paradoxical emboli.

These features are also seen in patients who have cyanotic congenital heart disease (i.e., where the lesion results in a right-to-left shunt from the outset).

PREGNANCY RISK ASSESSMENT

Pregnancy and delivery cause significant physiological changes and place increased demands on the cardiovascular system. During a singleton pregnancy, there is up to 50% increase in cardiac output, around 40% increase in circulating blood volume and 10%–20% increase in heart rate.

Female patients of child-bearing age with congenital heart disease or aortic disease should receive preconception counselling regarding the increased risk to the mother and foetus associated with pregnancy and, in appropriate cases, be referred to a specialist at a stage when they are considering starting a family. Ideally this is started in teenage years with age-appropriate information so that the patient can make decisions regarding contraception and understand the importance of assessment and management both before and during pregnancy. Medications may need to be modified prior to pregnancy to avoid teratogens. Genetic counselling is important to advise of any recurrence risk in the offspring. In low-risk cases, reassurance can be provided that most patients with congenital heart disease have uncomplicated pregnancies. In higher-risk patients, treatment may be advised prior to conception to optimize maternal health, or in a small group, pregnancy may be advised against altogether. Spontaneous vaginal delivery is usually recommended as first choice unless in very high-risk cardiac groups or for obstetric reasons.

The first step is to establish their cardiac status prior to pregnancy (with a detailed history, examination and appropriate investigations). This can help to identify any potential complications that may arise during pregnancy.

Patients with congenital heart disease may require additional monitoring and care (with close collaboration between obstetrician, cardiologists, etc.), as cardiac structural abnormalities and shunts may be worsened by the increased blood flow and pressure changes during pregnancy. These patients may also be at risk of arrhythmias and other cardiac complications.

Patients with other cardiac diseases (including valvular heart disease and ischaemic heart disease) may also require special attention during pregnancy, as they may be at risk for heart failure and other cardiac complications due to the increased circulating volume.

Regular prenatal care, including regular foetal surveillance and cardiac assessments, is essential for patients with cardiac disease during pregnancy. Patients may also require close monitoring during labour and delivery as well as careful management of postpartum care.

CONGENITAL DEFECTS WITH LEFT-TO-RIGHT SHUNTS

Left-to-right shunts do not cause cyanosis at birth because all the blood is passing through the pulmonary circulation and being

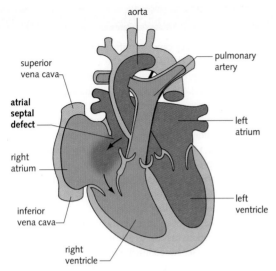

Fig. 17.2 Atrial septal defect. Blood flows from the higher-pressure left atrium to the lower-pressure right atrium. (Courtesy Lissauer T, Clayden G. *Illustrated textbook of paediatrics,* 2nd edn. London: Mosby, 2001.)

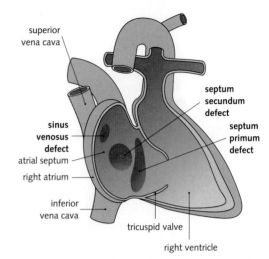

Fig. 17.3 Location of the three main types of atrial septal defect. The heart is viewed from the right side. The right atrial and ventricular walls have been omitted to reveal the septum.

oxygenated. Cyanosis may result eventually if shunt reversal occurs (see **Eisenmenger syndrome**).

Atrial septal defect

An ASD is an abnormal opening in the wall between the right and left atria (Fig. 17.2). Blood moves from the left atrium to the right atrium due to the pressure gradient. ASDs are common, accounting for roughly 10% of congenital heart disease, but are often not diagnosed early because they can be difficult to detect clinically.

There are three main types of ASD based on the location of the defect in the atrial septum (Fig. 17.3):

1. Septum primum (also called ostium primum ASD) – defect adjacent to the atrioventricular valves (which are often also abnormal and incompetent).
2. Septum secundum (also called ostium secundum ASD) – the most common form of ASD, it is mid-septal in location.
3. Sinus venosus ASD – rarer, high in the septum and may be associated with anomalous pulmonary venous drainage (where one of the pulmonary veins drains into the systemic venous system instead of the left atrium).

The magnitude of the left-to-right shunt seen in ASD depends upon the defect size and the relative pressures on the left and right sides of the heart.

History

In early life, patients are usually asymptomatic. In adult life, however, dyspnoea, fatigue and recurrent chest infections can occur.

Over time, increased pulmonary blood flow can result in pulmonary hypertension, eventually reversal of the shunt and Eisenmenger syndrome. Supraventricular arrhythmias may develop later.

Examination

The findings on examination of a patient with an ASD (Fig. 17.4) depend upon:

- Size of the ASD.
- Presence of pulmonary hypertension.
- Presence of shunt reversal.

The second heart sound is widely split because pulmonary valve closure is delayed due to increased pulmonary blood flow. The splitting is fixed in relation to respiration because the communication between the atria prevents the normal pressure differential between right and left sides that occurs during respiration.

The increased pulmonary blood flow causes a mid-systolic pulmonary flow murmur.

If pulmonary hypertension has developed, there is reduction of the left-to-right shunt and the pulmonary flow murmur disappears; instead, there is a loud pulmonary component to the second heart sound because the increased pressure causes the pulmonary valve to slam shut.

Patients may later develop Eisenmenger syndrome.

Investigation

Investigation includes:

- Electrocardiography (ECG) – patients with ostium secundum ASD usually have right axis deviation. Patients with ostium primum defect usually have left axis deviation.

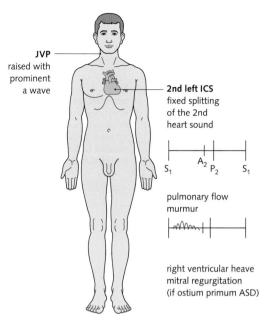

JVP
raised with
prominent
a wave

2nd left ICS
fixed splitting
of the 2nd
heart sound

S_1 A_2 P_2 S_1

pulmonary flow
murmur

right ventricular heave
mitral regurgitation
(if ostium primum ASD)

Fig. 17.4 Possible physical findings in a patient with an atrial septal defect (ASD). If the ASD is large and there is pulmonary hypertension, check for loud P_2 at the second left intercostal space (ICS) and for prominent right ventricular heave. If there is shunt reversal, you may find clubbing, central cyanosis and signs of congestive cardiac failure. A_2, aortic component of second heart sound; JVP, jugular venous pressure; P_2, pulmonary component of second heart sound; S_1, first heart sound.

- Chest X-ray (CXR) – the pulmonary artery may appear dilated with prominent branches. There may be enlargement of the right atrium seen at the right heart border and enlargement of the right ventricle causes rounding of the left heart border.
- Echocardiography – the right side of the heart and the pulmonary artery may be dilated. The ASD may be directly visualized and a jet of blood may be seen passing through it. Associated mitral or tricuspid valve incompetence may be seen. These findings are best seen on transoesophageal echocardiography.
- Cardiac catheterization – The ASD can be demonstrated by passing a catheter across it. Oxygen saturations can be measured at locations throughout the right side of the heart and this can be used to calculate the size of the shunt, which helps determine whether operative correction is required.
- CT angiography – allows for assessment of atrial anatomy, pulmonary veins and device closure planning.
- Magnetic resonance imaging (MRI) – offers excellent image quality and haemodynamic data without the use of ionizing radiation.

Management

If there are signs of congestive cardiac failure, diuretics and angiotensin-converting enzyme (ACE) inhibitors may be of benefit.

The primary aim in these patients is to diagnose and evaluate severity of the ASD early and to repair the defect (if necessary) before pulmonary hypertension occurs. Once the patient has developed pulmonary hypertension, repair does not stop its deterioration. All ASDs with pulmonary-to-systemic flow ratios exceeding 1.5:1 should be repaired. Surgical closure requires cardiopulmonary bypass and involves a median sternotomy scar. However, most ASDs are amenable to percutaneous closure, dependent on location and size. A device with two deformable discs connected by a narrow waist is inserted across the septal defect – this is introduced via a catheter inserted into the femoral vein and advanced up to the heart.

Patent foramen ovale

Around 25% of the population have a patent foramen ovale (PFO), which is a remnant of the foetal circulation that allows blood to bypass the lungs. In the remaining 75%, the foramen ovale closes with the increase in left atrial pressure that occurs during the neonate's first breaths. If present, a PFO may allow blood to cross (shunt) to the left atrium at all times or sometimes only during Valsalva.

If a patient with PFO has a venous thromboembolism, then there is a theoretic risk of paradoxical arterial embolism, e.g., an ischaemic stroke if the embolus travels to the brain.

Stroke of unknown aetiology in a young patient with a PFO may be an indication to undergo percutaneous device closure to prevent further paradoxical emboli. It has also been suggested that PFO might be associated with migraines, although trials of closure have had mixed results.

Ventricular septal defect

A VSD is a failure of fusion of the interventricular septum (Fig. 17.5). Blood shunts through a hole in the interventricular septum from the higher-pressure left ventricle to the right ventricle.

The ventricular septum is made up of two main components:

1. The membranous septum – situated high in the septum and relatively small. This is the most common site for a VSD.
2. The muscular septum – this is lower and defects here may be multiple.

History

In the neonate, a small VSD will be asymptomatic but a large VSD may result in the development of left ventricular failure (LVF). The signs of LVF in a neonate are as follows:

- Failure to thrive, feeding difficulties and sweating on feeding.

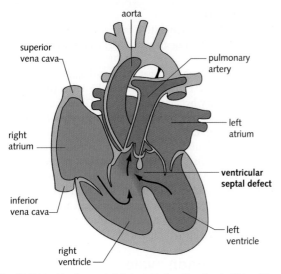

Fig. 17.5 Ventricular septal defect. Notice the shunt of blood from the left ventricle to the right ventricle. This results in oxygenated blood from the left ventricle reentering the pulmonary circulation. (Courtesy Lissauer T, Clayden G. *Illustrated textbook of paediatrics,* 2nd edn. London: Mosby, 2001.)

- Tachypnoea and intercostal recession.
- Hepatomegaly.

Adults with VSDs may be asymptomatic or may present with dyspnoea due to pulmonary hypertension or Eisenmenger syndrome.

Examination

The findings on examination of a patient with a VSD (Fig. 17.6) vary according to:

1. Size of the VSD – a small VSD causes a loud pansystolic murmur that radiates to the apex and axilla. A very large VSD causes a less loud pansystolic murmur but may be associated with signs of left ventricular and right ventricular hypertrophy.
2. Presence of pulmonary hypertension.
3. Presence of shunt reversal.

Investigation

Investigation of VSDs includes:

- CXR – may show an enlarged left ventricle with prominent pulmonary vascular markings. Pulmonary oedema may be seen in infants.
- Echocardiography – used to assess the VSD's size and location, and can help to evaluate the effects on cardiac function.
- MRI – can be used if further assessment is needed or if the VSD is not well seen on echocardiography.
- Cardiac catheterization – can be used if further assessment is required, as with ASD.

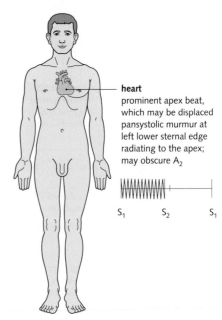

Fig. 17.6 Possible physical findings in a patient with a ventricular septal defect (VSD). If the VSD is large, the apex is displaced and pulmonary hypertension can develop. This results in a loud P_2 (pulmonary component of second heart sound) and right ventricular heave. Eisenmenger syndrome might also develop, with clubbing, cyanosis and disappearance of the pansystolic murmur. A_2, aortic component of second heart sound; S_1, first heart sound; S_2, second heart sound.

Management

Approximately 30% of cases close spontaneously, most of these by 3 years of age. Some do not close until 10 years of age. Defects near the valve ring or near the outlet of the ventricle do not usually close. Patients should be treated at an early stage to avoid development of pulmonary hypertension and Eisenmenger syndrome.

Operative closure is the treatment of choice (if there is a significant left-to-right shunt) and is recommended for all lesions that have not closed spontaneously. Some small lesions are managed conservatively; such patients have loud pansystolic murmurs (and may be seen in OSCE exams)!

Patients with VSDs are at higher risk of developing infective endocarditis.

Patent ductus arteriosus

In the foetus, most of the output of the right ventricle bypasses the lungs via the ductus arteriosus. This vessel runs from the pulmonary trunk to the aorta, connecting just distal to the left subclavian artery (Fig. 17.7). The ductus arteriosus normally closes about 1 month after birth in full-term infants and takes longer to close in premature infants.

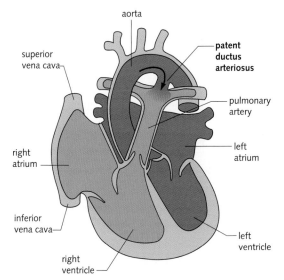

Fig. 17.7 Patent ductus arteriosus. This allows mixing of systemic and pulmonary blood. Movement of blood within the ductus can occur in both directions depending upon the relative pressures in the aorta and the pulmonary trunk. (Courtesy of Lissauer T, Clayden G. *Illustrated textbook of paediatrics*, 2nd edn. London: Mosby, 2001.)

Clinical features are determined by the same factors as in VSD and ASD (i.e., the size of the defect, the size of the shunt, the presence of pulmonary hypertension and the development of Eisenmenger syndrome).

A PDA is more likely in babies born at high altitude, probably due to the low atmospheric oxygen concentration. This lesion is also common in babies with congenital rubella syndrome.

History

A small PDA is asymptomatic but a large defect causes a large left-to-right shunt and may lead to LVF with pulmonary oedema, causing failure to thrive and tachypnoea.

Adults with undiagnosed PDA may develop pulmonary hypertension and present with dyspnoea.

In adults, reversal of the shunt may occur, with venous blood entering the systemic circulation. As blood enters below the subclavian arteries, this can result in cyanosis and clubbing of the lower extremities, whereas the arms remain pink. This is called differential cyanosis.

Examination

Classic findings in a patient with a PDA (Fig. 17.8) are:

- Collapsing high-volume pulses – due to run-off of blood back down the ductus.
- A loud continuous machinery murmur heard in the second left intercostal space – a palpable thrill may be associated.

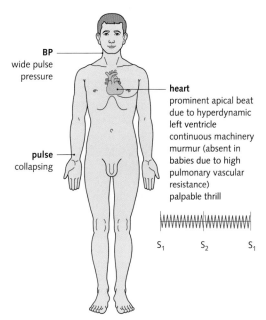

Fig. 17.8 Possible physical findings in a patient with patent ductus arteriosus (PDA). Patients with a large PDA have a loud pulmonary component of the second heart sound (P_2) due to pulmonary hypertension and the murmur is soft or absent. In those who have Eisenmenger syndrome, there is differential cyanosis and the toes are clubbed.

Management

The management of PDA involves:

1. Pharmacological closure in neonates – indomethacin may induce closure if given early (by inhibiting prostacyclin production).
2. Operative closure – can be performed as an open procedure where the PDA is ligated or divided. Alternatively, a percutaneous approach can be performed with the introduction of an occluding device via a cardiac catheter.

CONGENITAL DEFECTS WITH RIGHT-TO-LEFT SHUNTS

These conditions will generally cause cyanosis from early in life.

Tetralogy of Fallot

Tetralogy of Fallot (Fig. 17.9) is a congenital heart condition where the following four defects are seen:

1. Large VSD.
2. Pulmonary stenosis.
3. Right ventricular hypertrophy.
4. Aorta overriding the interventricular septum.

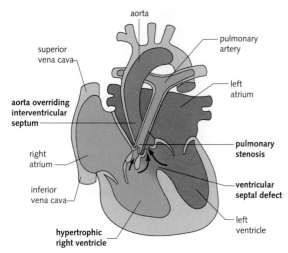

Fig. 17.9 Tetralogy of Fallot. The resulting right-to-left shunt causes cyanosis. (Courtesy Lissauer T, Clayden G. *Illustrated textbook of paediatrics,* 2nd edn. London: Mosby, 2001.)

Clinical features

Most children present within the first year of life with the following features:

- Central cyanosis (progressive hypoxaemia is the main feature and may not be present in the neonate if right ventricular pressure has not yet exceeded left ventricular pressure).
- 'Tet spells' and reduced exercise tolerance – intermittent cyanosis (and even syncope in some cases) can occur, characteristically after crying or feeding, due to increase in right-to-left shunt. Symptoms may be relieved by squatting or bringing the legs to the chest, which increases systemic resistance and reduces right-to-left shunt.
- Failure to thrive – difficulty feeding, behind on growth charts, etc.

Examination findings are described in Fig. 17.10.

After repair:

- Most patients are asymptomatic.
- Some may experience palpitations, as patients are prone to arrhythmias.
- Some may develop exertional dyspnoea (reoccurrence of right ventricular outflow tract obstruction or pulmonary regurgitation).
- There may be signs of residual right ventricular outflow tract obstruction, pulmonary regurgitation or VSD if incomplete repair.

Investigation

Investigations include:

- Blood tests – patients may be polycythaemic in response to prolonged hypoxia.
- ECG – may show signs of right ventricular hypertrophy.

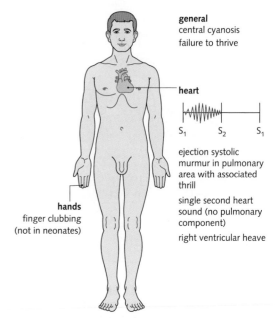

Fig. 17.10 Possible physical findings in a patient with tetralogy of Fallot. Central cyanosis may not be present in neonates if right ventricular pressure has not exceeded left ventricular pressure; finger clubbing takes time to develop and therefore is not seen in neonates.

- CXR – may show a 'boot shaped heart' due to right ventricular hypertrophy and a small pulmonary artery.
- Echocardiogram – visualization of abnormal anatomical features of tetralogy.
- CT/MRI – can provide additional information and three-dimensional (3D) reconstruction of abnormal anatomy if required.

Management

Corrective surgery is required, with total correction as the first-choice treatment. Surgery can be carried out at an early age (starting at 4–6 months). In very young infants with severe pulmonary atresia, a palliative operation (Blalock-Taussig shunt) may be undertaken to increase pulmonary flow. This is usually done by creating an anastomosis from the subclavian artery to the pulmonary artery with the intention that a definitive procedure can be carried out later.

Transposition of the great arteries

During development of the heart, the truncus arteriosus is divided by the aortic septum. This develops towards the proximal end of the truncus arteriosus, spiralling as it develops to meet what will become the ventricles. Transposition of the great arteries occurs when the truncus arteriosus develops normally but the normal spiral does not occur.

In complete transposition of the great arteries, the morphological left ventricle pumps blood into the pulmonary trunk and the morphological right ventricle pumps blood into the aorta, creating two closed systems (Fig. 17.11). There is also an ASD, VSD or PDA, allowing blood from the two systems to mix, otherwise this would be incompatible with life.

Clinical features

Symptoms are less severe in infants with a large communication between the two sides.

Early cardiac failure and cyanosis are the most common presenting features.

Examination findings are variable and dictated by the nature of the communication between the two sides – whether it is the result of PFO, ASD, VSD or PDA and the size of this communication.

Investigation

Diagnosis is made through:

- Echocardiography – can demonstrate abnormal anatomy, including the anatomy of the coronary arteries. Can also readily diagnose any additional associated lesions.
- Cardiac catheterization – can provide additional information if echocardiography imaging is insufficient, e.g., as part of surgical planning.
- CT/MRI – can provide additional information and direct 3D reconstruction of abnormal anatomy if required.
- CXR – not diagnostic but can demonstrate abnormal cardiac contour (classically described as an 'egg on a string').

Management

Management involves:

- Use of prostaglandin E1 to prevent postnatal closure of ductus arteriosus if this is the communication between the two sides.
- Operative management – surgical correction of the transposition is the definitive treatment. In some patients, arterial switch is not possible and an atrial switch operation is carried out instead. An operative procedure to create a large ASD may provide benefit in the short term while awaiting definitive corrective surgery.

OBSTRUCTIVE CONGENITAL DEFECTS

Coarctation of the aorta

In this condition, there is a congenital narrowing of the aorta, usually beyond the left subclavian artery around the area of the ductus arteriosus (Fig. 17.12). There are two main types:

1. Infantile type – presents soon after birth with heart failure.
2. Adult type – obstruction develops more gradually and presents in early adulthood. This type is associated with a high incidence of bicuspid aortic valve.

An adaptive response to the coarctation develops in those patients who do not present in infancy. This involves the development of collateral vessels, which divert blood from the proximal aorta to other peripheral arteries, bypassing the obstruction. These collaterals are seen around the scapula as tortuous vessels that can sometimes be palpated and as prominent posterior intercostal arteries that cause rib notching, visible on chest

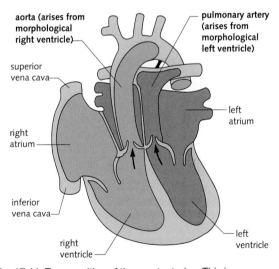

Fig. 17.11 Transposition of the great arteries. This is incompatible with life without a ventricular (VSD) or atrial septal defect (ASD) or a patent ductus arteriosus. (Courtesy Lissauer T, Clayden G. *Illustrated textbook of paediatrics,* 2nd edn. London: Mosby, 2001.)

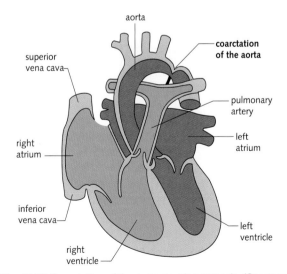

Fig. 17.12 Coarctation of the aorta, causing stenosis. (Courtesy Lissauer T, Clayden G. *Illustrated textbook of paediatrics,* 2nd edn. London: Mosby, 2001.)

radiography. These collaterals take years to develop and are rarely seen before 6 years of age.

History

Infants may present with failure to thrive and tachypnoea secondary to LVF. Alternatively, coarctation may present as rapid severe cardiac failure with the infant in extremis.

Adults whose condition is not diagnosed in childhood may present with:

- Hypertension – always consider coarctation in the young patient with hypertension.
- Symptoms of leg claudication.
- LVF.
- Subarachnoid haemorrhage – due to association with berry aneurysm.
- Angina pectoris due to premature heart disease.

Examination

Physical findings in patients with coarctation of the aorta are shown in Fig. 17.13. Check for:

- Blood pressure – measure this in both arms whenever performing the cardiovascular examination. Aortic dissection and coarctation both cause a pressure differential between the arms if the obstruction is proximal to the left subclavian artery. In coarctation, the blood pressure in the legs is also lower than in the arms.
- Radiofemoral delay and weak leg pulses.
- A heaving displaced apex beat due to left ventricular hypertrophy.
- Murmurs – often systolic but may be continuous if the narrowing is very tight. This is located below the left clavicle. The collaterals cause an ejection systolic murmur that can be heard over the scapulae. There may be a murmur associated with a bicuspid aortic valve, which is ejection systolic in nature and is located over the aortic area.

Investigation

Investigation of coarctation includes:

- ECG – may show left ventricular hypertrophy and often right bundle branch block.
- CXR – rib notching might be seen in children over 6 years of age. (Because the first and second intercostal arteries arise from the vertebral arteries, there is no rib notching on these ribs.) The aortic knuckle may be absent or a double knuckle may be seen (made up of the dilated subclavian artery above and the post-stenotic dilatation of the aorta below).
- Echocardiography – the coarctation and any associated lesion may be visualized but imaging the thoracic aorta can be difficult even with a transoesophageal echocardiogram. Coarctation is associated with a number of other congenital abnormalities (e.g., bicuspid aortic valve, transposition of the great arteries, septum primum ASD, VSD and mitral valve disease).
- Cardiac catheterization – localizes the coarctation accurately and also provides more information on associated lesions.
- CT/MRI – can identify any other congenital abnormalities, can provide 3D reconstruction of the coarctation and is a useful tool prior to treatment to correct the coarctation.

Management

First-line treatment is traditionally surgical, with a number of different procedures available, including resection of the coarctation and end-to-end anastomosis repair, bypass grafting, etc.

Balloon angioplasty and stenting may be carried out as an alternative first-line treatment, avoiding the need for sternotomy and cardiopulmonary bypass; these techniques can also be used to treat postoperative recurrence.

Without correction, the prognosis is extremely poor and most patients die before the age of 50.

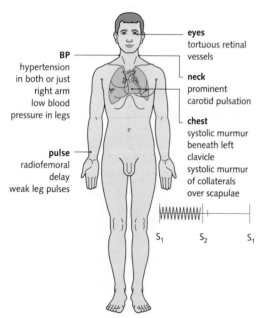

Figure 17.13 Possible physical findings in a patient with coarctation of the aorta. If the coarctation is severe, there may be a continuous murmur beneath the left clavicle and signs of left ventricular failure (bilateral basal crepitations and audible third heart sound).

OTHER LESIONS IN CONGENITAL HEART DISEASE

The conditions discussed above are those most likely to be seen. Several less common congenital cardiac abnormalities are detailed in Table 17.1.

Table 17.1 Other less common causes of congenital cardiac abnormalities

Congenital cardiac defect	Anatomical abnormality	Clinical features	Management
Congenital aortic stenosis (acyanotic)	• Stenosis may be valvular (most common), subvalvular, or supravalvular. • Note: Williams syndrome – an autosomal dominant condition with hypercalcaemia and supravalvular aortic stenosis.	• More common in males. • The child may be hypotensive, dyspnoeic and sweaty. • Increased incidence of angina and sudden death. • Ejection systolic murmur heard in the second right intercostal space. • May be signs of left ventricular strain (heaving apex) or failure (S3, tachycardia and bilateral basal crackles).	• Operative correction of stenosis is the treatment of choice. • In very small infants, valvuloplasty may be preferred initially.
Pulmonary artery stenosis (cyanotic only if severe)	• Stenosis at one or many points along the pulmonary arteries. • Note: associated with tetralogy of Fallot in some cases; also a complication of maternal rubella infection.	• If mild, the patient may be asymptomatic with signs of right ventricular hypertrophy (i.e., left parasternal heave) and a pulmonary ejection systolic murmur. • If severe, right-to-left shunt through the foramen ovale and the child is cyanosed and dyspnoeic.	• Diagnosis is confirmed by echocardiography. • Pulmonary angioplasty may provide a definitive cure. • If there is a recurrence or the lesion is not suitable for angioplasty, the obstruction may be removed surgically.
Hypoplastic left heart (cyanotic)	• Underdevelopment of all or part of the left heart – generally significant left ventricular hypoplasia, with atresia, hypoplasia or stenosis of the left heart valves. There may also be hypoplasia of the ascending aorta.	• The child is often cyanosed at birth. • Heart failure occurs in the first week of life. • Echocardiography is diagnostic.	• Surgical treatment is the only option – this can be done with staged reconstruction or transplantation. The mortality rate is extremely high. • Use of prostaglandin E1 to keep the ductus arteriosus open while awaiting surgery.
Ebstein anomaly (cyanotic if associated with PFO or ASD – occurs in 50%)	• Apical displacement of the tricuspid valve into the right ventricle, tricuspid regurgitation and 'atrialization' of the right ventricle. • Wide range of associated cardiac abnormalities. • Accessory pathway in 25%; high rate of arrhythmias.	• If severe, infants present with right heart failure and failure to thrive. • If moderate, may present in adolescence or adulthood with reduced exercise tolerance, palpitations, or heart failure. If right-to-left shunt present, may also present with cyanosis or paradoxical emboli. • Pansystolic murmur at tricuspid area, widely split S1 and S2 (due to RBBB). • If mild, may be asymptomatic.	• If intervention is required, tricuspid repair is preferable to tricuspid replacement.

Chapter Summary

- Congenital heart disease is associated with a number of genetic conditions (particularly chromosomal abnormalities) and environmental factors (particularly intrauterine exposure to alcohol/drugs/other toxins and maternal rubella).
- There are a number of complications associated with congenital heart disease (e.g., heart failure, arrhythmia, pulmonary hypertension, Eisenmenger syndrome and paradoxical emboli). Understanding the changes that occur in the cardiac cycle and which shunting mechanism occurs with each defect will aid understanding of how each condition presents.
- Some conditions present with a left-to-right-shunt (e.g., atrial septal defect, ventricular septal defect and patent foramen ovale). These conditions are the most common types of congenital heart disease and the patient will initially be acyanotic. These conditions can cause pulmonary hypertension and eventually shunt reversal, resulting in deoxygenated blood entering the arterial circulation, causing cyanosis. This is known as Eisenmenger syndrome.
- The aim should be to identify and correct left-to-right shunts before pulmonary hypertension has developed. By the time Eisenmenger syndrome has developed, the maladaptive changes are irreversible – definitive treatment requires either a lung transplant with correction of shunt or a heart-lung transplant.
- Some conditions result in a right-to-left shunt from birth (or soon after birth), such as tetralogy of Fallot or transposition of the great arteries. Infants with these conditions will be cyanosed.
- There are a number of methods of investigating congenital heart abnormalities but an echocardiogram is one of the most important. It can provide the vast majority of information required when planning treatment.
- Some patients with congenital heart disease will require palliative surgery while planning or awaiting definitive surgery.

UKMLA Conditions
Pulmonary hypertension

UKMLA Presentations
Cyanosis
Heart murmurs
Pregnancy risk assessment

A full explanation of vascular disease is not within the scope of this book; however, a summary of some important conditions is included due to the overlap and association of many of these conditions with cardiac disease.

ARTERIAL DISEASE

Aneurysms

An aneurysm is an abnormal, permanent dilatation of an artery or portion of an artery. True aneurysms involve all three layers of the vessel wall and can be classified morphologically as fusiform or saccular (Fig. 18.1). False (or pseudo-) aneurysms occur when blood leaks out of a vessel but is contained within the surrounding connective tissue rather than the vessel wall itself. Factors affecting aneurysm development:

- Hypertension and smoking: these risk factors are present in over 90% of patients.
- Atherosclerosis: this is very commonly associated with aneurysms. The migration of smooth muscle cells from the media into the intimal lesion weakens the wall, promoting aneurysm development. In addition, atherosclerosis affecting the vasa vasorum supplying the vessel wall can cause ischaemia/infarction of the wall, weakening it further. Interestingly, diabetes mellitus appears to be protective against aneurysm formation (likely due to a combination of the underlying disease process and effects of antidiabetic medications).
- Vasculitis: conditions such as Kawasaki disease (causes coronary artery aneurysms), giant cell arteritis (predisposes to ascending aortic aneurysms), and Takayasu arteritis all predispose to aneurysm development.
- Infection: tertiary syphilis can lead to the development of saccular aneurysms in the proximal aorta. These are referred to as luetic aneurysms.
- Congenital:
  o Marfan syndrome, Ehlers-Danlos syndrome and other connective tissue diseases – these patients are predisposed to aneurysms and dissections (particularly of the thoracic aorta). This occurs due to cystic medial degeneration (degeneration of the media and associated reduction in vascular elasticity).
  o Patients may have thoracic aortic aneurysms in association with other congenital heart disease (e.g., bicuspid aortic valve); see Chapter 17.
  o Small saccular aneurysms in the circle of Willis in the cerebral circulation called berry aneurysms. If these rupture, they cause a subarachnoid haemorrhage.

Aneurysms are often asymptomatic but can cause symptoms in the following situations:

- Rupture: likelihood of rupture increases with the degree of aneurysmal dilatation. Rupture can cause massive blood loss, particularly with the aorta, which can be rapidly fatal.
- Thrombosis: altered haemodynamics in the aneurysmal segment of a vessel can lead to thrombus formation within the aneurysm. This can extend and obstruct the vessel.
- Embolism: small pieces of thrombus can detach and occlude distal vessels, causing acute ischaemia. The calibre of vessel occluded depends on the size of the thrombus. Small emboli may lodge in small distal vessels causing digital ischaemia, whilst large emboli may occlude in larger vessels causing acute limb or bowel ischaemia.
- Pressure: as the aneurysm expands, it can compress adjacent structures. For example, an aneurysm in the aortic arch can compress the oesophagus causing dysphagia (difficulty swallowing).

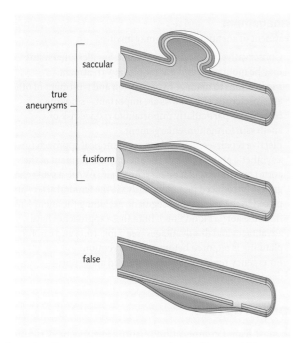

Fig. 18.1 Types of aneurysm: saccular, fusiform and false.

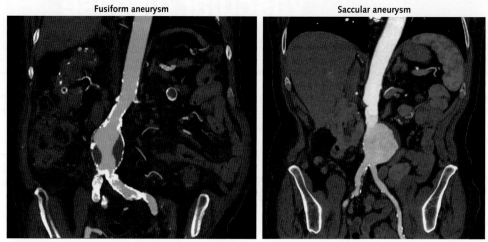

Fig. 18.2 Coronal CT images of two abdominal aortic aneurysms – on the left is an aneurysm with a fusiform morphology, and on the right is an aneurysm with saccular morphology. Often the lumen is partly occluded by thrombus (dark material within the aneurysm sac on the left).

An aneurysm can theoretically develop in any artery but are particularly common in the aorta, especially the abdominal aorta where they are a common finding in elderly men. The most common site for a peripheral aneurysm is the popliteal artery.

Aortic aneurysms

Abdominal aortic aneurysms (AAAs; see Fig. 18.2) are more common than thoracic aortic aneurysms (TAAs). AAAs are present in approximately 3% of men over 50, and affected patients often have a history of hypertension. AAAs can be asymptomatic and identified incidentally on physical examination with a pulsatile abdominal mass or during imaging studies for another purpose. Some will present with back pain due to compression of retroperitoneal structures, or abdominal pain.

Investigation

Investigation of aortic aneurysms includes:

- Ultrasound – to establish whether the patient has an aneurysm or not (and to measure the diameter) as part of the national screening programme. Ultrasound can be used acutely to rule in/out an aneurysm (to decide if the patient requires further imaging) or if the patient is unstable. Ultrasound is very useful with peripheral aneurysms, but visualization of the aorta is sometimes limited due to the overlying bowel.
- CT angiography – best test in the acute setting if the patient is stable enough. This gives detailed images of the aneurysm size and location and may identify signs of rupture or impending rupture.

- MR angiography can also be used for aneurysm follow-up but is less useful in the acute setting due to longer scan duration and limited scanner availability.
- Blood tests – may be relevant depending on the cause of the aneurysm (e.g., inflammatory markers may be raised if infective/inflammatory aetiology) or presurgically if operative repair is considered.

Management

Treatment of aortic aneurysms may involve:

- Conservative/medical management. Smaller aneurysms may be monitored and not require any treatment. Medications to manage hypertension and treatment of other atherosclerotic risk factors are important – smoking cessation is particularly important to reduce risk of aneurysm formation/enlargement.
- Elective repair – either with an open surgical approach (using a synthetic graft to replace the aneurysmal segment of the aorta) or endovascular aneurysm repair (EVAR; a synthetic graft is introduced percutaneously via the femoral artery and placed in the aneurysmal segment, excluding the aneurysm from the aortic blood flow). Both these approaches have advantages and disadvantages (see Table 18.1) and careful planning is required before any intervention.
- Emergency repair in leaking/ruptured aneurysm – described later.

Aortic rupture

The most feared complication of aortic aneurysms is rupture, leading to catastrophic blood loss and very high mortality.

Table 18.1 Advantages and disadvantages of endovascular versus open aneurysm repair

	Endovascular aneurysm repair	Open surgical repair
Advantages	Less invasive procedure – better in individuals who may not tolerate an open surgical approach.	More 'definitive' repair – if patient makes it through the immediate postoperative period, then long-term outcomes are generally better.
Disadvantages	Higher failure rate and possibility of leak developing around the stent into the aneurysm sac (called an 'endoleak'). Higher late mortality.	Higher initial morbidity and mortality – only appropriate in patients without multiple comorbidities.

Chance of rupture increases with aneurysm diameter and is increased in hypertensive individuals.

CLINICAL NOTES

Patients with known AAAs will usually undergo regular ultrasound to monitor aneurysm diameter. Surgical/endovascular repair is usually considered when the aneurysm diameter is >5.5 cm, as at this size, the risk of conservative management (and possible rupture) begins to outweigh the surgical risk.

The clinical presentation of aortic rupture may include sudden and severe chest or abdominal pain, shortness of breath and dizziness. Other symptoms may include weakness or numbness in the limbs and syncope. The patient may be profoundly shocked or in cardiac arrest.

Abdominal aortic rupture is most commonly retroperitoneal but if rupture occurs anteriorly, there can be haemorrhage into the peritoneal cavity. As this is a larger space than the retroperitoneum, blood loss is more profound/rapid and usually fatal.

Aortic rupture can also occur secondary to aortic dissection (described later) or trauma.

COMMON PITFALLS

In the elderly patient presenting with back pain, it is vital to consider the possibility of a leaking AAA, especially if the patient is presenting with other concerning features (e.g., hypotension or other features of shock).

Diagnostic evaluation for aortic rupture may involve a CT scan if patient is stable enough and is fit for urgent surgical repair. Treatment options are similar to that of nonruptured aneurysms – either open repair with a surgical graft to replace the diseased portion of the aorta or with an endovascular approach (EVAR). However, in the emergency setting, prognosis is much poorer than in elective repair, with very high morbidity and mortality.

Aortic dissection and acute aortic syndromes

Aortic dissection (Fig. 18.3) is the most well-known acute aortic syndrome. It is a medical emergency and potentially life-threatening condition resulting from a tear in the intima (innermost layer) of the aorta. This tear can cause blood to flow between the aorta's layers, separating the inner and outer layers of the vessel, creating a new 'false lumen' through which blood can flow. It usually occurs in the thoracic aorta due to the high physical forces exerted on the vessel wall.

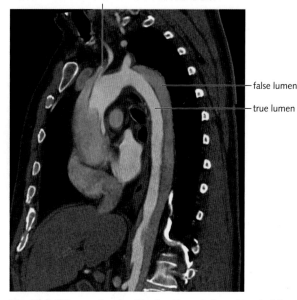
Dissection also often extends into the aortic branches

false lumen

true lumen

Fig. 18.3 CT scan showing Stanford type A dissection. In this patient, because there is less blood flow into/through the false lumen, this lumen contains less IV contrast and doesn't appear as bright. Organs are at risk of ischaemia/infarcts if the dissection affects the aortic branch vessels (the brachiocephalic artery is involved in this case).

The other two common acute aortic syndromes are:

- Intramural haematoma – contained haemorrhage within the aortic wall without obvious intimal tear.
- Penetrating atherosclerotic ulcer (PAU) – an atherosclerotic ulcer erodes through the intima and later into the media.

This section will mainly focus on aortic dissection but these other two acute aortic syndromes may present with similar symptoms and are worth remembering. Also, both of these can progress to aortic dissection or rupture.

Classification of aortic dissection

The most widely used classification of aortic dissection is the Stanford classification (type A – involving the ascending aorta; type B – only involves the descending aorta), with the DeBakey system less frequently used. These are detailed in Fig. 18.4.

Clinical presentation

Clinical presentation and management of aortic dissection/acute aortic syndrome will be determined by the location and extent of the acute aortic syndrome, summarized in Table 18.2. Patients may experience either chest or abdominal symptoms as well as symptoms relating to involvement/occlusion of aortic branches.

Pulmonary vascular disease

Pulmonary embolism

Pulmonary embolism (PE) is a potentially life-threatening condition that occurs when a blood clot or other material becomes lodged in a pulmonary artery (see Fig. 18.5). PE is most often due to embolism of a blood clot from the leg or pelvis to the lungs. To reduce the risk of deep vein thrombosis (DVT) and PE, patients with risk factors (generally all patients admitted to hospital!) should be given prophylactic anticoagulation (and graduated compression stockings or intermittent pneumatic compression devices if appropriate).

PE is common and can present as acute chest pain and breathlessness in an ill patient or as intermittent chest pain and breathlessness in a relatively well patient. For an overview of PE, see Table 18.3.

CLINICAL NOTES

D-dimer is a protein fragment that results from the breakdown of a blood clot within the body and is very sensitive for PE and DVT. It is, however, not specific and is elevated in many other conditions that may present similarly (e.g., it also may be elevated in infection and inflammation) – therefore, this is useful to rule out DVT or PE but not useful for ruling in these diagnoses.

Risk stratification in PE

Early risk stratification guides decisions regarding immediate treatment and hospitalization or early discharge. To help with this, the Pulmonary Embolism Severity Index (PESI) or the simplified version (sPESI) are validated tools to help evaluate the

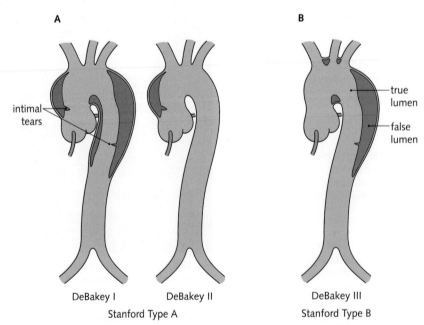

Fig. 18.4 Classification of aortic dissection: Stanford types A and B; DeBakey types I, II and III.

Table 18.2 Overview of dissection of the thoracic aorta

Predisposing factors	• Hypertension. • Atherosclerosis and associated risk factors (male gender, increased age, smoking, etc.). • Aortic aneurysm. • Aortitis (autoimmune diseases, syphilis). • Aortic trauma or instrumentation. • Connective tissue disorders – Marfan syndrome, Ehlers-Danlos syndrome. • Congenital heart disease – particularly aortic coarctation and bicuspid aortic valve. • Pregnancy. • Cocaine use.
Symptoms	• Severe sudden onset central tearing/ripping/sharp chest pain radiating to the back. • Pain can migrate when the dissection extends. • Further complications if the dissection involves branches of the aorta: coronary ostia – myocardial infarction; carotid arteries – focal neurological deficit; spinal arteries – paraplegia; renal arteries – oliguria/anuria and renal failure; mesenteric arteries – abdominal pain; iliac and femoral arteries – limb ischaemia.
Signs	• Shock, cyanosis, sweating. • Blood pressure and pulse difference between extremities. • If proximal extension, may cause aortic regurgitation or haemopericardium/cardiac tamponade. • Cardiac failure. • Signs associated with involvement of other aortic branches as above, including pulse deficit or reduced lower limb perfusion.
Investigation	• If renal arteries involved, may have renal dysfunction. • If coronary ostia involved, troponin may be raised and ECG may demonstrate ST elevation (classically involves right coronary artery). • CXR – widened mediastinum (absence does not exclude dissection). May demonstrate pericardial or pleural effusion. • CT aortogram – the investigation of choice, will accurately demonstrate aortic false and true lumens and their extent. The false lumen is often larger than the true lumen. Will help identify associated complications (e.g., infarcts). • Echocardiography – may demonstrate the intimal flap and the false and true lumens. Aortic regurgitation, pericardial effusion or tamponade may be seen.
Management	• Intravenous access. • Analgesia – morphine (and antiemetic – ondansetron). • If the patient is moribund, treatment is supportive with fluid/blood replacement and other aspects of resuscitation. • If the patient is more stable, strict blood pressure and heart rate control are essential – hypertension must be controlled urgently to reduce wall shear stress to avoid any further extension. First-line agents include intravenous infusions of labetalol ± nicardipine. This will require invasive monitoring; transfer to a coronary care/critical care/high dependency unit. • Seek early consultation with cardiothoracic and vascular surgeons. • Stanford type A dissections are treated with emergency surgery by replacing the affected aortic segment with a synthetic graft. • For Stanford type B dissections, medical management is the priority, with possible surgical or endovascular treatment. • Some patients with aortic dissection may have evidence of ST elevation myocardial infarction (due to coronary involvement). Thrombolysis is contraindicated in dissection due to risk of massive aortic haemorrhage. Therefore, it is important to decide whether the history is typical of infarction due to coronary artery disease before considering thrombolysis. • Lifestyle changes (e.g., smoking cessation) and risk factor management if patient survives acute presentation.
Prognosis	• Acute type A dissection has a mortality rate of 1%–2% per hour during the first 48 hours and a 90% mortality rate at 30 days if left untreated; therefore, urgent diagnosis and treatment is critical. • Acute type A dissection has a high risk of rupture, and type B dissection has a lower risk of rupture. If rupture occurs, this is almost always rapidly fatal.

CT, computed tomography; CXR, chest X-ray; ECG, electrocardiography; MRI, magnetic resonance imaging.

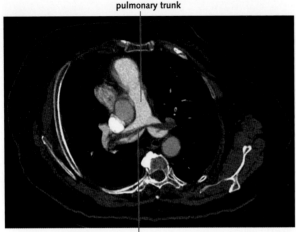

pulmonary trunk

filling defect (thrombus) that straddles the
bifurcation of the pulmonary trunk

Fig. 18.5 Axial oblique CT image showing the pulmonary trunk
and the main pulmonary arteries. There is a 'saddle' pulmonary
embolus – a thromboembolism that straddles the bifurcation of the
pulmonary trunk and extends into both main pulmonary arteries.

patient's mortality risk and combine factors related to PE severity
and the patient's comorbidity (see Table 18.4).

PE is risk stratified as follows:

- High risk (previously a 'massive PE') – a clinical diagnosis,
  defined as a PE large enough to cause circulatory collapse, either
  with a systolic BP <90 mmHg (or >40 mmHg below baseline)
  for 15 minutes, cardiac arrest, features of cardiogenic shock or
  requirement of vasopressors to maintain blood pressure.
- Intermediate-high risk (previously a 'submassive PE') – does
  not have features of high-risk PE but shows right heart strain
  on imaging **and** raised troponin.
- Intermediate-low risk – PESI class III–V or sPESI ≥1 point
  or right heart strain **or** raised troponin.
- Low risk – PESI class I–II or sPESI of 0 with no right heart
  strain and no elevation of troponin.

Risk is not entirely dependent on volume of pulmonary embolus (i.e., a 'massive PE' can't be diagnosed by imaging alone),
although high risk or massive PE is more common in patients with
a higher clot burden.

Pulmonary hypertension

Pulmonary hypertension is a condition associated with increased
pulmonary artery pressure.

The patient may present with shortness of breath, fatigue,
peripheral oedema, chest pain, dizziness, syncope or palpitations.

Occasionally pulmonary hypertension is idiopathic (most
frequently in young women) but usually there is an underlying
cause, including:

- Pulmonary artery disease – CTEPH in recurrent/chronic
  PE, pulmonary arteritis
- Left heart disease – left ventricular failure, mitral valve
  stenosis
- Right heart disease – increased pressure from longstanding
  left to right shunt (e.g., septal defects) and development of
  Eisenmenger syndrome
- Pulmonary disease – emphysema, asthma, cystic fibrosis
- Many other conditions including HIV, sickle cell disease,
  portal hypertension and certain connective tissue disorders
  (e.g., scleroderma)

Signs on examination include:

- Dominant a wave in the jugular venous pulse.
- Palpable and loud pulmonary component of second heart
  sound.
- Ejection systolic murmur in pulmonary area due to
  increased flow.
- Left parasternal (right ventricular) heave.
- Tricuspid regurgitation if the right ventricle dilates.

Investigation of pulmonary hypertension and underlying cause
may include:

- Chest X-ray – may show enlargement of the right atrium
  and pulmonary arteries, and elevation of the cardiac apex
  due to right ventricular hypertrophy.
- Echocardiography – assesses the probability of pulmonary
  hypertension; may show a high-velocity jet of tricuspid
  regurgitation, enlargement of right heart/pulmonary artery
  and may identify underlying causes (e.g., septal defect,
  mitral valve stenosis).
- Computed tomography (CT) – may show right heart/
  pulmonary artery enlargement or other features of right
  heart strain or evidence of chronic PE.
- Right heart catheterization – the gold standard test,
  pulmonary hypertension is diagnosed as a mean pulmonary
  arterial pressure (PAP) of ≥20 mmHg via right heart
  catheterization (normal systolic PAP is 15 to 30 mmHg and
  diastolic PAP is 6 to 12 mmHg).

Treatment will depend on the underlying cause and severity of
symptoms. Medications may include:

- Diuretics – symptomatic management of cardiac failure
- Oxygen – if patient is hypoxic
- Consider anticoagulation
- Digoxin if in atrial fibrillation
- Various other specialist medications including endothelin
  receptor antagonists (e.g., bosentan), phosphodiesterase
  5 inhibitors (e.g., sildenafil, tadalafil), prostaglandins
  (e.g., iloprost, epoprostenol), and calcium channel
  blockers (e.g., nifedipine, diltiazem)

Rarely, surgical/endovascular intervention may be required,
including pulmonary endarterectomy (to remove chronic PE),

Table 18.3 Overview of pulmonary embolus

Predisposing factors	• Hypercoagulable states – malignancy, oral contraceptive pill, thrombophilia (e.g., protein C/protein S deficiency), inflammatory states (e.g., inflammatory bowel disease). • Postoperative – abdominal/pelvic/hip/leg surgery. • Venous stasis – congestive cardiac failure, atrial fibrillation (right ventricular thrombus can cause PE). • Immobility – prolonged bed rest, long journeys. • Haemoconcentration – diuretics, polycythaemia. • Pregnancy – hypercoagulable state with possible immobility, venous stasis, haemoconcentration or surgery (Caesarean section).
Symptoms	• Chest pain – typically pleuritic but can be tight, can be anywhere in the chest. • Dyspnoea. • Dry cough. • Haemoptysis. • Hypotension/ autonomic features (patient may experience a 'sense of impending doom' or profound anxiety). • Syncope or cardiac arrest. • Sometimes incidental in relatively asymptomatic patient.
Signs	• Tachypnoea, tachycardia, hypotension. • Cyanosis (a late sign). • Signs of DVT (e.g., red, swollen calf). • Pleural rub – inflamed pleura due to adjacent pulmonary ischaemia/infarct.
Investigation	• Blood tests – assess for other cause of symptoms (e.g., infection), D-dimer (fibrin degradation product), ABG useful to demonstrate hypoxia. • CXR – low sensitivity for PE; can be used to rule out other cause of symptoms. • ECG – most frequently = sinus tachycardia. Classic 'S1Q3T3' pattern is not sensitive or specific for PE. In massive PE, there may be ventricular tachyarrhythmia or pulseless electrical activity in cardiac arrest. • Echocardiography – useful in unstable patients to decide about thrombolysis in suspected massive PE. May show right heart strain or an alternative cause of hypotension. • CTPA – high sensitivity/specificity for PE and any complications (e.g., right heart strain, pulmonary infarct) or other cause of symptoms. • Ventilation/perfusion (V/Q) scanning – rare, sometimes used in specific circumstances (e.g., CT contrast allergy). This is a nuclear medicine scan looking for perfusion defects. Provides limited information other than presence/absence of PE. • Invasive angiography – not commonly used unless catheter-directed targeted thrombolysis or mechanical thrombectomy is being considered. • No longer recommended by the National Institute for Health and Care Excellence (NICE) to offer routine further investigation for cancer in patients with unprovoked DVT or PE unless relevant symptoms/signs.
Management	• Anticoagulation – heparin (generally low molecular weight heparin) or oral anticoagulation (e.g., direct oral anticoagulants such as apixaban). Duration dependent on whether PE provoked/unprovoked and if patient has had previous DVT/PE. • In high-risk PE (see later), consider immediate thrombolysis if no contraindication and in specific cases consider percutaneous mechanical thrombectomy/clot-directed thrombolysis or surgical thrombectomy. • Intermediate-high-risk PE should be monitored closely for haemodynamic deterioration and consideration of rescue reperfusion therapy. • Intermediate-low-risk PE patients should be admitted to hospital. • Low-risk patients may be discharged home with anticoagulants if there is no other reason for hospitalization, there is sufficient family/social support and there is easy access to medical care.
Prognosis	• If untreated, mortality high at 23%–87%, reducing to 0.2%–6% with treatment (variation between studies). • Mortality higher in massive PE, estimated at 20% even with treatment. • Some may develop chronic thromboembolic pulmonary hypertension (CTEPH) with significant morbidity and mortality – may lead to progressive increased pulmonary arterial pressure and right heart failure.

CXR, chest X-ray; ECG, electrocardiography; CTPA, computed tomography pulmonary angiography.

Table 18.4 Original and simplified Pulmonary Embolism Severity Index

Parameter	Original version	Simplified version
Age	Age in years	1 point (if age >80)
Male sex	+10 points	–
Cancer	+30 points	1 point
Chronic heart failure	+10 points	1 point
Chronic pulmonary disease	+10 points	
Pulse rate ≥110 beats/minute	+20 points	1 point
Systolic BP <100 mmHg	+30 points	1 point
Respiratory rate >30 breaths/min	+20 points	–
Temperature <36°C	+20 points	–
Altered mental status	+60 points	–
Arterial oxyhaemoglobin saturation <90%	+20 points	1 point
Risk stratification	Class I: ≤65 points Class II: 66–85 points	0 points
	Class III: 86–105 points Class IV: 106–125 points Class V: >125 points	≥1 point

pulmonary artery angioplasty or transplantation (lung or heart and lung) in severe cases.

Prognosis is poor with a mean survival of approximately 3 years without treatment – patients usually die due to right heart failure.

Intestinal ischaemia

Intestinal ischaemia is where the blood supply to the large or small bowel is interrupted. This can result in necrosis of a section of the bowel and is associated with high morbidity and mortality.

It is important to understand the abdominal arterial anatomy and the bowel territory supplied by each artery:

- Coeliac trunk – foregut; distal oesophagus up to the second part of duodenum
- Superior mesenteric artery – midgut; second part of duodenum up to two-thirds of the way across the transverse colon
- Inferior mesenteric artery – hindgut; distal third of the transverse colon to upper two-thirds of the rectum

An overview of abdominal arterial and venous anatomy is in Figs. 18.6 and 18.7, respectively.

Intestinal ischaemia can occur acutely due to:

- Embolus into a mesenteric artery
- Thrombus formation within a mesenteric artery or mesenteric vein
- Insufficient blood flow due to hypovolaemia, hypotension, etc.

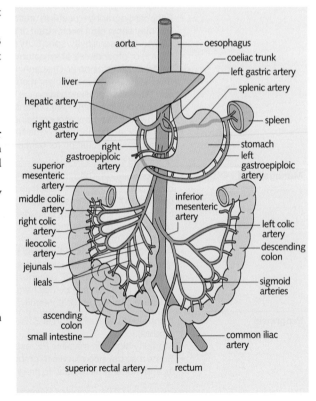

Fig. 18.6 Arterial supply of the abdomen.

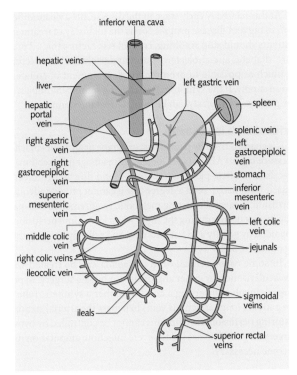

inferior vena cava
hepatic veins
liver
hepatic portal vein
right gastric vein
right gastroepiploic vein
superior mesenteric vein
middle colic vein
right colic veins
ileocolic vein
ileals
left gastric vein
spleen
splenic vein
left gastroepiploic vein
stomach
inferior mesenteric vein
left colic vein
jejunals
sigmoidal veins
superior rectal veins

Fig. 18.7 Venous drainage of the abdomen.

Intestinal ischaemia can also be chronic, with development of atherosclerotic disease within the mesenteric vasculature, which can lead to 'abdominal angina'. An overview of these conditions is included in Table 18.5.

Peripheral vascular disease

The term 'peripheral vascular disease' is often used to refer specifically to peripheral arterial disease (venous disease is discussed later). An overview of upper and lower limb arterial anatomy is in Figs. 18.8 and 18.9, respectively.

Chronic peripheral arterial disease

Peripheral arterial disease is caused by atherosclerosis in the major arteries supplying the lower limbs (rarely the upper limbs). As a result, the pathogenesis and risk factors for this disease are those that apply to atherosclerosis (see Chapter 11). People with coronary artery disease are more likely to have a degree of peripheral vascular disease and vice versa.

Intermittent claudication
This is characterized by a 'gripping', cramp-like pain in the calf or buttock on exercise which subsides at rest. Intermittent claudication is the lower limb equivalent of stable angina of the heart. It is due to an imbalance between oxygen supply and demand in the

Table 18.5 Overview of intestinal ischaemia	
Predisposing factors	• Risk factors for atherosclerosis (Chapter 11) • Atrial fibrillation (risk of embolization) • Underlying thrombophilia • Chronic renal failure
Symptoms	• Acute ischaemia – severe (often sudden) onset abdominal pain, abdominal distension, bloody diarrhoea; later confusion • Chronic ischaemia – abdominal angina (postprandial abdominal pain, anorexia, significant weight loss (reduced intake and poor digestion of food), nausea, vomiting)
Signs	• May have no abnormal findings (especially in chronic ischaemia) • Acute ischaemia – abdominal tenderness, distension, absent bowel sounds. Hypotension, tachycardia and other features of shock (e.g., cold peripheries, prolonged capillary refill time)
Investigation	• Blood tests – may be elevation of inflammatory markers or lactate in acute ischaemia; may be normal in chronic ischaemia • Abdominal X-ray – usually normal, may be findings in advanced cases (e.g., gas within the bowel wall, portal venous gas, perforation) • Computed tomography – will show above findings more clearly, may also show bowel wall thickening/oedema/reduced perfusion or free fluid • Invasive angiography – may show an arterial occlusion, can also allow endovascular intervention (as below).
Management	• Management of underlying risk factors in chronic ischaemia • Supportive treatments and resuscitation if nonocclusive ischaemia (e.g., if occurring due to hypotension) • Anticoagulation if thromboembolic cause of ischaemia • Surgical or endovascular revascularization (surgical thrombectomy, catheter-directed thrombolysis or angioplasty and stenting, bypass grafting, etc.) • If bowel has become necrotic, surgery is required to remove the infarcted segment of bowel

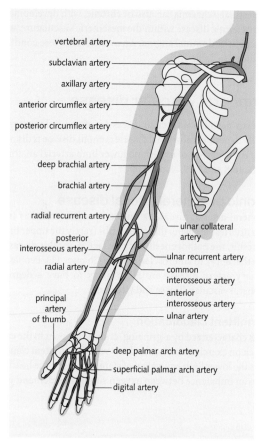

vertebral artery
subclavian artery
axillary artery
anterior circumflex artery
posterior circumflex artery
deep brachial artery
brachial artery
radial recurrent artery
posterior interosseous artery
radial artery
principal artery of thumb
ulnar collateral artery
ulnar recurrent artery
common interosseous artery
anterior interosseous artery
ulnar artery
deep palmar arch artery
superficial palmar arch artery
digital artery

Fig. 18.8 Arterial supply of the upper limbs.

skeletal muscle. Atherosclerotic plaques in the arteries supplying the leg cause a stenosis, preventing the normal metabolically mediated increase in blood flow during exercise. As oxygen demand subsides with rest to a level such that blood flow is adequate once again, pain subsides. If pain is felt in the calf muscle, the blockage is usually in the femoral artery or the popliteal artery. If pain is felt in the buttocks, the blockage is usually more proximal in the iliac artery.

CLINICAL NOTES

Erectile dysfunction can be associated with peripheral vascular disease, but other causes include neuropathy, hormonal imbalance, medications and psychosocial issues. Aortoiliac occlusive disease can affect blood supply to the penile arteries. The triad of bilateral claudication, erectile dysfunction and absent femoral pulses are known as Leriche syndrome.

At this relatively early stage in the disease, lifestyle modification to prevent disease progression is the mainstay of treatment. Patients should stop smoking, control risk factors (blood pressure, diabetes and cholesterol), and undertake aerobic exercise as much as possible to promote the development of collateral blood supply. If the symptoms are causing significant impact on the patient, angioplasty can be used to treat the stenosis.

Critical limb ischaemia

This is characterized by pain at rest, gangrene or an ankle–brachial pressure index (ABPI) (see Doppler ultrasonography section) of less than 0.5. Rest pain occurs when blood flow to the affected muscle is limited to such a degree that it cannot provide adequate perfusion to meet the resting metabolic requirements. Rest pain usually first occurs during the night when lower limb perfusion is not aided by gravity and patients may find relief by hanging their leg out of the bed.

In some cases, critical limb ischaemia can be treated with revascularization by either angioplasty or bypass surgery. Bypass surgery involves inserting a conduit (either a synthetic tube or the patient's long saphenous vein) to bypass the arterial stenosis, restoring perfusion. If symptoms cannot be controlled by bypass surgery or gangrene has led to severe infection, amputation may become necessary.

Arterial thrombosis/embolus and acute limb ischaemia

Unless there has been a history of chronic occlusive disease and a collateral circulation has developed, acute arterial occlusion causes blood flow to the distal tissues to be completely interrupted and acute limb ischaemia ensues.

Causes of acute ischaemia include:

- Embolism of thrombus from the heart in someone with atrial fibrillation, vegetations in someone with infective endocarditis or thrombus from an aneurysm sac.
- Thrombosis of a ruptured atherosclerotic plaque (equivalent of acute coronary syndrome).
- Raynaud syndrome: excessive vasoconstriction, often in response to cold; prevents tissue perfusion. Most commonly affects the fingers. Usually benign in primary Raynaud's but can be associated with tissue loss in secondary Raynaud's.
- Trauma.

Acute limb ischaemia presents with the 'six Ps' (three symptoms and three signs):

- Pain: due to skeletal muscle ischaemia.
- Paraesthesia: due to sensory nerve ischaemia.
- Paralysis.
- Pallor.
- Pulselessness.
- Perishing cold (to touch).

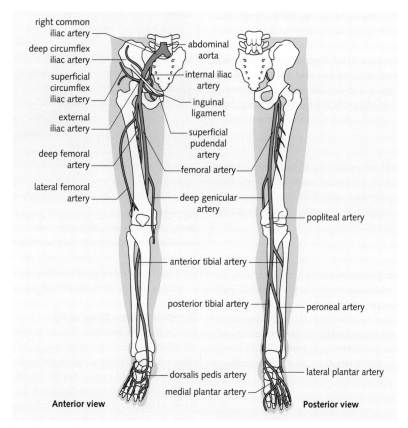

right common iliac artery
deep circumflex iliac artery
superficial circumflex iliac artery
external iliac artery
deep femoral artery
lateral femoral artery

abdominal aorta
internal iliac artery
inguinal ligament
superficial pudendal artery
femoral artery
deep genicular artery

popliteal artery

anterior tibial artery

posterior tibial artery
peroneal artery

lateral plantar artery
dorsalis pedis artery
medial plantar artery

Anterior view **Posterior view**

Fig. 18.9 Arterial supply of the lower limbs.

Examination

Begin with inspection, comparing the two legs. Features concerning for acute limb ischaemia include:

- Pallor.
- Skin mottling.

Signs of underlying chronic limb ischaemia include:

- Ulcers: see later.
- Hair loss.
- Scars (poor healing, previous ulcers and possibly previous surgery).

Next, palpate both legs from top to bottom with the back of the hands to assess for cold peripheries or any temperature difference between the limbs. Assess the capillary refill time in each foot by pressing firmly on the skin for 5 seconds, releasing your finger and observing the time it takes for the skin to return to its original colour. Normal capillary refill time is less than 2 seconds.

Palpate the abdominal aorta, then palpate and auscultate (for bruits) each peripheral pulse:

- Femoral pulse – just below the mid-inguinal point (halfway between the anterior superior iliac spine (ASIS) and the pubic symphysis). It is a strong pulse and should be easy to palpate.
- Popliteal pulse – in the popliteal fossae behind the knee and often difficult to palpate. The thumbs of both hands should be rested on either side of the patella and the fingertips should be placed deep into the popliteal fossa so that the popliteal artery is compressed against the posterior aspect of the tibia. The popliteals are best palpated with the knees flexed at about 120 degrees.
- Posterior tibial pulse – about 1 cm posterior and inferior to the medial malleolus of the tibia with the patient's foot relaxed.
- Dorsalis pedis pulse – against the tarsal bones on the dorsum of the foot, just lateral to the tendon of extensor hallucis longus.

The Buerger test is the final part of the examination. Start with the patient lying on the bed. Slowly lift each leg off the bed and observe the angle at which the leg goes pale, i.e., stops being adequately perfused. In normal individuals, the leg will remain perfused (and thus pink) to 90 degrees of hip flexion, but in patients with peripheral vascular disease, the leg may go pale at an angle of as little as 15 degrees. A Buerger angle of less than 20 degrees indicates severe ischaemia. Having identified the Buerger angle, lower the leg over the side of the bed and observe the colour change.

In a patient with severe peripheral arterial disease, there will be a delay in the restoration of blood flow, but once perfusion is restored, the leg will go a red-orange colour (sometimes described as sunset foot) due to profound metabolic vasodilatation before returning to normal colour (positive Buerger sign).

Arterial ulcers

Arterial ulcers (Fig. 18.10) are punched out, occasionally deep lesions of irregular shape on the lateral malleolus/lateral foot, between the toes and on pressure points. They may be associated with necrotic tissue or slough and are generally not exudative unless there is a coexisting infection.

Gangrene

In patients with critical limb ischaemia or an acute arterial occlusion where appropriate revascularization is not possible, gangrene may develop. Gangrene is tissue loss due to a lack of blood supply and is characterized by red-black skin discolouration, skin breakdown, pain, numbness and coolness. Treatment usually involves surgery to remove the necrotic tissue. Treat coexisting infection (if present) and attempt to treat the underlying cause.

HINTS AND TIPS

The type of gangrene seen with arterial disease is usually 'dry gangrene', as the tissue is dry and firm when no infection is present. If infection develops, the gangrene may become 'wet gangrene' (tissue becomes more swollen, oedematous and soft) or 'gas gangrene' (gas-forming organisms grow within the tissues). Both of these are associated with higher morbidity and mortality.

Investigation

Investigation of peripheral arterial disease includes:

- Doppler ultrasonography – described in detail below.
- CT angiogram – use of intravenous contrast to assess in detail the abdominal aorta and lower limb arterial system. This can be limited if vessels are heavily calcified (e.g., in diabetes mellitus or chronic renal disease). If there is concern regarding an embolic cause of acute limb ischaemia, then the heart and thoracic aorta may also be imaged.
- Echocardiography – if there is concern regarding intracardiac thrombus as a source of embolism, then this may be useful (as with CT).

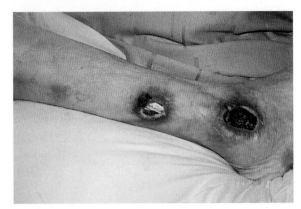

Fig. 18.10 Patient with peripheral arterial disease who has arterial ulcers of the lateral malleolus and distal and lateral portion of the leg. Ulcer is round, smooth and 'punched-out' in appearance.

- Blood tests – a range of baseline blood tests and coagulation screen may be useful as part of preoperative planning.

Doppler ultrasonography

This is used to measure flow in peripheral vessels to provide information about the arteries (e.g., in peripheral vascular disease) and the veins (e.g., in suspected deep venous thrombosis). It uses ultrasound to map out the vessel, highlighting any stenosis. Red blood cells move relative to the ultrasound beam. They create a Doppler shift, which is a change in the frequency of the ultrasound echo that returns to the transducer. The frequency shift is directly proportional to the velocity of the blood. The velocity of blood flow can be used to assess distal perfusion when flow is low or the severity of a stenosis where flow rates are high at the site of the narrowing (much like the flow of water when you pinch a hose pipe). It is commonly used to assess peripheral blood vessels before a site is selected for angiography.

Doppler can also be used to calculate the ABPI. The Doppler-derived systolic pressure from one of the foot pulses in the ankle (usually the dorsalis pedis) is divided into the Doppler-derived systolic pressure in the brachial artery recorded with the patient lying down (when the pressures should be equal). This ratio provides useful information about the severity of peripheral vascular disease:

- ABPI <0.5 indicates severe arterial disease. The patient may experience symptoms of ischaemia at rest, arterial ulceration or tissue loss – urgent vascular referral indicated.
- ABPI between 0.5 and 0.8 indicates a degree of peripheral vascular disease (the blood pressure in the feet is less than that in the arm due to atheroma formation or diabetic vessel changes) – routine vascular referral indicated.
- ABPI between 0.8 and 1.3 is normal.
- ABPI greater than 1.3 might suggest calcification of the vessels – common in diabetes, advanced renal failure, etc.

VENOUS DISEASE

The venous system of the limbs comprises a deep and superficial system. There are two important conditions of the veins to understand: varicose veins, affecting the superficial venous system, and DVT, affecting the deep venous system.

These conditions most commonly affect the lower limbs but are also possible in the upper limbs. An overview of upper and lower limb venous anatomy is included in Figs. 18.11 and 18.12, respectively.

In the lower limbs, the major superficial veins, the long and short saphenous veins join the femoral vein and popliteal vein (deep veins), respectively, as well as give off a number of small perforating veins to the deep veins. Blood flows into the deep veins and with the aid of the skeletal (primarily calf) muscle pump and the numerous valves, blood is returned to the central veins.

Deep vein thrombosis

DVT describes the presence of a thrombus within the deep veins, most commonly in the thigh or calf. Often DVT is asymptomatic but it can cause calf pain, unilateral leg swelling with raised skin temperature and dilated superficial veins. The major concern in a patient with a DVT is that thrombus will embolize to the pulmonary circulation, causing a pulmonary embolism.

Risk factors for thrombosis and clinical findings are used to formulate a Wells score (Table 18.6) but can be considered more broadly using Virchow triad:

- Stasis: this can be a result of obstruction to venous outflow from the legs caused by a pelvic mass or by a foetus in a pregnant woman.
- Hypercoagulable state: the oral contraceptive pill and malignancy are both factors that increase the coagulability of the blood.
- Endothelial damage.

CLINICAL NOTES

Leg swelling in DVT results from oedema due to alteration in the forces of fluid filtration. Increased venous pressure will increase the capillary hydrostatic pressure within the leg, increasing interstitial fluid.

Investigation of suspected DVT is usually with Doppler ultrasonography. D-dimer (fibrin degradation products) can also be measured. The 'gold standard' investigation is venography using intravenous contrast but this is rarely used. Initial treatment is

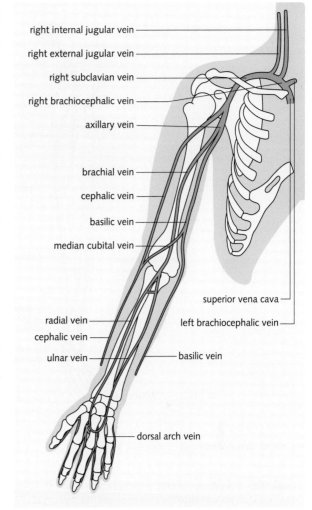

Fig. 18.11 Venous drainage of the upper limbs.

anticoagulation with low molecular weight heparin or oral anticoagulation.

In patients who suffer a pulmonary embolism and have a persistent DVT, an inferior vena cava (IVC) filter can be considered. As the name suggests, this is a fine filter that is placed in the IVC and prevents emboli from the leg veins reaching the pulmonary circulation.

Varicose veins

Varicose veins are tortuous, dilated superficial veins, usually of the lower limbs, caused by valvular incompetence. They occur in 10% to 20% of the normal population, and although more women present to hospital or their GP as a result of their varicose veins, the actual incidence is thought to be the same in men and women.

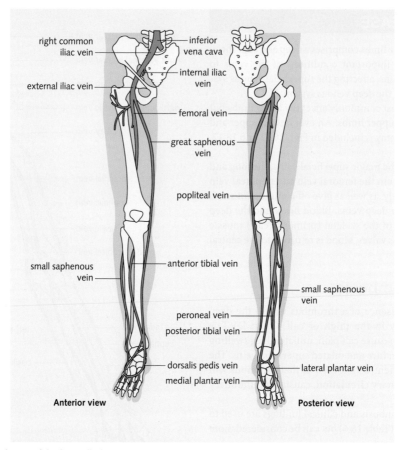

Fig. 18.12 Venous drainage of the lower limbs.

Table 18.6 Wells Score for DVT. A Wells Score <2 and a negative D-dimer can stratify patients as low risk and avoid the need for further testing.

Criteria	Score
Lower limb trauma, surgery or immobilization in a plaster cast	+1
Bedridden for more than three days or surgery within last twelve weeks	+1
Tenderness along line of femoral or popliteal veins	+1
Entire limb swollen	+1
Calf more than 3 cm greater in circumference compared to the other leg (measured 10 cm below tibial tuberosity)	+1
Pitting oedema, confined to the symptomatic leg	+1
Dilated collateral (nonvaricose) superficial veins	+1
Previous history of DVT (confirmed)	+1
Malignancy (within last 6 months)	+1
Alternative diagnosis as likely or more likely than DVT	–2

Risk factors include:

- Pregnancy.
- Obesity.
- Prolonged standing (important to ask the patient's occupation).
- Previous DVT.
- Pelvic masses compressing the deep veins.

If there is obstruction to deep venous flow (e.g., by thrombosis or pelvic mass) or incompetent valves in the perforating veins, then blood will move from the deep veins into the superficial veins. This will lead to distension and further valvular incompetence, resulting in stasis of blood. Oedema and skin changes develop, which fail to heal as a result of impaired circulation. Sequelae of varicose veins include:

- Bleeding: mild trauma can cause profuse bleeding because venous pressures are high and the walls of the vein are thin and distended.
- Thrombophlebitis: inflammation of the vessel wall that may be complicated by superficial thrombosis/bacterial

infection. Patients may present with a firm, tender, erythematous swelling along the course of the vein.

- Venous eczema: skin becomes thin and has a brown discolouration. It is caused by leakage of cells into the tissue due to the high venous pressure, which then break down, releasing haemosiderin into the skin. The ankle may be narrower with hardened skin (lipodermatosclerosis) and irregular white scars from poor healing (atrophie blanche).
- Venous ulcers: described later.

Varicose veins do not usually require treatment. Occasionally, patients complain of a dragging sensation or bleeding, or they are disturbed by the appearance of their legs. In these patients, varicose vein ablation or surgery may be appropriate to remove the distended veins.

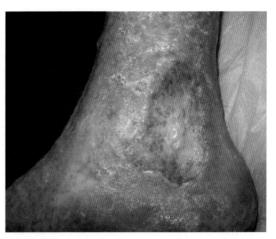

Fig. 18.13 Patient with lower limb venous disease and a typical venous ulcer – ulcer is shallow, with exudate and granulation tissue.

CLINICAL NOTES

Increased venous pressures can cause abnormal dilatation of veins elsewhere in the body, including:

- Haemorrhoids (piles) – distended submucosal veins in the anal canal that may protrude through the anus. Bleeding and pain may result from trauma, protrusion or spasm of the anal sphincter.
- Varicocele – distension of the veins of the pampiniform plexus in the spermatic cord.
- Oesophageal varices – distended veins at the oesophageal–gastric junction. They are caused by portal hypertension, usually due to liver cirrhosis.

Venous ulcers

Venous ulcers (Fig. 18.13) are generally shallow, sloughy, containing pink granulation tissue as they attempt to heal, and are located on the medial aspect of the calf in the gaiter area. There is often associated exudate, even without infection.

HINTS AND TIPS

Ulceration is usually on the lower limbs, and distinguishing between the different causes clinically is often difficult. As well as arterial and venous ulcers, some patients (usually diabetics) may also have neuropathic ulcers (usually painless and at pressure points). The key to detecting neuropathic ulceration is to test the sensation in the feet. Diabetic patients are also prone to arterial disease; therefore, diabetic ulcers tend to be a mixture of neuropathic and microangiopathic ulcers.

● Chapter Summary

- Aortic aneurysms are common, particularly in older males with a background of hypertension and smoking.
- Aortic dissection is a life-threatening condition where the wall of the aorta develops a tear and blood flows between the wall layers creating a 'false lumen'. This can be associated with organ ischaemia/infarction.
- Stanford type A aortic dissection (involving the ascending aorta) is usually treated with emergency surgery, whereas a type B aortic dissection (only involving the descending aorta) is usually initially medically managed, with possible later surgical/endovascular intervention.
- Aortic aneurysms and aortic dissection can both lead to aortic rupture – a condition that is often rapidly fatal.
- Repair of aortic dissection, aneurysms and rupture can include both endovascular and open surgical procedures.

- Vascular occlusion can be chronic, acute or acute-on-chronic. If there is chronic occlusion, then usually collateralization will develop. In acute occlusion, the patient will not generally have any collateral vessels and ischaemia/infarct is more likely to result unless the occlusion is identified and treated early.
- Intestinal ischaemia usually results from occlusion of the superior or inferior mesenteric artery (or one of their branches) or of one of the mesenteric veins – patients presenting with acute intestinal ischaemia have a high morbidity and mortality. Patients with chronic intestinal ischaemia often present with 'abdominal angina' – pain after eating, with nausea, anorexia and significant weight loss.
- Pulmonary embolus is another important differential in the patient presenting with chest pain, shortness of breath or collapse. Patients often have pleuritic pain, which can be located anywhere in the chest.
- Pulmonary hypertension (increased pressure within the pulmonary arteries) is a hard-to-treat condition that can result from several underlying conditions including previous pulmonary arterial disease (e.g., chronic PE – this is known as chronic thromboembolic pulmonary hypertension or CTEPH), respiratory disease (e.g., emphysema), or cardiac disease (e.g., left ventricular failure, mitral stenosis).
- Vascular disease of the limbs can be either arterial, venous or a combination of both.
- Chronic lower limb ischaemia often presents initially as intermittent claudication – leg pain on exertion that resolves with rest. Rest pain is more concerning and indicative of critical limb ischaemia.
- Patients who have an acute occlusion of a peripheral artery present with the 6 Ps – pain, paraesthesia, paralysis, pallor, pulselessness and perishing cold.
- Deep vein thrombosis is the most common cause of pulmonary embolus and is important to treat early with anticoagulation.
- Ulcers are common on the lower limbs in several conditions, including in arterial and venous disease – determining whether ulcers are arterial or venous can be tricky. Arterial ulcers may be deeper and 'punched-out' with generally little exudate (unless infected) and are often located at the lateral foot/ankle and at pressure areas. Venous ulcers are shallower, associated with exudate and granulation tissue, and usually located on the 'gaiter area' of the calf.

UKMLA Conditions
Aneurysms
Aortic aneurysm
Aortic dissection
Arterial thrombosis
Arterial ulcers
Deep vein thrombosis
Gangrene
Intestinal ischaemia
Ischaemic limb and occlusions
Peripheral vascular disease
Pulmonary embolism
Pulmonary hypertension
Venous ulcers

UKMLA Presentations
Acute abdominal pain
Cold, painful, pale, pulseless leg/foot
Erectile dysfunction
Painful swollen leg
Skin ulcers

SELF-ASSESSMENT

Key findings	Diagnoses
Central heavy chest pain occurring with exertion, resolves with rest and not associated with any elevation of troponin	Stable angina
Central heavy chest pain that occurs at rest without elevation of troponin	Unstable angina
Central heavy chest pain that occurs either at rest or on exertion, associated with elevation of troponin but no ST-elevation on ECG	Non-ST-elevation myocardial infarction (NSTEMI)
Central heavy chest pain that occurs either at rest or on exertion, associated with elevation of troponin and ST-elevation on ECG	ST-elevation myocardial infarction (STEMI)
ST-segment elevation in leads II, III and aVF	Inferior STEMI
ST-segment elevation in precordial leads (V1–V6)	Anterior STEMI (V1–V2 septal, V3–V4 anteroapical, V5–V6 more lateral)
ST-segment elevation in leads I, aVL, V5–V6	Lateral STEMI – if involvement of V1–V4 as well, then this would be considered extensive anterolateral MI
ST-segment elevation in leads V7–V9 (posterior chest) with reciprocal ST depression in V1–V2	Posterior STEMI
Atypical chest pain in female, diabetic or elderly patient with elevation of troponin	Myocardial infarction or acute myocardial injury
Burning chest pain worse after eating and lying flat, improved with sitting up and antacids, associated waterbrash	Gastro-oesophageal reflux disease
Chest pain after eating, may be relieved by GTN or associated with dysphagia and reflux symptoms	Oesophageal spasm
Chest pain and haemoptysis following multiple episodes of vomiting	Mallory-Weiss tear
Chest pain, subcutaneous emphysema, pleural effusion or signs of shock/sepsis following multiple episodes of vomiting	Boerhaave syndrome (oesophageal rupture)
Corneal arcus, tendon xanthomata and xanthelasma	Hypercholesterolaemia
Peripheral oedema, ascites, weight gain, loss of appetite	Right ventricular failure (or liver failure/renal failure/hypoalbuminaemia)
Hypoxia, orthopnoea, paroxysmal nocturnal dyspnoea	Left ventricular failure
Alveolar oedema, Kerley **B** lines, **C**ardiomegaly, Upper lobe venous **D**iversion, Pleural **E**ffusions	Pulmonary oedema
New ankle oedema in patient recently started on antihypertensive	Dihydropyridine calcium channel blocker therapy (e.g., amlodipine, nifedipine)
Elevated BNP/NT-proBNP	Heart failure (sensitive although not specific)
Pulsus paradoxus (exaggerated drop in systolic BP of >10 mmHg on inspiration)	Several conditions including cardiac tamponade, constrictive pericarditis, status asthmaticus
Pulsus alternans (alternating strong and weak pulses)	Severe heart failure

Continued

Key findings	Diagnoses
Added heart sound in early diastole (S3)	Due to rapid ventricular filling. May be seen in young adults/ athletes but can also be seen in heart failure.
Added heart sound in late diastole – just before the normal first heart sound (S4)	Due to forceful atrial contraction against a stiff ventricle. Always abnormal and may be seen in ventricular hypertrophy
Sudden onset pulmonary oedema in patient with new pansystolic murmur and recent myocardial infarction	Acute mitral regurgitation with flash pulmonary oedema (potentially secondary to papillary rupture following MI) or ventricular septal defect, but pulmonary oedema less prominent in this case
Acute breathlessness and bilateral crepitations following stroke/subarachnoid haemorrhage/seizures	Acute neurogenic pulmonary oedema (neurogenic stunned myocardium)
New onset dry cough following new heart failure/blood pressure medication	ACE inhibitor-related cough (inhibition of bradykinin/ substance P metabolism)
New gynaecomastia after starting on a new medication for heart failure or treatment-resistant hypertension	Side effect of spironolactone therapy (note that eplerenone does not cause gynaecomastia)
Bilateral crepitations and wheeze	Pulmonary oedema, bilateral pneumonia on a background of obstructive lung disease (if unilateral much more likely infection)
Every P wave followed by a QRS complex and every QRS complex preceded by a P wave, at a rate of between 60 and 100 beats per minute	Sinus rhythm
Sinus rhythm but rate increases with inspiration and decreases with expiration	Sinus arrhythmia
Collapse preceded by tingling sensation in the fingers or perioral region	Hyperventilation/anxiety
Cannon a wave in the JVP	Third-degree atrioventricular block
Absent a wave in the JVP	Atrial fibrillation
Normal sinus rhythm on ECG (or evidence of other organized electrical activity) in patient without a pulse	Pulseless electrical activity (PEA)
Prolonged PR interval (>200 ms)	First-degree atrioventricular block
Progressive prolongation of PR interval followed by QRS being dropped (with this cycle then repeating)	Second-degree atrioventricular block, Mobitz I (Wenckebach)
Dropped QRS complex that is not preceded by progressive PR interval prolongation	Second-degree atrioventricular block, Mobitz II
Complete dissociation of P waves and QRS complexes (often these are at different rates)	Third-degree atrioventricular block/complete heart block
WiLLiaM (W appearance of QRS complex in V1 and M appearance of QRS in V6)	Left bundle branch block
MaRRoW (M appearance of QRS complex in V1 and W appearance of QRS in V6)	Right bundle branch block
Irregularly irregular rhythm	Atrial fibrillation (can rarely be seen with other arrhythmias, e.g., atrial flutter with variable block)
Sawtooth P waves and heart rate of 300/x (e.g., 150, 100, 75, etc.)	Atrial flutter
Dizziness, nausea, flushing followed by collapse in context of stress, heat, venepuncture, noxious stimulus, etc.	Vasovagal syncope
Collapse following micturition, defaecation, coughing, lifting a heavy weight, etc.	Situational syncope

Key findings	Diagnoses
Collapse occurs shortly after standing up from a sitting or lying position (may be a history of volume depletion, e.g., vomiting, diarrhoea, blood loss)	Orthostatic hypotension
Sudden onset, rapid, regular palpitations that are relieved with vagal manoeuvres (e.g., Valsalva, carotid sinus massage) or adenosine administration	Atrioventricular nodal reentrant tachycardia
Short PR interval and slurred upstroke of QRS complex (delta wave)	Wolff-Parkinson-White syndrome (presence of an accessory conduction pathway)
Broad complex tachycardia with QRS complexes of consistent shape throughout	Monomorphic ventricular tachycardia
Broad complex tachycardia with QRS complexes of varying shapes (axis and amplitude of QRS complex vary over time), prolonged QTc prior to arrhythmia	Polymorphic ventricular tachycardia (torsades de pointes)
Palpitations and evidence of tachycardia in patient with medications known to prolong QT interval (a long list, including clarithromycin, methadone, antiemetics, antidepressants, antipsychotics, etc.)	Polymorphic ventricular tachycardia (torsades de pointes)
Palpitations in a young patient with sweating, flushing, significantly elevated (or labile) blood pressure	Phaeochromocytoma
Collapse associated with pressure on the neck (e.g., from shirt collar)	Carotid sinus hypersensitivity
Downsloping ST segment ('reverse tick' shape), T wave inversion	Digoxin therapy
J wave on ECG	Hypothermia
U wave on ECG	Hypokalaemia (can be seen on chest leads of a normal ECG)
Peaked T waves, PR prolongation or P wave flattening, QRS widening, 'sine wave' appearance on ECG	Hyperkalaemia
Ejection systolic murmur heard best at the aortic area, radiating to the carotids	Aortic stenosis
Chest pain, breathlessness and exertional syncope in patient with an ejection systolic murmur	Aortic stenosis
Slow-rising pulse with narrow pulse pressure	Aortic stenosis
Ejection systolic murmur heard best at the aortic area, without radiation, symptoms or evidence of left ventricular outflow obstruction	Aortic sclerosis
Early development of aortic stenosis	Bicuspid (or less commonly unicuspid) aortic valve
Pulsus bisferiens (pulse waveform with two systolic peaks per beat)	Mixed aortic disease
New murmur in a patient with sepsis/pyrexia	Infective endocarditis (or less commonly acute rheumatic fever)
Pansystolic murmur heard best at the apex and radiating to the axilla	Mitral regurgitation
Late systolic murmur with mid-systolic 'click'	Mitral valve prolapse
Pansystolic murmur heard best at the lower left sternal edge (without radiation)	Ventricular septal defect
Giant a wave in the JVP	Tricuspid stenosis

Continued

Key findings	Diagnoses
Large v waves in the JVP	Tricuspid regurgitation
'Water-hammer' or collapsing pulse (wide pulse pressure)	Aortic regurgitation
Several eponymous signs including Quincke's, Corrigan's, De Musset's, Duroziez's, Traube's and Müller's signs	Aortic regurgitation
Murmur louder on expiration	Left-sided heart murmur (aortic/mitral)
Murmur louder on inspiration	Right-sided heart murmur (pulmonary/tricuspid)
Continuous murmur in the supraclavicular area, increased in diastole, reduced by lying down and light pressure overlying the internal jugular vein	Venous hum (normal blood flow through the jugular veins, can be more prominent in high output states, e.g., anaemia, pregnancy)
Symptoms similar to myocardial infarction in a patient with normal coronaries and recent stressful/emotional episode	Takotsubo cardiomyopathy
Apical ballooning of the left ventricle in context of recent stressful/emotional episode	Takotsubo cardiomyopathy
Hypotension, muffled heart sounds, raised JVP	Beck's triad (in cardiac tamponade)
Saddle-shaped ST-elevation and PR depression on ECG across multiple coronary territories	Acute pericarditis
Sharp, pleuritic chest pain that is worse on lying down and relieved by sitting forward	Acute pericarditis
Globular or 'water bottle' shaped heart	Pericardial effusion
Electrical alternans (QRS amplitude alternating between beats) with small (low amplitude) QRS complexes	Large pericardial effusion/tamponade (heart 'swinging' in fluid)
Recent myocardial infarction, now hypotensive with elevated JVP on inspiration (Kussmaul sign)	Pericardial effusion/tamponade
Recent myocardial infarction, fever and sharp chest pain several weeks later	Dressler syndrome
A murmur with syncope or sudden cardiac death during a period of exertion	Hypertrophic obstructive cardiomyopathy
Elevated JVP on inspiration (Kussmaul sign), signs of right and left ventricular failure (low-output failure), pericardial calcification	Constrictive pericarditis
Elevated JVP on inspiration (Kussmaul sign), signs of right and left ventricular failure (low-output failure)	Restrictive cardiomyopathy
Cardiomegaly in patient with history of alcohol excess, thyrotoxicosis or recent viral infection	Dilated cardiomyopathy
Boot-shaped heart	Tetralogy of Fallot
Pulmonary stenosis, overriding aorta, ventricular septal defect, and right ventricular hypertrophy	Tetralogy of Fallot
Intermittent cyanosis in a young child, characteristically after crying or feeding symptoms may be relieved by squatting or bringing the legs up to the chest	'Tet spells' in tetralogy of Fallot
Box-shaped heart	Ebstein anomaly
Fixed splitting of the second heart sound	Atrial septal defect
Cyanosis that does not improve with increasing inspired oxygen	Right-to-left shunt (blood bypassing the lungs)

Key findings	Diagnoses
Prominent apex beat (which may be displaced), pansystolic murmur at left lower sternal edge radiating to the apex	Ventricular septal defect
A continuous 'machinery' murmur	Patent ductus arteriosus
'Egg-on-a-string' appearance of the heart on chest X-ray	Transposition of the great arteries
Notching of inferior surfaces of the ribs on chest X-ray	Coarctation of the aorta (notching occurs due to enlarged collateral vessels)
Left-to-right shunt with increasing pulmonary pressures and resultant reversal of shunt with systemic cyanosis	Eisenmenger syndrome
Absent or reduced volume femoral pulses	Coarctation of the aorta, aortic dissection or very rarely aortic occlusion
Radiofemoral delay	Coarctation of the aorta or aortic dissection
Widened mediastinum and pleural effusion (potentially following significant trauma)	Aortic rupture (thoracic)
Abdominal or lower back pain in older patient, limb numbness/weakness, syncope, shock, or cardiac arrest	Aortic rupture (abdominal)
Pain, pallor, pulselessness, paraesthesia, perishingly cold, paralysis (when referring to a limb)	Acute limb ischaemia
Cramp-like pain in the calf or buttock brought on by exercise and subsiding with rest	Intermittent claudication
Lower limb pain at rest ± gangrene ± ankle-brachial pressure index of less than 0.5	Critical limb ischaemia
Painful, white fingers in response to cold. Fingers then go blue and then later red as blood flow returns	Raynaud's phenomenon
Unilateral painful, swollen limb with distended collateral veins (may be history of risk factors for venous thromboembolism such as immobility, recent surgery, malignancy, or history of previous DVT/PE)	Deep vein thrombosis
New breathlessness, hypoxia, chest pain and collapse. ECG may show sinus tachycardia ± evidence of right heart strain (anterior T wave inversion) or S1Q3T3 pattern	Pulmonary embolism
Wedge-shaped opacification on chest X-ray (or CT) in patient with confirmed pulmonary embolus	Pulmonary infarct
Tearing or ripping chest pain that radiates through to the back in an unwell patient, may be associated with difference in blood pressure between arms or organ ischaemia/infarction	Aortic dissection
Aortic dissection involving the ascending aorta	Stanford Type A aortic dissection
Aortic dissection involving the descending aorta only	Stanford Type B aortic dissection
Chest pain in patient with known Marfan syndrome	Aortic dissection (or possibly pneumothorax)
Patient presents with stroke or other arterial embolus with evidence of acute/recent DVT	Paradoxical embolus in context of a right-to-left shunt (e.g., septal defect)
Multiple coronary artery aneurysms	Kawasaki disease
Pulsatile central abdominal mass	Abdominal aortic aneurysm

Continued

Key findings	Diagnoses
Sudden onset abdominal pain with diarrhoea/PR bleeding and elevated lactate	Intestinal ischaemia (less likely diverticulitis, etc., if onset sudden)
Punched out, deep, irregular ulcer on the lateral malleolus/ lateral foot or pressure point, without significant exudate	Arterial ulcer
Shallow, sloughy ulcer containing pink granulation tissue on the medial aspect of the calf in the gaiter area, often associated with exudate	Venous ulcer

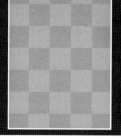

UKMLA Single Best Answer (SBA) Questions

Chapter 1 Cardiac anatomy, physiology and development

1. During your cardiothoracic surgery attachment, the consultant asks about the mediastinum and its contents. Which of these links the mediastinal compartment to the contents correctly?
   A. Anterior mediastinum – sympathetic chain.
   B. Anterior mediastinum – trachea.
   C. Middle mediastinum – oesophagus.
   D. Posterior mediastinum – internal thoracic artery.
   E. Superior mediastinum – thymus.

2. Which of the following statements regarding the coronary vessels is true?
   A. From the coronary veins, blood drains into the coronary sinus and then into the right atrium.
   B. In the majority of people, the SA node and the AV node are supplied with blood from the left coronary artery.
   C. The coronary arteries arise just distal to the pulmonary valve.
   D. The left coronary artery usually gives rise to the posterior descending artery.
   E. The right coronary artery usually gives rise to the circumflex artery.

3. Which of the following statements regarding cardiac myocytes is true?
   A. They are longer than skeletal muscle fibres.
   B. They are multinucleated.
   C. They have a branched structure.
   D. They never have the ability to generate a spontaneous action potential.
   E. Troponin is contained within the thick filaments.

4. Which of these most accurately describes the circulation changes occurring after birth?
   A. Pulmonary vascular resistance increases.
   B. There is increased blood flow through the umbilical vessels.
   C. The foramen ovale immediately closes and fuses between the two atria.
   D. The ductus arteriosus closes and becomes the ligamentum arteriosum.
   E. Foetal haemoglobin continues to be produced for 3 months.

5. Which of these is true of the cardiac vasculature?
   A. A branch of the right coronary artery usually supplies the sinoatrial node.
   B. The coronary arteries usually are contained within the myocardium.
   C. The coronary arteries usually arise just inferior to the aortic valve cusps.
   D. The coronary sinus usually drains into the right ventricle.
   E. The diagonal branches arise from the left circumflex artery.

Chapter 2 The cardiac cycle, control of cardiac output and haemodynamic regulation

1. Regarding hormonal control of the cardiovascular system, which of the following statements is correct?
   A. Angiotensin-converting enzyme is predominately found in the vascular bed of the gastrointestinal tract.
   B. Antidiuretic hormone is released when a rise in osmolarity is detected.
   C. Adrenaline is secreted from the adrenal cortex.
   D. Adrenaline/epinephrine causes vasodilatation in skeletal muscle by acting on β_1 receptors.
   E. Renin is converted to angiotensin I by angiotensinogen.

2. Which of the following is true of the baroreceptor reflex?
   A. Baroreceptors in the carotid body are innervated by the glossopharyngeal nerve.
   B. Constriction of cutaneous arterioles brought about by the baroreceptor reflex can be overcome by thermoregulatory changes in vascular tone.
   C. Decreased loading of baroreceptors increases venous tone by reducing parasympathetic activity.
   D. Increased stretch in the arterial wall causes a decrease in baroreceptor firing.
   E. It is central to the long-term regulation of blood pressure.

3. A tall, thin 38-year-old man attends the GP with progressive breathlessness on exertion and when lying down at night. He is noted to have a blood pressure of 185/68 mmHg and a heart rate of 55 beats per minute. What is the most likely cause of his wide pulse pressure?
   A. Aortic regurgitation.
   B. Aortic stenosis.
   C. Cardiac tamponade.
   D. Hypovolaemia.
   E. Sepsis.

4. A 75-year-old woman attends her GP for some routine blood tests after feeling generally lethargic for a number of weeks. Her haematocrit is noted to be 0.61. Her blood tests were normal 6 months ago. What is the most likely diagnosis?
   A. Acute myeloid leukaemia.
   B. Asthma.
   C. Cardiac failure.
   D. High altitude living.
   E. Polycythaemia rubra vera.

5. Which of the following cardiovascular reflexes results in an increased parasympathetic outflow and can be used to terminate supraventricular tachycardia?
   A. Alerting response.
   B. Baroreceptor reflex.
   C. Chemoreceptor reflex.
   D. Diving reflex.
   E. Hepatojugular reflex.

6. A 48-year-old woman presents with episodes of a broad complex tachycardia that is diagnosed as polymorphic VT. She is noted on her ECG to have a QTc of 528 ms. In long QT syndrome, which one of these may be abnormal?
   A. Gap junction.
   B. L-type Ca^{2+} channels.
   C. Na^+/K^+ ATPase.
   D. Voltage-gated K^+ channels.
   E. Voltage-gated Na^+ channels.

Chapter 3 ECG interpretation

1. A 72-year-old man is brought into the hospital after a fall and lying for 8 hours outside in the cold overnight. His observations on arrival include a temperature of 33.9°C, a heart rate of 48 beats per minute and a blood pressure of 104/56 mmHg. Which of these abnormalities might be found on the ECG?
   A. Downsloping ST segment.
   B. J waves.
   C. Raised ST segment.
   D. 'Tented' T waves.
   E. U waves.

2. A 56-year-old man with a history of hypertension and a smoking history of 40 to 50 pack years presents with a 6-hour history of central chest pain. His ECG shows 3 mm ST elevation in leads II, III and aVF. What is the likely diagnosis?
   A. Anterior ST elevation myocardial infarction.
   B. Inferior ST elevation myocardial infarction.
   C. Lateral ST elevation myocardial infarction.
   D. Posterior ST elevation myocardial infarction.
   E. Septal ST elevation myocardial infarction.

3. A 32-year-old woman undergoes a period of cardiac monitoring as the result of a number of episodes of transient loss of consciousness. During the monitoring, the following arrhythmia is seen. What abnormality is most likely to be seen on the resting ECG?
   A. Broad QRS complexes.
   B. Delta waves.
   C. Long PR interval.
   D. Long QT interval.
   E. 'Tented' T waves.

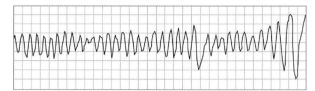

4. A 72-year-old woman is admitted to the acute medical unit following a fall at home. As part of the clerk-in process, an ECG is carried out. This shows a cardiac axis of −45 degrees. Which one of the following might cause this abnormality?
   A. Chronic lung disease.
   B. Left ventricular hypertrophy.
   C. Pulmonary embolus.
   D. Right bundle branch block.
   E. Ostium secundum atrial septal defect.

5. A 75-year-old man is admitted to the respiratory ward with a lower respiratory tract infection. He has prominent Q waves on his admission ECG. Which of the following is true of Q waves?
   A. In leads I and aVL, they suggest old inferior myocardial infarction.
   B. They are always pathological.
   C. They are usually transient.
   D. They may suggest transmural myocardial infarction.
   E. They are due to depolarization current towards the lead.

6. Which of the following is true regarding findings on an ECG?
   A. PR interval may be shortened with accessory pathways.
   B. QT interval is prolonged in bundle branch block.
   C. ST segment represents phase 3 (the repolarization phase) of the cardiac action potential.
   D. U wave represents ventricular repolarization.
   E. Upsloping ST depression may be seen in patients on digoxin.

Chapter 4 Other cardiac investigations

1. What is the gold standard investigation for assessment of the vessel lumen in obstructive coronary artery disease?
   A. Invasive coronary angiogram.
   B. CT coronary angiogram.
   C. Dobutamine stress echocardiogram.
   D. Electrocardiogram.
   E. Exercise tolerance test.

2. A 57-year-old male smoker with a history of hypertension and dyslipidaemia presents to the chest pain clinic with 3 months of exertional chest pain. This occurs predictably when he runs 3 miles (previously able to run 5 miles twice a week). His father had an MI aged 50 and his brothers have had MIs aged 48 and 59. His GP started aspirin, amlodipine, bisoprolol and atorvastatin last week with little improvement. What investigation is most appropriate?
   A. Invasive coronary angiogram.
   B. CT coronary angiogram.
   C. Exercise ECG test.
   D. Dobutamine stress echocardiogram.
   E. Myocardial perfusion MRI scan.

3. A 24-year-old man who is an IV drug user is admitted with a 1-month history of fevers, night sweats and rigors. On examination, he has splinter haemorrhages, a raised jugular venous pressure, a pansystolic murmur and mild pedal oedema. Which investigation below is most likely to give a definitive diagnosis?
   A. Blood cultures.
   B. ECG.
   C. Chest X-ray.
   D. Routine blood test.
   E. Urine sample.

4. A 67-year-old woman was referred to the cardiology clinic when her GP incidentally found a murmur. She is in good health without any cardiac symptoms and still regularly goes country dancing. There are no known ischaemic risk factors. On examination, she has an ejection systolic murmur, but there are no signs of cardiac failure. ECG is unremarkable. Which investigation would be most appropriate?
   A. Cardiac MRI scan.
   B. CT coronary angiogram.
   C. Echocardiography.
   D. Exercise ECG.
   E. MUGA scan.

5. A 61-year-old man presents to the emergency department with chest pain and breathlessness and has a chest X-ray. Which of the following features on the X-ray are matched to the underlying diagnosis?
   A. Boot-shaped heart – ventricular septal defect.
   B. Continuous diaphragm sign – pneumothorax.
   C. Double density sign – right atrial enlargement.
   D. Egg-on-a-string sign – Ebstein anomaly.
   E. Water bottle sign – pericardial effusion.

Chapter 5 History and examination

1. Which of these is the third stage of finger clubbing?
   A. Clubbed or 'drumstick appearance' of the fingertip.
   B. Increased convexity of the nail bed.
   C. Increased fluctuation of the nail bed only.
   D. Loss of the normal angle at the base of the nail.
   E. Painful, red swelling on the finger pulp.

2. Which clinical sign and diagnosis are correctly matched?
   A. Flame-shaped haemorrhages – retinal haemorrhages seen in thyrotoxicosis.
   B. Roth spots – retinal haemorrhages with a pale centre, seen in hypertensive retinopathy.
   C. Osler nodes – septic emboli within the skin of the hands and feet in infective endocarditis.
   D. Corneal arcus – brown rings encircling the cornea of the eye in Wilson disease.
   E. Absent x descent in the JVP – seen in atrial fibrillation.

3. A 72-year-old lady with fatigue and dyspnoea is noted to have a very thickened and calcified pericardium on a CT scan of her chest. Which of the following pulse characters might you expect in this condition?
   A. Bisferiens pulse.
   B. Collapsing (water hammer) pulse.
   C. Pulsus alternans.
   D. Pulsus paradoxus.
   E. Slow-rising pulse.

Chapter 6 Chest pain

1. A 28-year-old man is admitted with sharp chest pain that is eased by lying down. An ECG showed ST elevation in all leads. What is the most likely diagnosis?
   A. Pericarditis.
   B. Pleurisy.
   C. Pneumothorax.
   D. Pulmonary embolus.
   E. ST elevation myocardial infarction.

2. A 45-year-old man presents acutely unwell to the emergency department. He is pale and sweaty. He complains of chest pain going through to between the shoulder blades. He has a difference in blood pressure of 50/30 mmHg between left and right arms. What is the most likely diagnosis?
   A. Acute aortic regurgitation.
   B. Acute myocardial infarction.
   C. Aortic dissection.
   D. Pulmonary embolus.
   E. Tension pneumothorax.

3. A 63-year-old man presents to the emergency department with chest pain 4 weeks after presenting with an ST elevation myocardial infarction (STEMI). He complains of a sharp pain that is worse on deep breaths and eased on sitting forward. Temperature is 38.1°C. ECG shows ST elevation in all leads. What is the most likely diagnosis?
   A. Aortic dissection.
   B. Dressler syndrome.
   C. Further ST elevation myocardial infarction.
   D. Pulmonary embolus.
   E. Unstable angina.

4. A 45-year-old woman is admitted with chest pain and ST elevation in all leads of her ECG 1 week after a viral illness. What is the most appropriate treatment?
   A. Aspirin 300 mg and clopidogrel 300 mg.
   B. Ibuprofen.
   C. Paracetamol.
   D. Primary percutaneous coronary intervention.
   E. Thrombolysis.

5. Which of the following statements regarding cardiac enzymes/biomarkers is correct?
   A. A negative troponin at the time of presentation and 12 hours later excludes myocardial infarction.
   B. Elevated high-sensitivity troponin is always due to myocardial infarction.
   C. Creatine kinase, lactate dehydrogenase and troponin are all raised in unstable angina.
   D. If a patient presents 48 hours after onset of chest pain, it is too late to measure troponin.
   E. Troponin is found in cardiomyocyte cell membranes.

6. A 36-year-old man presents with heavy central chest pain that started 1 hour after taking cocaine. He is a smoker but has no other known atherosclerotic risk factors. He is pale and sweaty, but examination is otherwise normal. Anterolateral ST elevation is seen on the ECG, and troponin is positive. What is the most likely diagnosis?
   A. Aortic dissection.
   B. Myocardial infarction.

C. Myocarditis.
D. Pulmonary embolus.
E. Takotsubo cardiomyopathy.

7. A 16-year-old with no past medical history is admitted to A&E with 1 day of chest pain and 3 days of fatigue, dyspnoea and orthopnoea. During your systemic enquiry, he reports a flu-like illness 2 weeks ago which he felt was unrelated, as it had already resolved. On examination, he has a tachycardia of 108 bpm, a tachypnoea of 22 breaths/min, a raised JVP, a third heart sound and bilateral crepitations. ECG demonstrates sinus tachycardia with inferior T wave flattening, and troponin is mildly raised. What is the most likely diagnosis?
   A. Indigestion.
   B. Myocardial infarction.
   C. Myocarditis.
   D. Pericarditis.
   E. Pulmonary embolus.

8. A 26-year-old gentleman has a 1 day history of severe vomiting and presents with severe sudden-onset central chest pain and breathlessness. On admission, he is tachycardic at 117 bpm with otherwise normal observations. Examination reveals a dull left base, a left lateral rasping sound and subcutaneous emphysema. What is the most likely diagnosis?
   A. Boerhaave syndrome.
   B. Mallory-Weiss tear.
   C. Myocarditis.
   D. Pericarditis.
   E. Pneumothorax.

Chapter 7 Breathlessness and peripheral oedema

1. Cardiovascular system examination is a common OSCE station in finals. Which of the following is true when examining the jugular venous pressure (JVP)?
   A. A JVP with a vertical height greater than 2 cm above the manubriosternal angle is abnormal.
   B. Gentle pressure over the abdomen elicits the hepatojugular reflex and causes a transient increase in the JVP.
   C. The height of the JVP above the manubriosternal angle gives an estimate of right atrial pressure in mmHg.
   D. The internal jugular vein should be visualized and is usually located just lateral to the sternocleidomastoid.
   E. The patient should be lying flat with their head turned slightly away from the examiner.

2. A 72-year-old woman attends the clinic with isolated ankle swelling over the past 3 months. She is not troubled by breathlessness. She has a history of hypertension, indigestion and migraine. She has been started on a

number of medicines recently. She has a normal echocardiogram that day. Which medication is most likely to blame?

A. Amlodipine.
B. Bendroflumethiazide.
C. Furosemide.
D. Lansoprazole.
E. Propranolol.

3. A 71-year-old woman presents with dyspnoea and a cough. She has a past medical history of hypertension and two previous myocardial infarctions. Her observations include a heart rate of 110 bpm, blood pressure of 96/64 mmHg, oxygen saturations of 91% on room air and a temperature of 38.6°C. She has left basal consolidation on her chest X-ray. ECG shows new atrial fibrillation. What is the most appropriate immediate management?

A. Antibiotic therapy as per local guidelines.
B. Oral digoxin loading.
C. Oxygen therapy, aiming for saturations 94%–98%.
D. Intravenous fluid administration.
E. Referral to cardiology for urgent assessment.

4. A 64-year-old man presents to the hospital with a syncopal episode and ongoing dyspnoea. He has a sharp left-sided chest pain that is pleuritic in nature. Pulmonary embolism (PE) is suspected. Which of these chest radiograph features is associated with PE?

A. Bat's wing shadowing.
B. Increased cardiothoracic ratio.
C. Oligaemic lung fields.
D. Kerley B lines.
E. Upper lobe venous diversion.

5. A 74-year-old woman comes to the emergency department complaining of breathlessness. She is distressed and tachypnoeic at 28 breaths per minute, but her other observations are normal. On examination, her chest sounds clear and she has mild bilateral pitting oedema up to the ankles. She has an arterial blood gas (ABG) which shows the following results (on room air):

$$H^+ = 32 \text{ nmol/L, } PO_2 = 13 \text{ kPa,}$$
$$PCO_2 = 3.4 \text{ kPa, } HCO_3^- = 24 \text{ mmol/L}$$

What is the most likely diagnosis?

A. Acute left ventricular failure (LVF).
B. Exacerbation of chronic obstructive pulmonary disease (COPD).
C. Exacerbation of interstitial lung disease.
D. Psychogenic hyperventilation.
E. Pulmonary embolism.

6. An 81-year-old lady presents with an approximately 4-month history of right leg swelling and abdominal bloating. Despite this, she reports approximately two stone weight loss over the past year. She has a past medical history of asthma and hypertension. Blood tests show a microcytic anaemia with a haemoglobin level of 98 g/dL but no other abnormalities. An echocardiogram from 6 weeks ago showed good ventricular function and no valvular abnormalities. What is the most likely cause of her right leg swelling?

A. Anaemia related.
B. Arterial insufficiency.
C. Cardiac failure.
D. Renal failure.
E. Venous compression.

Chapter 8 Palpitations

1. A 28-year-old man comes into the emergency department with palpitations and breathlessness. He has a past medical history of irritable bowel syndrome and brittle asthma. He has a heart rate of 180 bpm and his ECG confirms an AV nodal reentrant tachycardia (AVNRT). Which of the following is an appropriate first-line treatment?

A. Rapid bolus of intravenous adenosine.
B. Intravenous verapamil infused over 2 minutes.
C. Ocular pressure.
D. Defibrillation.
E. Isoprenaline infusion.

2. A 64-year-old woman presents with a number of episodes of rapid palpitations over the preceding 4 weeks. Which clinical feature allows differentiation between atrial fibrillation and AV nodal reentrant tachycardia (AVNRT)?

A. Association with chest pain.
B. Irregularly irregular pulse.
C. Normal resting ECG.
D. Palpitations are less severe and less frequent.
E. Precipitation by excessive coffee drinking.

3. A 75-year-old woman complains of palpitations. There are no P waves on her ECG. Which of the following conditions is associated with this ECG finding?

A. Atrial fibrillation.
B. Atrial flutter.
C. Sick sinus syndrome.
D. Third-degree atrioventricular block.
E. Ventricular tachycardia.

4. On a routine ECG, a 67-year-old man is found to have a prolonged PR interval. Which of the following is a common cause of this abnormality?

A. ACE inhibitors.
B. β-Blockers.

C. Left bundle branch block.

D. Pericarditis.

E. Wolff–Parkinson–White syndrome.

5. A 46-year-old man presents to the emergency department with a collapse and a 30-minute history of sudden-onset palpitations. He is clammy, sweaty and looks unwell. ECG shows a narrow complex tachycardia. Which one of the following is an indication for urgent DC cardioversion?

A. A blood pressure of 95 mmHg systolic.

B. Central heavy chest pain.

C. A rate of >200 bpm.

D. Breathlessness at rest.

E. Peripheral oedema.

6. A 24-year-old lady is studying for her final exams at university. She has recently broken up with a long-term partner. She has had a number of episodes of rapid palpitations over the preceding three days. Which of the following features would be least concerning?

A. Associated with fever and productive cough.

B. Associated with recent history of dark stool.

C. Metabolic acidosis.

D. Paraesthesia around the mouth.

E. Slurred upstroke of QRS complex on ECG.

Chapter 9 Syncope, blackout and faints

1. A 28-year-old woman presents to the emergency department following a faint. Which of the following is the most classic feature of cardiac syncope?

A. Gradual onset.

B. Precipitated by sudden turning of the head.

C. Rapid recovery.

D. Residual neurological deficit.

E. Warning symptoms.

2. A 71-year-old man is brought in by ambulance. He complains of a collapse and sudden-onset, severe 'ripping' pain in his chest and upper back. He looks pale and his systolic blood pressure is 110 mmHg in his right arm and 70 mmHg in his left arm. Auscultation of his chest is unremarkable. ECG shows ST depression and T wave changes in leads II, III and aVF. What is the most likely underlying diagnosis?

A. Aortic dissection.

B. Myocardial infarction.

C. Pericarditis.

D. Pulmonary embolism.

E. Tension pneumothorax.

3. A 26-year-old man who is otherwise fit and well presents to the GP a couple of days after collapsing whilst playing basketball. It

occurred suddenly and without warning symptoms. He recovered quickly and feels back to normal. This has happened to him twice in the past and his father and uncle have also had similar problems. What condition might be suspected?

A. Acute coronary syndrome.

B. Hypertrophic cardiomyopathy.

C. Orthostatic hypotension.

D. Takotsubo cardiomyopathy.

E. Vasovagal syncope.

4. An 81-year-old woman who is on holiday presents to the hospital in the evening complaining of ongoing, fast palpitations and a number of episodes of feeling faint that day (without loss of consciousness). She had been out at a party the previous night and has little recollection of events but does remember drinking alcohol. What is the most likely cause of her symptoms?

A. Atrial fibrillation.

B. Complete heart block.

C. Ongoing intoxication.

D. Sinus tachycardia.

E. Ventricular tachycardia.

5. A 67-year-old woman presents to the hospital reporting a number of events of presyncope over the last few days. She does not report any other symptoms. She had a non-ST elevation myocardial infarction around 3 months ago and was started on a number of medications following this, including aspirin, bisoprolol, ramipril and atorvastatin. Her blood pressure is 104/67 mmHg. ECG shows sinus bradycardia at a rate of 45 bpm but is otherwise unremarkable. Which of the following options is most appropriate initially?

A. Insertion of temporary pacing wire.

B. List patient for permanent pacemaker.

C. Start digoxin for its positive inotropic effect.

D. Treat bradycardia with intravenous atropine.

E. Withhold bisoprolol and ramipril.

6. A 54-year-old lady with a background of depression and previous intravenous drug use is admitted for treatment of pneumonia. She has a number of episodes on the ward of rapid palpitations associated with light-headedness and one 'faint'. ECG during one of these episodes shows a polymorphic ventricular tachycardia. Which medication is least likely to be contributing?

A. Amoxicillin.

B. Citalopram.

C. Clarithromycin.

D. Methadone.

E. Ondansetron.

Chapter 10 Heart murmurs

1. A 45-year-old woman is found to have a pansystolic murmur. Which of the following causes this?
   A. Aortic regurgitation.
   B. Aortic stenosis.
   C. Atrial septal defect.
   D. Mitral regurgitation.
   E. Tricuspid stenosis.

2. A 45-year-old woman presents with a fever. She has not had any recent illnesses. On examination, she has digital clubbing, and auscultation reveals a mid-diastolic murmur and a diastolic 'plop'. What is the most likely diagnosis?
   A. Atrial myxoma.
   B. Infective endocarditis.
   C. Mitral valve prolapse.
   D. Pericarditis.
   E. Rheumatic fever.

3. A keen medical student examining a patient on the ward palpates a tapping apex beat. What is the cause?
   A. Mitral regurgitation.
   B. Mitral stenosis.
   C. Left ventricular aneurysm.
   D. Left ventricular hypertrophy.
   E. Pericardial effusion.

4. A 35-year-old man presents with fever, clubbing, haematuria and a murmur. What is the most likely diagnosis?
   A. Haemolytic uraemic syndrome (HUS).
   B. Infectious mononucleosis.
   C. Infective endocarditis.
   D. Rheumatic fever.
   E. Tetralogy of Fallot.

5. Which of the following is correct with respect to the character of the arterial pulse?
   A. Collapsing pulse can be a feature of mitral regurgitation.
   B. Pulsus alternans is a feature of atrial fibrillation.
   C. Pulsus paradoxus may be found in restrictive cardiomyopathy.
   D. Radiofemoral delay occurs in atrial septal defect.
   E. Slow rising pulse is a feature of aortic regurgitation.

6. At a neonatal check, the paediatrician hears a loud systolic murmur at the lower left sternal edge. The baby seems otherwise well. Which of the following is most likely to be the cause?
   A. Acute mitral regurgitation.
   B. Congenital aortic stenosis.
   C. Hypertrophic cardiomyopathy.
   D. Large ventricular septal defect.
   E. Small ventricular septal defect.

7. A 25-year-old woman who is being investigated for exertional shortness of breath is found to have a pulmonary venous pressure of 48 mmHg on echocardiography. Which of the following is a feature of pulmonary hypertension?
   A. Corrigan's pulse.
   B. Heaving apex beat.
   C. JVP not visible.
   D. Mid-diastolic murmur.
   E. Palpable second heart sound.

8. Which of the following is a correct association?
   A. Continuous murmur – atrial septal defect.
   B. Early diastolic murmur – aortic stenosis.
   C. Mid-diastolic murmur – tricuspid regurgitation.
   D. Pansystolic murmur – mitral stenosis.
   E. Physiological splitting of the second heart sound – inspiration.

Chapter 11 Atherosclerosis and its risk factors

1. A previously fit 55-year-old male smoker presents with sudden-onset central chest heaviness and breathlessness. Troponin is raised and his ECG demonstrates sinus rhythm 55 bpm with new inferior T wave inversion. What is the diagnosis?
   A. Pulmonary embolus (PE).
   B. NSTEMI.
   C. Stable angina.
   D. STEMI.
   E. Unstable angina.

2. The following patients have presented on a busy day in the emergency department. Which of these is most likely due to embolus rather than atherosclerotic plaque rupture?
   A. A 45-year-old male smoker with a history of hypertension, type 1 diabetes and severe deforming rheumatoid arthritis, who presents with sudden severe central chest pain.
   B. A 76-year-old man with previous ischaemic stroke and angina, with normal heart sounds and ECG, who attends with a suddenly painful left leg that is cold and pale.
   C. An 82-year-old female smoker with sudden-onset severe abdominal pain, nausea and diarrhoea. Pain is out of keeping with abdominal examination findings, cardiovascular examination is normal and CT demonstrates bowel ischaemia.
   D. A 34-year-old woman with a new diagnosis of atrial fibrillation and ischaemic stroke.
   E. A 63-year-old man with hyperlipidaemia and a strong family history of MI presents with change from predictable exertional angina to prolonged chest pain at rest.

3. A 62-year-old man with a history of hypertension, type 2 diabetes and intermittent claudication presents to A&E with a 1-hour history of crushing central chest pain. An ECG shows ST segment elevation in the anterior leads. Which of the following is likely to be responsible?
   A. 45% stenosis of the left main coronary artery by a stable atherosclerotic plaque.
   B. Complete occlusion of the circumflex artery following erosion of an atherosclerotic plaque.
   C. Complete occlusion of the left anterior descending artery following rupture of an atherosclerotic plaque.
   D. Complete occlusion of the right coronary artery following rupture of an atherosclerotic plaque.
   E. Severe anaemia.

4. Which of these would be most suitable for primary prevention in a patient with hypercholesterolaemia and a 16% 10-year risk of a cardiovascular event?
   A. Atorvastatin 20 mg nocte.
   B. Cholestyramine 4 g daily.
   C. Niacin 1 g.
   D. Pravastatin 20 mg nocte.
   E. Simvastatin 20 mg nocte.

5. A 56-year-old Caucasian woman visits her GP for an asthma review. The GP opportunistically checks her blood pressure and finds it to be 182/110 mmHg. She feels well and full examination including fundoscopy is normal. What should the GP do next?

A. Arrange ambulatory or home BP monitoring.
B. Blood test and urinalysis.
C. Send to hospital for an urgent assessment.
D. Start an ACE inhibitor.
E. Start amlodipine.

6. A 28-year-old Caucasian man has a BP of 198/110 mmHg on his mother's BP machine at home. He visits his GP and his BP is 224/126 mmHg. He says he is probably just more nervous today as he has been worrying about his blood pressure and has been having palpitations and headaches as a result. The GP notes that he has a background of anxiety and looks tremulous. It is difficult to visualize his fundi in a bright room with no blinds. What should the GP do?
   A. Ask for a detailed family history.
   B. Blood test and urinalysis.
   C. Send to hospital for an urgent assessment.
   D. Start an ACE inhibitor.
   E. Tell him it is likely due to anxiety, not to worry and to come back for a repeat BP.

7. Your colleague comes to you to ask you about a pre-operative ECG for a patient attending for elective knee replacement. She is 76 years old with a background of hypertension for 30 years. She has never had any chest pain and currently feels entirely well. You cannot find any previous ECGs to compare. What do you advise?

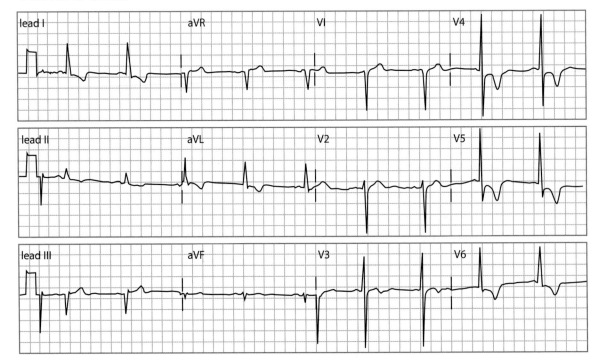

A. She has had a lateral MI in the past.
B. She is having a heart attack.
C. This demonstrates an electrolyte abnormality.
D. This is a normal variant.
E. This is likely due to hypertension.

8. A 54-year-old man with autism is diagnosed with essential hypertension by his GP. He has always been terrified of needles and does not wish to have regular blood tests. Which antihypertensive would be most suitable?
   A. Amlodipine.
   B. Bendroflumethiazide.
   C. Candesartan.
   D. Indapamide.
   E. Ramipril.

9. Which of the following medications used in the treatment of acute coronary syndrome is correctly matched with its mechanism of action?
   A. Aspirin – activation of cyclooxygenase (COX).
   B. Fondaparinux – GPIIb/IIIa inhibitor.
   C. Ticagrelor – irreversible platelet ADP receptor P2Y12 antagonist.
   D. Tirofiban – directly inhibits factor Xa.
   E. Unfractionated heparin – antithrombin III enhancer.

10. A 30-year-old man was started on an ACE inhibitor for hypertension a month ago. His BP today is 145/90 mmHg, but since repeating his blood test, his creatinine has risen from 80 to 130 μmol/L and his K+ has risen to 5.7 mmol/L. His ACE inhibitor is stopped immediately. What should be done next?
    A. Refer for specialist assessment.
    B. Refer urgently to emergency department.
    C. Start an angiotensin-receptor blocker (ARB).
    D. Start calcium channel blocker.
    E. Start sacubitril/valsartan combination.

Chapter 12 Acute coronary syndromes and stable angina

1. Which of the following drugs should be used in the management of STEMI but not NSTEMI?
   A. β-Blocker.
   B. Thienopyridine.
   C. Recombinant tissue plasminogen activator (tPA).
   D. Aspirin.
   E. Glyceryl trinitrate.

2. A 68-year-old woman with central dull chest pain has a raised troponin and anterolateral T-wave inversion on her ECG. She has no past medical history or allergies and otherwise normal blood test. Which treatment combination would be best to reduce thrombus extension?

A. Aspirin and clopidogrel.
B. Aspirin, ticagrelor and fondaparinux.
C. Aspirin, ticagrelor and metoprolol.
D. Aspirin, clopidogrel and oxygen.
E. Clopidogrel, ticagrelor and tirofiban.

3. A 56-year-old man with a history of hypertension is complaining of central chest pain on exertion that resolves with rest. He is currently taking an ACE inhibitor for his hypertension and a salbutamol inhaler for asthma. His doctor makes a diagnosis of angina pectoris and wants to start him on a medicine to decrease frequency of angina attacks. His heart rate is 88 bpm and his BP is 140/85 mmHg. What would be the most appropriate drug for this patient?
   A. Atenolol.
   B. Digoxin.
   C. Diltiazem.
   D. GTN spray.
   E. Nifedipine.

4. A 73-year-old woman who presented 24 hours after developing chest pain was diagnosed with an anterior STEMI and received percutaneous coronary intervention with standard medical care. She was a smoker but had no other risk factors. You see her in clinic 4 months later. She has not had any further chest pain but tells you she has not been walking as far after the heart attack. On palpation of her precordium, she has a slight rocking or dyskinetic cardiac impulse but examination is otherwise unremarkable. Routine ECG shows anterior Q waves and ST elevation, with no other abnormalities. What is the most likely complication?
   A. Further ST elevation myocardial infarction.
   B. Left ventricular aneurysm formation.
   C. Left ventricular hypertrophy.
   D. Pericarditis.
   E. Ventricular septal defect.

5. An 81-year-old man underwent percutaneous coronary intervention for an inferior NSTEMI 3 days ago. Whilst having breakfast, he suddenly collapses. He is found to have no pulse. CPR and airway management have been started by your colleagues and a resuscitation team is on its way. Which of the following is next most urgent?
   A. Arterial blood gas (ABG).
   B. Blood glucose.
   C. Application of defibrillator pads.
   D. Portable chest X-ray (CXR) urgently.
   E. Urgent bedside echocardiography.

6. A 74-year-old man was admitted with a late presentation of inferior STEMI 3 days ago. He had been initially stable on the cardiology ward but has suddenly become breathless at rest. His oxygen saturations have fallen from 98% to 92% on air, and you start him on oxygen therapy. BP has fallen slightly to 110/75 mmHg. Examination reveals a quiet pansystolic murmur radiating to the left axilla, third heart sound and bilateral crepitations. There is nothing of note on the recent cardiac monitor trace, and 12-lead ECG demonstrates sinus rhythm at 99 bpm and anterior Q waves and T wave inversion. What is the most likely complication?
   A. Acute mitral regurgitation.
   B. Arrhythmia.
   C. Myocardial free wall rupture.
   D. Complete heart block.
   E. Ventricular septal rupture.

Chapter 13 Heart failure

1. A 65-year-old man develops worsening ankle swelling and is found to have right ventricular failure. Which other clinical sign is most likely to be elicited on examination?
   A. Bilateral basal crepitations.
   B. Hepatomegaly.
   C. Hypertension.
   D. Mid-diastolic murmur.
   E. Wheeze.

2. A 74-year-old man is admitted with shortness of breath. On examination, crepitations are heard up to the mid-zones. A diagnosis of acute left ventricular failure is made. Which of the following treatments would be started first?
   A. β-Blockers.
   B. Continuous positive airway pressure (CPAP).
   C. Diuretics.
   D. Morphine.
   E. Oxygen.

3. A 72-year-old woman who is breathless on even mild exertion attends the cardiology clinic. Her ECG shows sinus rhythm with a left bundle branch block (LBBB) pattern and QRS duration of 155 ms. Echocardiogram shows severe left ventricular systolic dysfunction (LVSD). She is already on appropriate medications. Which of the following treatments is most likely to be considered?
   A. Biventricular pacemaker.
   B. Dual chamber pacemaker.
   C. Left ventricular assist device.
   D. Single lead atrial pacemaker.
   E. Single lead ventricular pacemaker.

4. A 54-year-old man with heart failure develops diarrhoea and vomiting. Which of the following medications is it most important to withhold?
   A. Amlodipine.
   B. Aspirin.
   C. Atorvastatin.
   D. Bisoprolol.
   E. Candesartan.

5. An 81-year-old woman with worsening breathlessness is referred for an echocardiogram and diagnosed with moderate left ventricular systolic dysfunction. Which one of the following is classic of left ventricular failure?
   A. Ascites.
   B. Bilateral pitting peripheral oedema.
   C. Dyspnoea due to poor pulmonary perfusion.
   D. Nocturia.
   E. Paroxysmal nocturnal dyspnoea.

6. Which of these is a side effect of sodium-glucose cotransporter 2 (SLGT2) inhibitors?
   A. Euglycaemic ketoacidosis.
   B. Hypertension.
   C. Long-term renal toxicity.
   D. Urinary hesitancy.
   E. Weight gain.

Chapter 14 Arrhythmias

1. A 72-year-old man on the cardiology ward complains of palpitations and light-headedness. An ECG is performed and a diagnosis of ventricular tachycardia is made. Which of the following is correct regarding ventricular tachycardia?
   A. It is a life-threatening condition.
   B. It is a narrow complex tachycardia.
   C. It should always be treated with immediate defibrillation.
   D. It should be treated with atropine.
   E. Ventricular tachycardia with a pulse may be treated with a synchronized DC cardioversion with an energy of 50 J.

2. An 81-year-old woman is prescribed digoxin for atrial fibrillation. Which of the following is correct regarding digoxin?
   A. It acts to slow conduction of the sinoatrial node.
   B. It is contraindicated in Wolff–Parkinson–White syndrome.
   C. Its main route of excretion is by the liver.
   D. It has a very short half-life.
   E. Its effects are enhanced by hyperkalaemia.

3. A patient suffers a cardiac arrest whilst on the cardiology ward. Resuscitation is unfortunately unsuccessful. Which of the following is true regarding advanced life support?

A. Pulseless ventricular tachycardia (pVT) requires an immediate synchronized DC shock.

B. Adrenaline is administered at a dose of 1 µg every 3 to 5 minutes of CPR.

C. Atropine is given in cases of PEA/asystole.

D. Pulseless VT/ventricular fibrillation cardiac arrest has a better prognosis than asystole.

E. A defibrillator energy setting of 75 J should be used in the first instance for adults with ventricular fibrillation.

4. A 67-year-old man is admitted in extremis to the emergency department. His ECG shows a broad complex tachycardia. The staff are unsure whether this represents VT or SVT with aberrancy. Which of the following features/treatments are correct?

A. Concordance is present in VT.

B. Capture beats are present in SVT with aberrancy.

C. Fusion beats are seen in SVT with aberrancy.

D. Intravenous verapamil can safely be used to differentiate between the VT and SVT with aberrancy.

E. If in doubt, treat as SVT.

5. A 57-year-old man on the medical ward is struggling with his breathing. He has an elevated jugular venous pressure and crepitations bilaterally to the mid zones on auscultation. Blood pressure is 92/55 mmHg and his ECG shows atrial fibrillation at a rate of 160 beats/min. He was admitted for treatment of cellulitis and noted to be in sinus rhythm the previous day. Which of the following is the most appropriate initial management?

A. Oral bisoprolol and warfarin.

B. Oral digoxin.

C. Intravenous furosemide.

D. Intravenous amiodarone.

E. Urgent synchronized direct current cardioversion.

6. In terms of the out-of-hospital management of cardiac arrest in a paediatric patient, what is the most appropriate sequence of events in management by a single rescuer (as per BLS guidelines)?

A. Call 999 using speaker function if phone is available. If no phone is available, continue CPR for 1 minute seeking help. Open airway and deliver five rescue breaths.

B. Call 999 using speaker function if phone is available. If no phone is available, open airway, deliver five rescue breaths and continue CPR until help arrives.

C. Carry out CPR for 1 minute. Call 999 using speaker function if phone is available. If no phone is available, open the airway and deliver five rescue breaths before leaving the patient to seek help.

D. Leave patient to find automated external defibrillator and deliver immediate defibrillation on return, as the majority of arrhythmias in children are pulseless ventricular tachycardia or ventricular fibrillation.

E. Open airway, deliver five rescue breaths, and call 999 using speaker function if phone is available. If no phone is available, continue CPR for 1 minute before leaving the patient to seek help.

7. With regards to the adult advanced life support (ALS) algorithm, which of the following is true?

A. Peripheral oedema seen in a patient indicates severe heart failure (a life-threatening feature of arrhythmia) and warrants urgent synchronized DC cardioversion.

B. In patients with shockable rhythms, adrenaline 1 mg IV should be given every 3 to 5 shocks.

C. In patients with shockable rhythms, amiodarone 300 mg IV should be given after the third shock.

D. In patients with shockable rhythms, there should be a rhythm check immediately after shock is delivered.

E. Lidocaine 100 mg IV may be used as an alternative to adrenaline if adrenaline is not available or a local decision has been made to use lidocaine instead of adrenaline.

8. A 49-year-old man experiences a cardiac arrest on the medical ward. In cardiac arrest, it is important to rule out a reversible cause of cardiac arrest. Which of the following is true of reversible causes of cardiac arrest?

A. Consider continuing CPR for 60 to 90 minutes after administering thrombolysis.

B. Drug-induced hypotension does not usually respond well to IV fluids.

C. If tension pneumothorax is felt to be the cause of cardiac arrest, then carry out immediate needle decompression with a large bore cannula in the second intercostal space in the midaxillary line.

D. In cardiac arrest due to pulmonary embolism (PE), the most common rhythm is ventricular tachycardia.

E. Mechanical chest compression devices are contraindicated if prolonged CPR is needed due to increased potential for causing chest trauma.

9. Which of the following would be the most suitable treatment for atrial fibrillation with rapid ventricular response in Wolff–Parkinson–White (WPW) syndrome?

A. Adenosine.

B. Beta-blocker.

C. Calcium channel blocker.

D. Amiodarone.

E. Flecainide.

Chapter 15 Valvular disease

1. A 62-year-old woman is reviewed in clinic. She is known to have previous rheumatic fever. Which of the following is a feature of the disease?
   A. It only affects mitral and aortic valves.
   B. It is by far the most common cause of mitral regurgitation.
   C. It is caused by valve infection with group B streptococci.
   D. Requires antibiotic prophylaxis to prevent endocarditis.
   E. Results in cusp and commissural fusion.

2. A 67-year-old man goes to his GP with exertional shortness of breath and chest tightness and is found to have an ejection systolic murmur. Which of the following is a feature of severe aortic stenosis?
   A. Fixed splitting of S2.
   B. Loud S2.
   C. S4.
   D. Thrusting displaced apex beat.
   E. Wide pulse pressure.

3. A 45-year-old woman is found to have mitral stenosis on an echocardiography. Which of the following is a feature of the condition?
   A. A displaced apex beat.
   B. A pansystolic murmur heard best at the apex.
   C. An early diastolic murmur best heard with the diaphragm of the stethoscope.
   D. An end-diastolic murmur best heard with the bell of the stethoscope.
   E. Malar flush.

4. Which of the following statements is true regarding mitral valve prolapse?
   A. Affects 0.1% of the population.
   B. Frequently leads to severe heart failure.
   C. It is always associated with mitral regurgitation.
   D. It is associated with a mid-diastolic click.
   E. More common in women.

5. A 63-year-old man is reviewed in the cardiology clinic. On examination, he has a median sternotomy scar. Which of the following operations would fit with his scar?
   A. Aortic valve replacement.
   B. Closed mitral valvotomy.
   C. Implantable cardiac defibrillator (ICD) insertion.
   D. Mitral valvuloplasty.
   E. Temporary pacemaker insertion.

6. Which is correct regarding causative organisms in infective endocarditis?
   A. A negative blood culture rules out infective endocarditis.
   B. Enterococci are very rare.
   C. Fungal infections are common causes of infective endocarditis.
   D. *Staphylococcus aureus* is associated with severe and destructive infection.
   E. The most common causative organisms in developed countries are the *Streptococcus viridans* group.

7. A 74-year-old woman is admitted with a 2-week history of fever, malaise and progressive breathlessness. During assessment, findings include an ejection systolic murmur, an early diastolic murmur and bibasal crepitations. She had a prosthetic aortic valve replacement 4 years ago. Which clinical sign is most likely to be found on examination?
   A. First-degree AV block.
   B. Janeway lesions.
   C. Microscopic haematuria.
   D. Roth spots.
   E. Splenomegaly.

8. A 28-year-old IV drug user is thought to have endocarditis. Which of the following is a minor criterion for the diagnosis of infective endocarditis?
   A. Erythema multiforme.
   B. Growth of *Staphylococcus aureus* in sputum culture.
   C. IV drug use.
   D. Prolonged QRS duration.
   E. Vegetations visualized on echocardiography.

Chapter 16 Diseases of the myocardium and pericardium

1. A 63-year-old man presents to the emergency department with chest pain 3 weeks after presenting with an ST elevation myocardial infarction (STEMI). He complains of a sharp left-sided chest pain that is worse when lying flat. ECG shows ST elevation in all territories. What is the most likely diagnosis?
   A. Aortic dissection.
   B. Dressler syndrome.
   C. Further ST elevation myocardial infarction.
   D. Pneumothorax.
   E. Unstable angina.

2. A 32-year-old man with hypertrophic cardiomyopathy attends the cardiology clinic. He is thinking of starting a family and is asking about the risk of passing on the condition to his children. What is the most common mode of inheritance of hypertrophic cardiomyopathy?
   A. Autosomal dominant.
   B. Autosomal recessive.
   C. Non-Mendelian.

D. X-linked dominant.

E. X-linked recessive.

3. A 32-year-old woman attends the emergency department with sharp chest pain. Pericarditis is suspected. Which of these clinical signs is associated with pericarditis?

A. Clubbing.

B. Conjunctival haemorrhages.

C. Janeway lesions.

D. Pericardial rub.

E. Parasternal heave.

4. A man has been involved in a road traffic accident and is brought in by ambulance to the emergency department with suspected cardiac tamponade. What does Beck's triad of signs in tamponade consist of?

A. Hypoxia, decreased level of consciousness and impalpable apex beat.

B. Low arterial blood pressure, jugular venous distension and muffled heart sounds.

C. Poor capillary refill, tachycardia and decreased level of consciousness.

D. Narrow pulse pressure, exaggerated reduction in systemic blood pressure during inspiration and presence of gallop rhythm.

E. Raised jugular venous pressure which drops with inspiration, pericardial friction rub and impalpable apex beat.

5. A 58-year-old woman is admitted with chest pain a week after the death of her mother. As part of the investigation of her condition, she has an echocardiogram which shows ballooning of the left ventricular apex and a diagnosis of Takotsubo cardiomyopathy is made. Which of the following is true regarding this condition?

A. It carries a 30% mortality rate in the acute phase.

B. It is more common in young men.

C. It should be treated with fluid resuscitation.

D. It may be misdiagnosed as ST elevation myocardial infarction (STEMI).

E. It was first described in Japanese lobster fishermen.

6. A 24-year-old man is referred for an echocardiogram after attending the emergency department with chest pain. His ECG at the time showed changes consistent with left ventricular hypertrophy. Which of the following statements is true of hypertrophic cardiomyopathy (HCM)?

A. Disopyramide is contraindicated.

B. It does not present after the third decade.

C. It may be treated with percutaneous myomectomy.

D. Prognosis is worse if diagnosed at an earlier age.

E. It is approximately three times more common in men than women.

Chapter 17 Congenital heart disease

1. A baby is noted to have a murmur at the 6-week post-natal check. The GP suspects congenital heart disease. Which of these cardiac malformations is most common?

A. Atrial septal defect (ASD).

B. Ebstein anomaly.

C. Patent ductus arteriosus (PDA).

D. Tetralogy of Fallot.

E. Ventricular septal defect (VSD).

2. A mother brings her 6-week-old baby boy to see her GP as she is concerned his lips, hands and feet look blue. Which of the following congenital heart defects causes cyanosis early in life?

A. Atrial septal defect (ASD).

B. Coarctation of the aorta.

C. Patent ductus arteriosus (PDA).

D. Tetralogy of Fallot.

E. Ventricular septal defect (VSD).

3. A 62-year-old woman reports a 3-year history of worsening breathlessness to her GP. She is found to be significantly cyanosed and is known to have a ventricular septal defect. Which one of the following may occur in Eisenmenger syndrome?

A. Anaemia.

B. Reversal of longstanding right-to-left shunt.

C. Paradoxical emboli.

D. Decreased pulmonary vascular resistance.

E. Splinter haemorrhages.

4. A 28-year-old woman presents with sudden-onset left-sided weakness. As part of her investigations, her echocardiography raised a suspicion of a patent foramen ovale (PFO). About a quarter of the population have a PFO. Which of the following may be associated?

A. Left bundle branch block.

B. Migraine.

C. Mitral prolapse.

D. Mitral stenosis.

E. Right axis deviation.

5. A worried mother takes her 6-month-old baby to the GP as she is worried he looks blue. The GP hears a murmur and wonders whether this might be Tetralogy of Fallot. Which of the following is true of this condition?

A. Feeding improves symptoms.

B. It includes patent ductus arteriosus.

C. Left ventricular hypertrophy is a feature.

D. Pulmonary hypertension is a prominent feature.

E. Squatting helps ease symptoms.

6. A 28-year-old man is found to have mild Ebstein anomaly on an echocardiography during a private medical assessment. Which of the following describes Ebstein anomaly?
   A. Apical displacement of the tricuspid valve.
   B. Overriding aorta.
   C. Pulmonary stenosis.
   D. Right ventricular hypertrophy (RVH).
   E. Ventricular septal defect (VSD).

Chapter 18 Vascular disease

1. A 56-year-old man is brought to the ED following a collapse. Bystanders reported he looked blue at the time and was briefly unconscious. He describes 1 week of breathlessness and left leg swelling, with brief chest heaviness and blurred vision prior to collapse. His heart rate is 110 bpm, SpO$_2$ is 95% on 2 L oxygen but observations are otherwise within normal limits. ECG shows anterior T wave inversion, and high sensitivity troponin is 63 ng/L. His only past medical history is a hernia operation 1 month ago. What is the most appropriate investigation?
   A. 24 hour tape.
   B. CTPA.
   C. Echo.
   D. Erect and supine BP.
   E. Urgent PCI.

2. A 71-year-old man presents with pain in his left buttock when walking/exercising. He has no symptoms on the right. The pain resolves with rest and returns when he continues exercising. He is otherwise well. A Doppler ultrasound demonstrates a single flow-limiting stenosis. Where is this most likely to be?
   A. Abdominal aorta.
   B. Lateral circumflex femoral artery.
   C. Left common iliac artery.
   D. Left peroneal artery.
   E. Left profunda femoris artery.

3. An 81-year-old woman presents to the emergency department with sudden-onset left-sided abdominal pain, diarrhoea and red PR bleeding. She reports losing 10 kg over the last 2 years and has had a myocardial infarction 6 years ago. She looks pale and is tachycardic at 120 bpm. Her abdomen is soft but tender. Her lactate is raised at 7.2 mmol/L but initial blood tests are otherwise unremarkable. What is the most likely diagnosis?
   A. Appendicitis on background of caecal tumour.
   B. Diverticulitis.

C. Inferior mesenteric artery occlusion.

D. Inflammatory bowel disease.

E. Sigmoid flexure mass.

4. Which of these findings in relation to peripheral arterial/venous disease is correctly matched with the diagnosis?
   A. Arterial ulcer – a shallow, sloughy ulcer over the lateral malleolus.
   B. Dry gangrene – cool, white, dry, firm tissue on the feet.
   C. Positive Buerger's sign – when patient is lying on the bed, elevating their leg off the bed causes it to go pale. Hanging this leg off the bed will then, after a delay, cause the leg to turn a reddish colour.
   D. Superficial thrombophlebitis – firm, nontender swelling along the course of a vein.
   E. Venous ulcer – a deep, punched-out ulcer in the 'gaiter area' of the calf.

5. A 58-year-old man presents to the emergency department with a tearing central chest pain. He has a history of hypertension and hypercholesterolaemia but does not comply well with his prescribed medications. He is hypertensive at 178/98 mmHg and looks distressed and sweaty. He has sinus tachycardia on his ECG. Chest X-ray appears normal. A CT scan shows two lumens within the aorta, one of these arising just distal to the left subclavian artery and extending down to the level of the aortic bifurcation. A tear in the intima can be seen in the mid-descending thoracic aorta. What is the most appropriate immediate management?
   A. Immediate cardiothoracic surgery in theatre.
   B. Immediate endovascular repair.
   C. Primary percutaneous coronary intervention.
   D. Resuscitative thoracotomy in the emergency department.
   E. Tight blood pressure and heart rate control.

6. A 67-year-old woman presents to her GP due to a pulsatile abdominal mass. She is otherwise asymptomatic. She has a history of psoriatic arthritis and hypertension (which is controlled at present), and is an ex-smoker. She is referred for an ultrasound which demonstrates a 57 mm infrarenal abdominal aortic aneurysm. What is the most appropriate first management?
   A. Refer to vascular service for regular ultrasound monitoring.
   B. Send to emergency department for immediate vascular review.
   C. Refer to vascular service for planning of aneurysm repair.
   D. Start a beta-blocker to reduce aortic wall shear stress.
   E. Optimize blood pressure and cholesterol control, with clinic review in 6 to 8 weeks.

Chapter 1 Cardiac anatomy, physiology and development

1. E. The thymus is contained within the superior and anterior mediastinal compartments and can extend up into the neck; however, it involutes (becomes smaller) after puberty and may be hardly identifiable in old age. The sympathetic chain is part of the autonomic nervous system and sits to either side of the spinal cord. As the trachea travels posteriorly, it bifurcates at the border of the superior and inferior mediastinal compartments and therefore does not extend into the posterior mediastinum. The oesophagus sits behind the trachea and travels through both the superior and posterior mediastinal compartments and through the diaphragm to join the stomach. The internal thoracic arteries arise from the subclavian arteries, travel down the interior surface of the anterior chest wall and through the anterior mediastinum.

2. A. The coronary veins drain via the coronary sinus into the right atrium. In most people, the SA and AV nodes are supplied by the right coronary artery. The coronary arteries arise from the aorta just distal to the aortic valve. The right coronary artery usually gives rise to the posterior descending artery, but a small proportion of patients have a left dominant circulation where the circumflex also supplies the posterior descending artery. The left coronary artery gives rise to the circumflex artery.

3. C. Cardiac myocytes have a branched structure, are shorter than skeletal muscle fibres and have a single central nucleus. Pacemaker cells exist in the SA node, AV node, Purkinje fibres and ventricular cardiomyocytes, and unlike other cardiomyocytes, these do not require external stimulation to initiate their action potential but are capable of self-generating rhythmic depolarization – this is known as automaticity. Troponin is a complex of proteins which are present at intervals along the thin actin filaments.

4. D. The ductus arteriosus is maintained by prostaglandin E during pregnancy and closes after birth to become the ligamentum arteriosum. Pulmonary vascular resistance decreases immediately after birth. The umbilical vessels vasoconstrict during and after birth, and the cord is then clamped; therefore, blood flow stops. The foramen ovale quickly closes (functionally) between the atria due to the shift in atrial pressures when the pulmonary circulation opens up with the first breaths after birth – however, fusion only occurs about 3 months later, and interestingly, anatomic closure is incomplete (known as patent foramen ovale) in about a quarter of the normal population. Foetal haemoglobin continues to be produced for around 6 months.

5. A. The right coronary artery supplies the sinoatrial node in approximately 60% of individuals and the left circumflex coronary artery in approximately 40% (very rarely has anomalous origin from elsewhere). The coronary sinus usually drains into the right atrium. The coronary arteries usually run along the epicardium (on the outer surface of the heart) – occasionally the arteries may dip into the myocardium (called 'myocardial bridging') but this is not the usual location. The coronary arteries arise just superior to the aortic valve cusps. The diagonal branches are important branches of the left anterior descending artery.

Chapter 2 The cardiac cycle, control of cardiac output and haemodynamic regulation

1. B. Increased plasma osmolarity will stimulate antidiuretic hormone release. Angiotensin-converting enzyme (ACE) is predominantly found in the endothelium of the pulmonary vascular bed. Adrenaline is secreted from the adrenal medulla. Adrenaline causes vasodilatation in skeletal muscle by acting on β_2 receptors. Renin converts angiotensinogen to angiotensin I.

2. B. The baroreceptor reflex is important in the cutaneous circulation if the temperature is neutral but can be overcome if there is peripheral vasodilation due to high temperature. The carotid sinus, not the carotid body, contains baroreceptors; these are innervated by a branch of the glossopharyngeal nerve. Decreased baroreceptor loading increases venous tone by increasing sympathetic activity. Increased stretch in arterial walls increases baroreceptor firing. The baroreceptor reflex is important for minute-to-minute control of the blood pressure but little use for long-term regulation (as it adjusts to the new set point in chronic hypertension/hypotension).

3. A. Aortic regurgitation is the most likely cause of this gentleman's symptoms, as he has a wide pulse pressure. All of the other options are causes of a narrow pulse pressure.

4. E. Polycythaemia rubra vera is a well-documented cause of an elevated haematocrit. Acute myeloid leukaemia will generally cause a reduction in haematocrit. Chronic hypoxia can cause an elevated haematocrit but the asthmatic patient should not be chronically hypoxic. Cardiac failure

does not generally cause an elevated haematocrit (although may cause lethargy). Haematocrit may be elevated in high altitude living, but this is unlikely to be the cause in this case!

5. D. The diving reflex causes intense vagal (parasympathetic) inhibition decreasing the slope of the pacemaker action potential and slowing heart rate, possibly terminating supraventricular tachycardias (SVTs). The alerting (fight or flight) response will increase heart rate. The baroreceptor reflex acts to maintain blood pressure at a set point and is not involved in the treatment of SVTs. Under normal circumstances, chemoreceptor activation (via hypoxaemia or hypercapnia) will increase heart rate (and respiratory rate). The hepatojugular reflex is used to augment the jugular venous pressure, not to treat SVT.

6. D. Long QT syndrome is most frequently caused by defects in voltage-gated K^+ channels – defective K^+ channels delay the repolarization phase of the action potential and lengthen the QT interval. The gap junction is an intercellular connection between adjacent cells – these allow rapid conduction of action potentials through the myocardium. L-type Ca^{2+} channels are responsible for the plateau phase of the action potential. Na^+/K^+ ATPase is responsible for maintaining intracellular and extracellular Na^+ and K^+ concentrations which determine the resting membrane potential. Voltage-gated Na^+ channels are responsible for phase 0 of the action potential – rapid Na^+ influx occurs after the threshold potential is reached.

Chapter 3 ECG interpretation

1. B. J waves may be seen in hypothermia. A downsloping ST segment or 'reverse tick' may be seen in digoxin therapy. A raised ST segment is most commonly associated with myocardial infarction (but may be seen in other conditions such as pericarditis). 'Tented' T waves are a common finding in hyperkalaemia, as are U waves in hypokalaemia.

2. B. Inferior ST elevation myocardial infarction (STEMI) is classically seen as ST elevation in leads II, III, and aVF. Anterior STEMI may be seen on the ECG as ST elevation in leads V3–V4. A lateral STEMI would be seen as ST elevation in leads I, aVL and leads V5–V6. Posterior STEMI may be seen as ST elevation in leads placed on the posterior chest wall (V7–V9) or as reciprocal depression in leads V1–V2. Septal MI would be seen as ST elevation in leads V1–V2. Infarcts may commonly cover more than one of these territories, such as with anteroseptal or anterolateral infarcts.

3. D. This ECG rhythm strip shows torsades de pointes, a polymorphic ventricular tachycardia. Episodes of torsades are generally self-terminating but occasionally may lead to ventricular fibrillation and death. The ECG in between these episodes typically shows a long QT interval. Broad QRS complexes are generally seen in bundle branch block and ventricular rhythms – they are seen here during the arrhythmia but are unlikely to be present between arrhythmias in a woman of this age. Delta waves (a slurred upstroke of QRS complex) are seen in Wolff–Parkinson–White syndrome, a common cause of supraventricular tachycardia. A long PR interval describes first-degree heart block and is not associated with torsades de pointes. 'Tented' T waves are a common feature of hyperkalaemia – this can predispose to arrhythmia but generally not torsades de pointes.

4. B. This lady has left axis deviation. One of the possible causes of this is left ventricular hypertrophy. All the other conditions above are potential causes of *right* axis deviation.

5. D. Small Q waves represent normal left-to-right depolarization of the interventricular septum and small Q waves are often seen in the left-sided leads (I, aVL, V5, V6). Pathological Q waves are wider than two small squares (0.08 s) and/or >25% of the corresponding R wave. Pathological Q waves suggest previous transmural infarction. Pathological Q waves in leads I and aVL suggest an old high lateral infarct, whereas previous inferior myocardial infarction is suggested by pathological Q waves in II, III and aVF. They are usually permanent and are due to ventricular depolarization away from the lead (resulting in a negative deflection).

6. A. The PR interval may be short in patients with accessory pathways (e.g., in Wolff–Parkinson–White syndrome) due to more rapid conduction of action potential through the abnormal pathway. ST segment represents phase 2 (the plateau phase) of the cardiac action potential. It is the QRS interval that is prolonged in bundle branch block. The T wave represents ventricular repolarization; U waves are seen in hypokalaemia. Downsloping ST depression ('reverse tick') may be seen with digoxin treatment; upsloping ST depression is a normal variant.

Chapter 4 Other cardiac investigations

1. A. Although CT coronary angiography (CTCA) is arguably now the gold standard (and first line) investigation for patients presenting with angina, invasive coronary angiography is still the most sensitive and specific test for assessing the vessel lumen and diagnosing obstructive coronary artery disease, as it allows direct visualization of the coronary arteries with higher temporal and spatial resolution in order to demonstrate the location and extent of any stenosis or obstruction. Fractional flow reserve (FFR) can also be used to demonstrate pressure changes on either side of a stenosis to determine level of obstruction. With invasive angiography, there may be serious

complications, although these are rare. CT coronary angiograms (CTCA) provide an excellent assessment of the coronary arteries but can be limited in situations where there is extensive vessel calcification and in patients with high heart rates. CTCA is better than invasive angiography for assessing disease in the wall of the artery (which may be occult on invasive angiography) as well as assessment of chamber size, myocardial thickness and other noncoronary cardiac findings. Stress tests may indirectly demonstrate reduced perfusion in a coronary artery territory. An ECG may demonstrate evidence of reduced perfusion during chest pain, or evidence of a previous MI.

2. B. An exercise ECG is unlikely to demonstrate symptoms, as the Bruce protocol does not achieve the level of workload his symptoms are occurring at. This man presents with typical angina and, as per the NICE guidelines, should be initially investigated with a CT coronary angiogram.

3. A. This is a classic description of infective endocarditis (IE) with signs of right heart failure. Blood cultures are crucial to identify the causative organism and its antimicrobial sensitivities, both for diagnosis and to ensure effective treatment. Ideally, three sets of cultures should be taken prior to starting antibiotics urgently. All of the other investigations will also be helpful. An ECG may demonstrate atrioventricular block if there is aortic root abscess formation or occasionally MI secondary to septic emboli. A chest X-ray (CXR) may demonstrate cardiac failure or spread of septic emboli to the lungs from right heart IE. A urinalysis may demonstrate microscopic haematuria. Both a CXR and urine culture will look for other sources of infection. Routine bloods include inflammatory markers and renal function, which may be deranged if there is associated glomerulonephritis (a minor Duke's criteria). Echocardiogram is not mentioned here but will be required to demonstrate vegetations as the source of infection (in this case most likely affecting the tricuspid valve given the presentation and history of IV drug use).

4. C. This lady is likely to have asymptomatic aortic stenosis (or aortic sclerosis). An echocardiogram will assess myocardial function, as well as demonstrate presence and severity of valvular disease. If there was suspicion of hypertrophic cardiomyopathy, an echocardiography would still be the first-line investigation and would confirm the diagnosis, but in certain cases, an MRI can provide more information. There is no suggestion of coronary artery disease here; therefore, CT coronary angiography and exercise testing are not indicated. A MUGA scan is a test using radionuclides to evaluate ventricular function.

5. E. The water bottle sign is seen in pericardial effusion, referring to the heart's shape looking like an old-fashioned water bottle. The double density sign (or double right heart border) occurs as the result of left atrial enlargement. Continuous diaphragm sign is seen in

pneumomediastinum, pneumoperitoneum or (rarely) pneumopericardium. Boot-shaped heart is a term used to describe the appearance of the heart in Tetralogy of Fallot (due to elevation of the cardiac apex). Egg-on-a-string sign is the appearance of the heart in transposition of the great arteries (another congenital pathology); in Ebstein anomaly, the heart is described as 'box-shaped'.

Chapter 5 History and examination

1. B. The stages of fingernail clubbing are as follows:
   • 1st stage – Increased fluctuation of the nail bed only.
   • 2nd stage – Loss of the normal angle at the base of the nail.
   • 3rd stage – Increased convexity of the nail bed.
   • 4th stage – Clubbed or 'drumstick appearance' of the fingertip.
   Painful, red swellings on the finger pulp are a description of Osler nodes (seen in infective endocarditis).

2. E. Absent x descent is seen in atrial fibrillation, as the x descent corresponds to atrial relaxation. The a wave will also be absent, as this correlates with atrial contraction. Flame-shaped haemorrhages are classically seen in hypertensive retinopathy. Roth spots are a feature of infective endocarditis. Osler nodes are due to immune complex deposition rather than septic emboli (Janeway lesions are due to septic emboli). Corneal arcus is a pale ring encircling the cornea seen in hypercholesterolaemia; the description in D is of Kayser-Fleischer rings.

3. D. The description is of constrictive pericarditis. Pulsus paradoxus is a pulse that is weaker (or even absent) with inspiration and can be diagnosed if the blood pressure drops by more than 10 mmHg with inspiration – it is seen in constrictive pericarditis, tamponade and tension pneumothorax. Bisferiens pulse is seen in mixed aortic valve disease (aortic stenosis and regurgitation). Collapsing pulse is seen in aortic regurgitation (and patent ductus arteriosus). Pulsus alternans is alternating strong and week pulses, seen with severe left ventricular dysfunction. A slow-rising pulse suggests severe aortic stenosis.

Chapter 6 Chest pain

1. A. Pericarditis classically causes saddle-shaped ST elevation in all leads of a 12-lead ECG. Pleurisy, pneumothorax, and pulmonary embolus are not recognized causes of ST elevation. PE can cause the 'classic' but rare S1Q3T3; however, it most commonly demonstrates sinus tachycardia. ST elevation myocardial infarction could be rare in this age group and would not cause ST elevation in multiple unrelated anatomical territories.

2. C. Aortic dissection causes a difference in blood pressure between arms due to involvement of the brachiocephalic or

left subclavian arteries lowering the BP in the right or left arm, respectively. Dissection can cause acute aortic regurgitation, but regurgitation alone would not account for this presentation. Myocardial infarction, pulmonary embolus and tension pneumothorax are not associated with blood pressure differences between arms. Other causes of a blood pressure differential between the arms include peripheral vascular disease (including subclavian steal) and unilateral neuromuscular abnormalities. Coarctation usually occurs after the left subclavian artery and causes higher BP in both arms in comparison to the legs and radiofemoral delay; however, if the coarctation occurs before the left subclavian artery, it can cause a BP differential between the arms and radioradial delay.

3. B. Dressler syndrome is an immune-mediated pericarditis that usually occurs weeks to months after acute myocardial infarction. Aortic dissection can be associated with STEMI if the ostia are involved, and rarely pericarditic ECG changes, but you would then expect the patient to be more unwell, and dissection risk is not increased following MI. Further STEMI would cause regional rather than widespread ST elevation. Pulmonary embolus may cause pleuritic chest pain and pyrexia but would usually present with cough and dyspnoea and would not cause widespread ST elevation. Unstable angina would not cause ST elevation.

4. B. This lady is presenting with pericarditis, which causes saddle-shaped ST elevation in all ECG leads. First-line treatment of pericarditis is with a nonsteroidal anti-inflammatory drug, such as ibuprofen. ST elevation myocardial elevation causes ST elevation only within coronary artery territories; therefore, treatments for acute coronary syndrome are inappropriate. Paracetamol may be helpful but is less likely to be beneficial than ibuprofen.

5. A. A negative troponin at the time of presentation and 12 hours later excludes myocardial infarction. Troponin may also be raised for many other reasons (e.g., arrhythmia, heart failure, etc.). There is not muscle damage (by definition) in unstable angina; therefore, cardiac biomarkers would not be elevated. Troponin levels may be elevated for at least 1 week postmyocardial infarction. Troponin is found in the thin filaments of the myofibrils, not on cell membranes.

6. B. Although cocaine use is a risk factor for drug-induced myocarditis and aortic dissection, myocardial infarction is by far the most likely cause given the presentation and prevalence – this can be secondary to plaque rupture or severe coronary vasoconstriction secondary to cocaine. In myocarditis, nonspecific ECG changes and raised troponin may also be seen. Aortic dissection is rare in itself and can rarely be associated with STEMI (inferior more likely than anterior); it would need to be ruled out if there is a high clinical suspicion. Not surprisingly, Takotsubo cardiomyopathy is possible with cocaine use given it is

thought to be due to a catecholamine surge, and cocaine is a potent sympathomimetic. It can also cause a raised troponin but is less common than myocardial infarction and is associated with apical left ventricular dyskinesis in a territory unrelated to a single coronary artery. Cocaine is not known to be a risk factor for pulmonary embolism.

7. C. This story is typical of heart failure caused by viral myocarditis with the flu-like prodrome, although the presentation varies widely. ECG changes are variable and commonly demonstrate nonspecific ST segment changes. Myocarditis can involve the pericardium (myopericarditis) and can result in widespread concave ST elevation on the ECG. Pericarditis by itself would not cause these clinical features or elevation of troponin. At this young age, myocardial infarction is very unlikely (and is not associated with a viral prodrome). Indigestion does not explain features of cardiac failure, ECG changes or elevation of troponin. Features of left ventricular failure (orthopnoea, pulmonary oedema) would not be expected in pulmonary embolus (and again, this would not explain the flu-like illness).

8. A. Boerhaave syndrome describes a full-thickness oesophageal tear which occurs as a result of severe vomiting and is thought to occur due to uncoordinated forceful ejection of gastric contents against a closed glottis when the oesophagus is not relaxed. This allows caustic gastric contents to empty into the mediastinum and can leak into the pleural space causing pleural effusion and/or pneumothorax. The presentation is varied, and the classic Mackler's triad (vomiting, chest pain, and subcutaneous emphysema) is uncommon. The crunching/rasping sound in time with cardiac cycle due to pneumomediastinum is known as Hamman's sign. Aspiration pneumonia would be within the differential, as would pneumothorax given the subcutaneous emphysema (although pneumothorax is rare with vomiting and does not explain the other examination findings). Mallory-Weiss tear is a partial thickness oesophageal tear that presents with haematemesis following vomiting but doesn't cause subcutaneous emphysema or other chest findings on examination. The findings here are not in keeping with myocarditis or pericarditis – neither would cause subcutaneous emphysema and are not associated with vomiting. Boerhaave syndrome is the best unifying diagnosis and is important to diagnose early – untreated, it usually leads to severe sepsis and death.

Chapter 7 Breathlessness and peripheral oedema

1. B. If identification of the JVP is difficult, the hepatojugular reflex may be helpful. The JVP is considered raised if >4 cm above the manubriosternal angle. Height of the JVP above the manubriosternal angle gives an estimate of right atrial

pressure in cm H_2O (not mmHg). The internal jugular vein lies deep to the medial aspect of the sternocleidomastoid; the external jugular vein may be visualized lateral to sternocleidomastoid but is less reliable for assessing right atrial pressure. The patient should be lying at approximately 45 degrees with their head turned slightly away.

2. A. Calcium channel blockers of the dihydropyridine class (amlodipine, nifedipine, etc.) commonly cause ankle swelling as a side effect. Bendroflumethiazide and furosemide are diuretics and may be used in the treatment of ankle swelling/oedema. Ankle swelling is not a common side effect of propranolol or lansoprazole.

3. C. This lady is dyspnoeic and has low oxygen saturations and her presentation is in keeping with a pneumonia. Always perform an A–E assessment on unwell patients. She will likely need antibiotics and intravenous fluids but oxygenation is the first priority. Digoxin treatment for atrial fibrillation if it persists is not unreasonable but, again, is not the priority. Despite her cardiac history, there is nothing to indicate she warrants urgent assessment by a cardiologist.

4. C. Oligaemic lung fields (decreased pulmonary vascular markings) may occasionally be seen on chest X-rays in patients presenting with PE. X-rays are, however, often normal in PE. All of the other radiograph features mentioned are characteristic of pulmonary oedema/left ventricular failure.

5. D. Psychogenic hyperventilation is the most likely option, as she is hyperventilating despite normal oxygenation. She has an alkalaemia secondary to loss of CO_2. She does have pitting oedema, which may fit with a degree of cardiac failure, but this is a common finding and a clear chest on auscultation with normal oxygen saturations would not support a diagnosis of acute LVF. Exacerbation of COPD or interstitial lung disease would be seen as hypoxia +/− hypercapnoea on the ABG. Pulmonary embolism may be seen as a low CO_2 and resultant alkalosis but is unlikely given her entirely normal oxygenation.

6. E. The description here is suggestive of pelvic malignancy – bloating and weight loss is a classic presentation of ovarian cancer, especially given the anaemia and leg swelling. Leg swelling occurs due to pelvic venous compression by the mass and/or deep vein thrombosis. Anaemia, if very severe, can cause high-output heart failure. Arterial insufficiency would not cause leg swelling, abdominal bloating or microcytic anaemia – you might, however, get weight loss if there is intestinal arterial insufficiency. Cardiac failure and renal failure both cause fluid retention. This may include ascites (and associated abdominal distension), however in these cases lower limb swelling is usually bilateral and the patient would have weight gain rather than weight loss. Cardiac failure is very

unlikely given her recent normal echocardiogram. Severe renal failure may also cause a normocytic anaemia.

Chapter 8 Palpitations

1. B. Intravenous verapamil is an appropriate choice of treatment in this circumstance. Adenosine slows conduction through the AV node and is a valid treatment of AVNRT, but it should be avoided in asthma as it may precipitate bronchospasm. Ocular pressure is a vagotonic procedure but should not be used as it carries a risk of retinal detachment. Defibrillation is inappropriate here; if the patient shows adverse features of arrhythmia, then sedation and synchronized DC cardioversion may be appropriate. Isoprenaline is used in the treatment of bradycardia, not tachycardia.

2. B. AVNRT (often referred to under the umbrella term SVT) is generally rapid but regular, whereas AF is irregularly irregular. Both AF and AVNRT may cause chest pain. In both cases, resting ECG may be normal (apart from in patients with Wolff–Parkinson–White syndrome, which has characteristic resting ECG changes). AF with a fast ventricular response may be similar to AVNRT with respect to frequency and severity of the palpitations. Both AF and AVNRT may be precipitated by coffee.

3. A. Atrial fibrillation is the only condition where P waves are absent. Although sometimes difficult to see, P waves are still present in atrial flutter and ventricular tachycardia. Intermittent P waves are seen in sick sinus syndrome. P waves are independent of the QRS complexes in complete heart block and ventricular tachycardia.

4. B. β-Blockers (and calcium channel blockers) are well-recognized causes of first-degree heart block (long PR interval), whereas ACE inhibitors are not. Although left bundle branch block and first-degree heart block may be the result of the same underlying process (e.g., age-related fibrosis), left bundle branch block itself does not cause first-degree heart block. Pericarditis may result in PR segment depression but is not a common cause of prolonged PR interval unless in association with myocarditis. Wolff–Parkinson–White syndrome classically causes a short PR interval rather than a prolonged one.

5. B. The four life-threatening (or 'adverse') features that would warrant urgent DC cardioversion are shock (systolic BP <90 mmHg), syncope, myocardial ischaemia and severe heart failure. Typical ischaemic chest pain would warrant synchronized DC cardioversion. Other means of reverting his arrhythmia can be trialled while this is arranged. This blood pressure is not low enough to warrant DC cardioversion. A rate of >200 bpm is not an indication for DC cardioversion unless the rapid rate results in other adverse features. Breathlessness at rest and peripheral oedema are not necessarily adverse features; pulmonary

oedema is, however, as this is considered a sign of severe heart failure. The peripheral oedema is also unlikely to be secondary to the arrhythmia given the short duration.

6. D. The paraesthesia around the mouth is generally an innocent finding seen in hyperventilation which might imply her palpitations are the result of anxiety, particularly in the context of other social stressors. However, patients with palpitations of any other cause may find them distressing (and subsequently may hyperventilate); therefore, it is important to keep an open mind about the causes. Fever and productive cough may suggest palpitations are due to infection (e.g., a pneumonia) and resultant high-output state. Recent history of dark stool implies GI bleeding and potentially palpitations due to anaemia. Acidosis on blood gas analysis would not be usually seen with anxiety-related palpitations (although a respiratory alkalosis may be). Acidosis can predispose to arrhythmia as well as potentially be the result of arrhythmia (lactic acidosis may occur if organ perfusion has been insufficient). A slurred upstroke of the QRS complex is seen with accessory conduction pathways such as in Wolff–Parkinson–White syndrome, which can predispose to dangerous tachyarrhythmias.

Chapter 9   Syncope, blackout and faints

1. C. Classic cardiac syncope (due to a paroxysmal arrhythmia, for example) is of sudden onset and with rapid recovery. Patients generally have no warning symptoms and no neurological deficit. Persistent neurological deficit may indicate an intracranial event. Syncope precipitated by sudden turning of the head may indicate carotid sinus hypersensitivity.

2. A. A sudden onset 'tearing' or 'ripping' chest pain that radiates to the back with a difference in blood pressure between arms is classical of aortic dissection. A variety of ECG changes may be seen in dissection, including T wave inversion, ST depression or even ST elevation (the inferior territory is most commonly affected) due to dissection extending into the right coronary artery; the ECG changes here are much more likely to be indicative of this than an acute myocardial infarction. The typical history in pericarditis is a sharp stabbing pain that is relieved by sitting forward; the ECG findings and blood pressure discrepancy are not consistent with pericarditis. Pulmonary embolism (PE) would not be associated with a blood pressure discrepancy between arms; in PE, you might expect a sharp, pleuritic pain and hypoxia. Examination of the chest would not be unremarkable in tension pneumothorax and again, pain is more likely to be sharp and pleuritic.

3. B. The family history and exertional syncope that sounds cardiac (sudden onset without warning, rapid recovery) in a young person has to raise suspicion of hypertrophic cardiomyopathy (HCM). This man may have had dynamic obstruction from HCM or paroxysmal arrhythmia and requires urgent investigation. There is little to suggest that this is an acute coronary syndrome. Orthostatic (postural) hypotension generally occurs shortly after standing. Takotsubo cardiomyopathy is a sudden, transient weakness and ballooning of the ventricular myocardium (often in response to stress) and can mimic myocardial infarction – it does not fit with this history. This patient's episodes are not in keeping with vasovagal syncope as they are occurring suddenly and without warning.

4. A. Alcohol (especially when drinking to excess) is a very well-recognized trigger of atrial fibrillation and this seems the most likely cause of her symptoms given her ongoing rapid palpitations. Complete heart block may cause presyncope but not rapid palpitations. She is unlikely to still be intoxicated and this does not explain her symptoms (plus she probably wouldn't appreciate the suggestion)! Alcohol is associated with sinus tachycardia but this is not likely to persist for this length of time and is also unlikely to be the cause of presyncope. Alcohol generally predisposes to supraventricular arrhythmias rather than ventricular arrhythmias.

5. E. Withholding her medications is the most sensible first option out of those listed – both these medications will lower blood pressure and the bisoprolol will slow her heart rate. Given she is bradycardic, hypotensive and is having episodes of presyncope, these should be withheld (and perhaps later restarted at a lower dose). There are no adverse features of bradycardia (myocardial ischaemia, shock, heart failure and syncope) to suggest she requires atropine and there is no indication for pacing at this stage. Digoxin *is* positively inotropic but is also negatively chronotropic and likely to slow her heart rate further; it should not be given to such patients.

6. A. Amoxicillin does not affect the QT interval. The other medicines may all prolong the QT interval, which predisposes to torsades de pointes. QT prolongation is usually multifactorial – there may be a genetic tendency, plus electrolyte disturbance (e.g., hypokalaemia), plus medications that all act to prolong the QT interval. Drug culprits include some antibiotics, antifungals, antidepressants, antipsychotics, antiemetics, antihistamines and anticonvulsants.

Chapter 10   Heart murmurs

1. D. Mitral regurgitation is a classical cause of a pansystolic murmur. Aortic regurgitation is associated with an early diastolic murmur. Aortic stenosis is associated with an ejection systolic murmur. Atrial septal defects cause fixed splitting of the second heart sounds and possibly an ejection systolic pulmonary flow murmur. Tricuspid stenosis is associated with a mid-diastolic murmur.

2. A. Atrial myxoma is very rare; however, it is the most common cardiac tumour and is almost always benign. It is characteristically associated with a 'tumour plop' due to tumour impacting on the endocardial wall and can cause a mitral stenosis murmur if the tumour obstructs the mitral valve. It can present with fever (and other constitutional symptoms) and heart failure due to tumour obstruction. The 'plop' is not associated with any of the other conditions above. All except mitral valve prolapse can cause fever; mitral valve prolapse also produces a systolic murmur. Cardiac causes of clubbing are Atrial myxoma, Bacterial endocarditis and Cyanotic congenital heart disease (ABC). Infective endocarditis more often causes regurgitant murmurs (due to valve destruction or distortion) rather than stenotic murmurs (due to obstruction). Pericarditis is classically associated with a pericardial rub and chest pain. Rheumatic fever characteristically occurs 2 to 3 weeks after a streptococcal sore throat and can be associated with multiple organ involvement, including joints, skin and brain.

3. B. When the first heart sound is loud and palpable in mitral stenosis, this is described as a tapping apex beat. Mitral regurgitation is associated with a thrusting, displaced apex beat. Left ventricular aneurysm may cause diffuse asynchronous or double apex beat, as the aneurysm can cause a second outward bulge in systole. Left ventricular hypertrophy is associated with a heaving nondisplaced apex beat, which can be seen due to hypertension, aortic stenosis and HCM. In pericardial effusion, the apex beat may be reduced or impalpable. Other causes of an impalpable apex beat include anything that increases the distance between your fingers and the apex (e.g., obesity, emphysema, pneumothorax, massive pleural effusion) or because the apex is not where you expect it. Therefore, it is important to check not only for lateral and inferior displacement, but if still impalpable, also check the other side – the patient may have dextrocardia!

4. C. In a patient with clubbing, haematuria, fever and a murmur, suspect subacute bacterial endocarditis (clubbing takes time to develop). HUS is a thrombotic microangiopathy which tends to occur in children, often secondary to infection. Thrombosis occurs in the damaged microcirculation of the kidney to cause haemolytic anaemia, thrombocytopenia and acute kidney injury. Fever and microscopic haematuria are expected; a murmur due to increased cardiac output in sepsis may be found, but clubbing is not associated. Infectious mononucleosis (glandular fever) is due to Epstein-Barr virus infection and typically presents in young adults with a sore throat, lymphadenopathy, fever and fatigue, with later hepatomegaly and splenomegaly. Complications are most commonly haematological or neurological, but carditis and renal complications are rare. Rheumatic fever is a delayed immune reaction to Streptococcus A throat infection and can affect any valve; therefore, it can cause a range of murmurs along with fever, arthritis and skin manifestations. However, it is not associated with clubbing or haematuria. Tetralogy of Fallot is a congenital heart condition which presents within the first few years of life and survival to adulthood is rare without surgery. Clubbing can develop, but it is not associated with fever or haematuria.

5. C. Systolic blood pressure normally falls with inspiration, but an exaggerated fall of >10 mmHg is termed pulsus paradoxus. This can occur in cardiac tamponade, restrictive cardiomyopathy, constrictive pericarditis and severe obstructive lung disease. In most of these conditions, Kussmaul's sign may also be observed, where the JVP paradoxically rises with inspiration due to impaired right ventricular filling. These terms can be misleading and confusing, as pulsus paradoxus is an exaggeration of the normal trend, whereas Kussmaul's sign is a reversal of the normal fall in JVP during inspiration. Collapsing pulse can be a feature of aortic regurgitation, large arteriovenous malformations/fistulas or marked peripheral vasodilatation. Pulsus alternans is associated with severe heart failure. Radiofemoral delay can be found in aortic coarctation or dissection. Slow rising pulse is a feature of aortic stenosis.

6. E. A small VSD produces a louder murmur than a larger one (due to high velocity of flow through a narrow defect). Small VSDs are unlikely to cause significant haemodynamic derangement and are more likely to close spontaneously without requiring intervention. Acute mitral regurgitation is likely to present with heart failure or cardiogenic shock, and the baby is unlikely to be so well; the murmur is loudest at the apex and radiates to the left axilla. Aortic stenosis typically causes a murmur in the second right intercostal space (upper left sternal edge). Hypertrophic cardiomyopathy does not usually present until later in life.

7. E. A loud palpable second heart sound is a feature of pulmonary hypertension. A parasternal right ventricular heave can be found in pulmonary hypertension, but the apex beat is not affected. Other features include an elevated JVP and an early diastolic murmur. Corrigan's pulse is a feature of aortic regurgitation.

8. E. Physiological splitting of the second heart sound increases on inspiration and disappears on expiration. A continuous 'machinery' murmur may be due to patent ductus arteriosus. Aortic stenosis and atrial septal defect both cause an ejection systolic murmur. Early diastolic murmur may be due to aortic or pulmonary regurgitation. Tricuspid regurgitation can cause a pansystolic murmur. Mid-diastolic murmurs may be due to mitral or tricuspid stenosis.

Chapter 11 Atherosclerosis and its risk factors

1. B. This fulfils the criteria of non-ST elevation myocardial infarction (NSTEMI). Inferior MI is frequently associated with bradycardia. A massive pulmonary embolus may give similar symptoms and can cause troponin rise in right ventricular strain, but it tends to cause more anterior T wave or ST changes and tachycardia, and is less likely without other known additional PE risk factors. If there is any doubt, urgent bedside echocardiography may be helpful to differentiate between evidence of right heart strain (PE) or localized hypokinetic segment (MI). Angina alone would not cause a rise in troponin.

2. D. Atrial fibrillation suggests an embolic source to the stroke, and as a 34-year-old female, patient D is unlikely to have significant enough atherosclerosis to cause a stroke. This is therefore the best answer. Patient A has multiple established risk factors for MI. Patient B has known atherosclerotic disease and is at high risk of peripheral arterial disease.
   With patient C, although acute mesenteric ischaemia is more frequently due to embolus than thrombosis-in-situ, there is no obvious source of embolus and she clearly has a higher risk of atherosclerotic disease than the lady in answer D.
   Patient E's presentation is in keeping with unstable angina or MI.

3. C. The anterior myocardium is supplied by the left anterior descending artery, and complete occlusion will cause an anterior MI. 45% stenosis of the left main coronary artery would not be sufficient to cause myocardial infarction. The circumflex supplies the lateral wall, and the right coronary supplies the posterior/inferior surfaces. Severe anaemia can cause decompensation from preexisting stenosis but is very unlikely to cause ST elevation. It tends to cause worsening angina, or very rarely, type 2 MI (defined as myocardial injury resulting from imbalance of myocardial supply and demand rather than an acute coronary artery event).

4. A. NICE recommends a high-intensity statin treatment for both primary and secondary prevention (high-intensity statin treatment is defined as a dose that can achieve a >40% reduction in LDL). This dose of atorvastatin falls into this category and is appropriate for primary prevention.

   Cholestyramine is a bile acid-binding resin, which binds bile acids in the intestine, and as these are synthesized from cholesterol, they reduce plasma LDL.

   However, bile-acid binding resins can aggravate hypertriglyceridaemia, and there is no clear evidence

that these show benefit; therefore, they are no longer recommended for primary or secondary prevention.

   Niacin was thought to inhibit adipose tissue breakdown, thereby decreasing free fatty acid and therefore plasma cholesterol levels. However, large studies have not shown any benefit, and there is increased risk of statin side effects when used in combination. Preparations have been withdrawn.

   This dose of pravastatin is considered to be low-intensity cholesterol lowering and would not be recommended.

   This dose of simvastatin is medium-intensity cholesterol lowering.

5. B. Bloods and urinalysis are the next steps. With this level of hypertension, the first step is to assess for any end-organ damage and this includes blood testing and urinalysis. Ambulatory or home BP monitoring may be required to confirm diagnosis (with clinic review within 7 days) but this requires end-organ damage to be excluded first. There are no signs of a hypertensive emergency that would require urgent hospital assessment. At this level of blood pressure, you would be keen to start an oral antihypertensive quickly and arrange prompt review. If blood tests and urinalysis suggest the patient is diabetic, then, as per the National Institute for Health and Care Excellence (NICE)/British and Irish Hypertension Society guidelines, the patient should be started on an ACE inhibitor or angiotensin receptor blocker; otherwise, she should be started on a calcium channel blocker such as amlodipine.

6. C. This patient requires a full assessment including fundoscopy, as his blood pressure is very high. It should not be put down to anxiety without further assessment for hypertensive emergency; therefore the most appropriate place for ongoing monitoring and careful treatment of blood pressure is a hospital. Given he is under 40, he will need to be investigated for secondary causes of hypertension, and indeed anxiety, palpitations and headache may be symptoms of phaeochromocytoma.

7. E. This ECG meets the voltage criteria for LVH. The lateral ST depression and asymmetric T wave inversion are typical of the strain pattern seen in LVH (ST change in the opposite direction of the QRS complex), as expected in longstanding hypertension. It is not a normal ECG, but there is no suggestion of a current or previous MI. This is not typical of any electrolyte abnormality.

8. A. Calcium channel blockers do not require blood test monitoring. They are also first-line treatment in patients 55 and over, which this patient nearly is. ACE inhibitors,

angiotensin II receptor blockers, thiazide and thiazide-like diuretics all require monitoring of renal function and electrolytes.

9. E. Unfractionated heparin inhibits thrombin and factor Xa through an antithrombin III-dependent mechanism. Inactivation of thrombin prevents thrombin-induced platelet activation and activation of multiple coagulation factors. Aspirin irreversibly inactivates cyclooxygenase. Fondaparinux directly inhibits factor Xa. Ticagrelor is a reversible platelet ADP receptor P2Y12 antagonist. Tirofiban is a GPIIb/IIIa inhibitor.

10. A. This is an immediate indication to stop his ACE inhibitor, and he will require repeat blood tests – his renal function and mild hyperkalaemia will hopefully improve with cessation. Dramatic renal function decline after starting an ACE inhibitor can suggest renovascular hypertension, and the appropriate next step is a specialist review. There is no indication for immediate referral to the emergency department.

Chapter 12 Acute coronary syndromes and stable angina

1. C. tPA (thrombolysis) is only used in STEMI in the absence of contraindications and when primary percutaneous coronary intervention is not available within 90 minutes. The other treatments are used in both NSTEMI and STEMI. Thienopyridines are a class of irreversible P2Y12 inhibitors including clopidogrel and prasugrel (but not ticagrelor, which is a reversible P2Y12 inhibitor with a different chemical structure).

2. B. To prevent thrombus extension, patients should be started on dual antiplatelet therapy and an anticoagulant (assuming no contraindications) and therefore option B is correct. Options A, C and D are missing anticoagulants. A β-blocker is important in NSTEMI to minimize myocardial demand but will not help with thrombus extension. Oxygen may be appropriate if the patient is hypoxic to minimize ischaemia but will not impact on thrombus size. Option E includes two separate P2Y12 antagonists; this should be avoided due to bleeding risk, and there are no high-risk features suggested to warrant an additional GPIIb/IIIa inhibitor.

3. C. Diltiazem would be the most appropriate choice in reducing heart rate and myocardial demand. β-blockers (e.g., atenolol) are contraindicated due to asthma. Digoxin is not used to treat angina. A GTN spray would be useful during attacks or to prevent attacks before exercise but would not have as much effect on decreasing frequency of angina attacks as diltiazem. Nifedipine is likely to cause reflex tachycardia without a concurrent β-blocker, which would increase myocardial demand when his heart rate is already higher than desirable.

4. B. Left ventricular aneurysm is the most likely reason for persistent ST elevation in the anterior territory alone, explains the paradoxical cardiac impulse in systole, and will increase her risk of heart failure, ventricular arrhythmias and mural thrombus. Although she is at risk of further cardiac events, this is very unlikely without chest pain or sudden deterioration. Left ventricular hypertrophy is unlikely here given the history; however, it can give a 'strain pattern' of ST depression in the lateral leads and ST elevation in the anterior leads almost similar to left bundle branch block. There would be excessively high left ventricular voltages, however. Pericarditis is unlikely without symptoms or signs and given the timeframe after the initial STEMI, plus her ECG would show widespread concave ST elevation rather than in a single coronary artery territory. There is no murmur or signs of right heart failure to suggest ventricular septal defect.

5. C. Whilst all of these will be required, remember ABCDE and your basic life support/advanced life support training. Remember that arrhythmia is one of the most common post-MI complications. Application of defibrillator pads is required to determine whether arrhythmia is shockable or nonshockable. ABG will be helpful to determine whether there are any reversible causes (e.g., hypoxia, electrolyte abnormalities). Blood glucose can be checked very quickly and is easily treatable if abnormal. CXR may demonstrate pulmonary oedema and helps rule out other reversible causes (e.g., tension pneumothorax); however, you would look for clinical signs of these initially. Urgent echo may demonstrate other post-MI complications that can cause collapse (e.g., myocardial free wall rupture and cardiac tamponade, rupture of the interventricular wall, acute mitral regurgitation), as well as demonstrate evidence for other causes of collapse, e.g., pulmonary embolus.

6. A. Whilst both acute mitral regurgitation (due to rupture of chordae tendineae or papillary muscles) and ventricular septal defect can cause a pansystolic murmur and haemodynamic compromise, acute mitral regurgitation is much more frequent and often causes pulmonary oedema. Ventricular septal defect, however, is more associated with right heart failure and a pansystolic murmur radiating to the right sternal border. In practice, this is often difficult to differentiate; in any case, diagnosis will require Doppler echocardiography for confirmation. The ECG changes are normal evolving changes after anterior STEMI and although arrhythmia is a common complication, there is no evidence for it on the cardiac monitor. Heart block is not demonstrated on the ECG and is usually temporary if it occurs after inferior MI. Free wall rupture can present with signs of cardiac tamponade (hypotension, raised JVP, muffled heart sounds) or sudden cardiac death.

Chapter 13 Heart failure

1. B. Hepatomegaly occurs in right ventricular failure due to hepatic congestion. Bilateral basal crepitations and wheeze are signs of left ventricular failure and pulmonary congestion (or possibly respiratory disease). The patient is more likely to be hypotensive than hypertensive; right ventricular failure (with reduced right ventricular stroke volume) leads to poor filling of the left ventricle, reduced cardiac output and therefore, reduced blood pressure.

   Mid-diastolic murmur suggests mitral stenosis (which may lead to right ventricular failure) but is not a sign of right ventricular failure as such; mitral stenosis is also uncommon and almost always the result of rheumatic heart disease.

2. E. Remember to assess patients presenting with left ventricular failure in an A–E manner. The patient is breathless and therefore, oxygen is the priority. They will more than likely require intravenous diuretics but this takes longer to prepare (and to act) than giving oxygen. ß-Blockers should not be started until the patient is stable (no longer requiring intravenous diuretics). CPAP may be required in some patients (but certainly not all); consider if the patient is severely dyspnoeic and acidaemic. Opiates are no longer routinely recommended in acute left ventricular failure due to limited evidence of benefit and some evidence of increased harm.

3. A. Patients like this lady with heart failure secondary to severe LVSD and LBBB on an ECG may be candidates for biventricular pacing (also known *as cardiac resynchronization therapy;* CRT), sometimes using a device that has a defibrillator function in addition (CRT-D). Biventricular pacing has a lead into both ventricles and one to the right atrium. The other types of pacemaker are used in the treatment of atrioventricular blocks, sinus node dysfunction and certain other causes of bradycardia; they are unlikely to be helpful here. A left ventricular assist device (LVAD) is an implantable pump that assists left ventricular function – it is not likely to be considered at this stage, as LVADs are used as a 'bridge' e.g., to transplantation or recovery (if the issue is a transient one).

4. E. Candesartan is an angiotensin II receptor blocker and, as with ACE inhibitors, should be withheld during intercurrent illness, especially diarrhoea and vomiting, due to risk of renal impairment and hyperkalaemia. None of the other medications would be expected to cause significant harm if continued in this setting.

5. E. Paroxysmal nocturnal dyspnoea (PND) is classically seen in left ventricular failure. It is thought to be the result of pulmonary oedema due to gradual resorption of interstitial fluid overnight and nocturnal depression of respiratory function. All of the other options are more typical of right ventricular failure than left ventricular failure; the dyspnoea in left ventricular failure is the result of pulmonary oedema rather than poor pulmonary perfusion.

6. A. Diabetic ketoacidosis (DKA), including ketoacidosis with a relatively normal glucose level (euglycaemic ketoacidosis) can occur, and it can be difficult to recognize if the blood sugar is normal or if DKA is occurring unusually in type 2 diabetes; therefore, symptoms of nausea/vomiting/abdominal pain should prompt checking of ketones and blood gases. SGLT2 inhibitors reduce reabsorption of glucose at the proximal renal tubule. This results in increased renal excretion of glucose, lowering blood glucose, polyuria and modest weight loss as a result. Whilst the initial intravascular depletion and lowered blood pressure may cause a transient decrease in eGFR when SGLT2 inhibitors are started, in the long term, they have been found to reduce the risk of chronic kidney disease progression and are recommended in those patients with mild to moderate chronic kidney disease and albuminuria.

   Urinary hesitancy is difficulty starting to urinate and is not a recognized side effect, although SGLT2 inhibitors increase the risk of urinary tract infections (may present with dysuria/frequency) and fungal genital infections due to glycosuria.

Chapter 14 Arrhythmias

1. A. Ventricular tachycardia (VT) is a life-threatening arrhythmia. If the patient is conscious with no haemodynamic compromise, treatment may be with antiarrhythmic drugs. In cases of conscious patients with evidence of compromise, urgent synchronized DC cardioversion is used. In the unconscious patient without a pulse (pulseless VT), immediate unsynchronized cardioversion (defibrillation) is indicated. VT is a broad-complex tachycardia. Atropine may be given as part of the treatment of certain patients with bradycardia but not tachycardia. VT with a pulse should be treated with synchronized DC cardioversion at an energy level of 120–150 J.

2. B. Digoxin use in Wolff–Parkinson–White can result in rapid conduction through the accessory pathway and resultant haemodynamic compromise. Digoxin acts to slow conduction through the atrioventricular node. Digoxin's main route of excretion is renal. The half-life of digoxin is long, approximately 36 to 48 hours. The effects of digoxin are enhanced by *hypo*kalaemia and, as such, hypokalaemic patients are at increased risk of digoxin toxicity.

3. D. The 'shockable' rhythms have a better prognosis than 'nonshockable rhythms'. For pulseless VT, a *nonsynchronized* DC shock (i.e., defibrillation) is administered. Adrenaline is given at a dose of 1 mg every 3 to 5 minutes of CPR. Atropine is no longer routinely used in a cardiac arrest situation. In the case of ventricular fibrillation,

the defibrillator initial energy setting should be at least 150 J; synchronized DC cardioversion (e.g., in supraventricular tachyarrhythmias) uses lower energy settings.

4. A. Concordance means precordial leads with entirely positive (R) or entirely negative (QS) complexes, with no RS complexes seen. Capture and fusion beats are pathognomonic of VT. Verapamil can be hazardous in VT and should never be used to differentiate between SVT with aberrancy and VT. If in doubt, always treat as VT.

5. E. In a patient with an arrhythmia, elevated JVP is considered an indicator of severe heart failure, one of the life-threatening (or 'adverse') features of arrhythmia. This suggests an unstable rhythm, warranting urgent synchronized direct current cardioversion. The other treatments may all have a part to play in management of atrial fibrillation or heart failure but are not the priority in an unstable patient.

6. E. The correct sequence of events is to open the airway, deliver five rescue breaths and call 999 if a phone is available (using the speaker function). If no phone is available, then continue with CPR for 1 minute before finding a phone to call the emergency services. Cardiorespiratory arrest in paediatric patients is due to hypoxia in the majority of patients and early rescue breaths can improve outcomes. In the majority of arrests, the rhythm will be asystole or pulseless electrical activity and therefore, the rescue breaths and getting help are the immediate priority.

7. C. In patients with shockable rhythms, amiodarone 300 mg IV should be given after the third shock. Peripheral oedema is not considered a feature of severe heart failure in the ALS guidelines – although pulmonary oedema is. With shockable rhythms, adrenaline 1 mg IV should be given every 3 to 5 minutes (not 3–5 shocks). After delivering a shock, CPR should immediately recommence and a rhythm check then carried out at 2 minutes. Lidocaine 100 mg IV may be used as an alternative to amiodarone but not to adrenaline.

8. If thrombolytic drugs are administered (e.g., if PE is the suspected cause of arrest), then consider continuation of CPR for at least 60 to 90 minutes – mechanical chest compression devices are not superior to manual chest compressions but are helpful in situations where prolonged CPR is needed or if high-quality CPR is difficult (e.g., in an ambulance). Drug-induced hypotension does usually respond to IV fluids. Needle decompression of tension pneumothorax should be carried out in the second intercostal space in the midclavicular line, not midaxillary line. In cardiac arrest due to PE, the most common rhythm seen is pulseless electrical activity (PEA).

9. E. Flecainide can be used in WPW syndrome patients without structural or ischaemic heart disease. Adenosine, beta-blockers, calcium channel blockers and digoxin all slow AV node conduction, which can encourage conduction through the accessory pathway (at a more rapid rate, known as preexcited AF) and degenerate into ventricular fibrillation (VF). Therefore, AV node blocking drugs are all contraindicated in WPW. Amiodarone is also to be avoided, as it may cause deterioration into VF. If a patient with WPW syndrome is haemodynamically compromised, the treatment of choice is synchronized DC cardioversion. Ablation of the accessory pathway may provide definitive treatment.

Chapter 15 Valvular disease

1. E. Rheumatic fever is an autoimmune process triggered by pharyngeal infection with group A β-haemolytic streptococci; the Aschoff nodules with initial inflammatory infiltrate are gradually replaced by fibrous tissue and scarring, which leads to distortion of the cusps and commissures. Rheumatic fever can affect all heart valves, although the mitral and aortic are most frequently affected. It is not the most common cause of mitral regurgitation but is the cause of the vast majority of mitral stenosis. Antibiotic prophylaxis for infective endocarditis is no longer recommended; however, patients often are treated with long-term antibiotics to prevent recurrent rheumatic fever.

2. C. A fourth heart sound is heard when blood from atrial contraction strikes the noncompliant hypertrophied left ventricle, which can develop in severe aortic stenosis. Left ventricular hypertrophy also gives rise to a heaving nondisplaced apex beat. Severe aortic stenosis is associated with paradoxical splitting of S2 (not present if aortic closing sound is absent); fixed splitting is found in atrial septal defect. S2 becomes quieter in severe aortic stenosis as the thickened valves become less pliable and less able to coapt forcefully. Severe stenosis also limits stroke volume and is associated with a narrow pulse pressure. Other severity markers include a thrill, a slow-rising or low-volume pulse, a later-peaking murmur and signs of left ventricular failure.

3. E. Malar flush (a red/purple discolouration across the cheeks) is classically associated with mitral stenosis. Mitral stenosis causes a mid-diastolic murmur best heard with the bell of the stethoscope. It may result in a 'tapping' apex beat but in pure mitral stenosis, the apex beat will not be displaced.

4. E. Mitral valve prolapse affects around 2% to 3% of the population and has a female preponderance. Patients are usually asymptomatic, and it is often found incidentally on examination due to a mid-systolic click. This can be followed by a systolic murmur if there is associated mitral regurgitation. Mitral valve prolapse tends to follow a benign course and does not tend to progress towards severe mitral regurgitation or heart failure in the majority of cases.

5. A. Aortic valve replacement is performed through a median sternotomy incision. Closed mitral valvotomy is performed through a left thoracotomy incision. Mitral valvuloplasty, ICD insertion and temporary pacemaker insertion are performed percutaneously.

6. D. *Staphylococcus aureus* is associated with destructive infections and higher complication and mortality rates. It has overtaken Viridans streptococci as the most common causative organism in developed countries. Enterococci are the third most common cause of bacterial endocarditis. Fungal infections remain rare and are usually seen in immunocompromised patients, IV drug abusers, and after valve surgery. A significant proportion of cases will be culture-negative (~5% of infective endocarditis affecting native valves); this may be due to fastidious organisms that do not grow in normal blood cultures or antibiotic therapy prior to blood cultures. Other components of the modified Duke criteria may be present to make the diagnosis.

7. C. Whilst a systolic flow murmur is present in all prosthetic aortic valves, the early diastolic murmur of aortic regurgitation is not normal. This presentation of prolonged fever and new heart failure should ring alarm bells, as infective endocarditis of prosthetic valves has a poor prognosis – this must be identified and treated early. The most common findings in infective endocarditis are a murmur, pyrexia and microscopic haematuria (~90%). Splenomegaly is common (30%–40%), and finger clubbing is less so (~10%); both are only present in subacute endocarditis. The well-known signs such as Osler nodes, Janeway lesions and Roth spots are much less common (5% or less). Heart failure complicates ~50% of cases; conduction disorders are a less common complication (10%–20%). Stroke is a complication in ~20% of cases, but more subtle neurological abnormalities may be found in 30% to 40% of patients.

8. C. Predisposition to infective endocarditis is a minor criterion. Others are fever, vascular phenomena, immunological phenomena and microbiological evidence not meeting a major criterion. Blood culture (not sputum culture) growth of *Staphylococcus aureus* and vegetations seen on echo are major criteria. Endocarditis may be associated with prolonged PR interval and occasionally AV dissociation; however, prolonged PR interval and erythema multiforme are criteria for rheumatic fever (revised Jones criteria), not infective endocarditis (modified Duke criteria).

Chapter 16 Diseases of the myocardium and pericardium

1. B. Dressler syndrome is a pericarditis that usually occurs 2 to 8 weeks (although it can be as late as 3 months) after myocardial infarction or cardiac operation. Pericarditis frequently causes widespread ST elevation in a distribution that does not fit with coronary artery territories. The description of his pain is classic for pericarditic pain. In contrast, the pain of an aortic dissection is classically 'ripping' or 'tearing' in nature, is sudden in onset, often radiates to the back and is not normally positional; the ECG in aortic dissection may be normal or may show signs of STEMI if the dissection involves the coronary ostium. His pain is not classic for ischaemic pain and therefore not likely to represent further STEMI or unstable angina; there would also not be ST elevation in all territories in these conditions. Pneumothorax may cause sharp left-sided chest pain but will generally be worsened by inspiration rather than lying flat and it would not be associated with widespread ST elevation.

2. A. Hypertrophic cardiomyopathy (HCM) is inherited in the vast majority of cases in an autosomal dominant pattern (there are exceptions) and is attributed to mutations in a number of genes coding for sarcomere proteins. One could expect 50% of his children to inherit the mutation. Family members of affected patients are often offered screening. Some very rare, nonsarcomeric causes of HCM may follow other modes of inheritance.

3. D. Pericardial friction rubs are scratching sounds heard on auscultation and are associated with pericarditis. Janeway lesions, clubbing and conjunctival haemorrhages are features of endocarditis. Parasternal heave is a sign suggestive of right ventricular hypertrophy and pulmonary hypertension.

4. B. Beck's triad consists of muffled heart sounds (due to effusion), along with raised jugular venous pressure and low arterial blood pressure. Other signs such as delayed capillary refill, hypoxia, reduced consciousness, absent apex beat and pulsus paradoxus may occur in tamponade but these are not part of the classical triad. A friction rub may be heard if there is coexisting pericarditis.

5. D. Takotsubo cardiomyopathy is often initially misdiagnosed, as ECG features may mimic those of STEMI. Takotsubo cardiomyopathy is also known as 'broken heart syndrome'. It affects far more women than men and treatment is generally supportive in nature. Fluid resuscitation may be indicated in some cases but patients frequently have evidence of fluid overload due to systolic dysfunction. Long-term prognosis is generally very good, with a low mortality rate and up to 95% of patients achieving full recovery. The name 'Takotsubo' comes from the Japanese word for a kind of octopus trap because of the shape the left ventricle takes on rather than it being first described in Japanese fishermen.

6. D. Those diagnosed as children have a poorer prognosis and a higher risk of sudden cardiac death, whereas those who remain asymptomatic and are diagnosed at a later age, as adults, generally have a better prognosis.

Disopyramide is sometimes used in patients with obstruction to reduce resting pressure gradients and improve symptoms. HCM has many variants and can present at any age. Myomectomy may be indicated in some patients with HCM but this is not a percutaneous procedure. HCM affects men and women roughly equally.

Chapter 17 Congenital heart disease

1. E. VSD is the most common of the traditional congenital cardiac abnormalities (or second most common if bicuspid aortic valve is included).

2. D. Tetralogy of Fallot presents with progressive cyanosis early in life. ASD, VSD and PDA do not present initially with cyanosis, as the shunt is from left to right; however, cyanosis can occur later if Eisenmenger syndrome develops. Coarctation is not associated with cyanosis.

3. C. Eisenmenger syndrome develops when a longstanding left-to-right shunt reverses into a cyanotic right-to-left shunt due to increased pulmonary vascular resistance and therefore, there is the potential for paradoxical emboli. It is associated with polycythaemia and fingernail clubbing but not anaemia or splinter haemorrhages.

4. B. PFO is thought to be associated with migraine, along with paradoxical emboli causing stroke/transient ischaemic attack and decompression sickness. The other conditions listed here are not believed to have a positive association with PFO.

5. E. Squatting may relieve symptoms, as it increases systemic vascular resistance, thereby decreasing right-to-left shunting. Exertion, such as feeding or crying, may worsen right ventricular outflow obstruction and precipitate a 'tet' spell, where cyanosis worsens and syncope may even occur. Pulmonary artery pressure is usually low because pulmonary stenosis protects the pulmonary circulation. Patent ductus arteriosus and left ventricular hypertrophy are not included in the four defects seen in Tetralogy of Fallot.

6. A. Downward/apical displacement of the septal tricuspid leaflet is common to all cases of Ebstein anomaly. In around half of patients with Ebstein anomaly, PFO or ASD is associated, and accessory conduction pathway is seen less commonly. VSD and right ventricular outflow tract obstruction are infrequently associated; however, these, along with overriding aorta and RVH, are the four features of Tetralogy of Fallot.

Chapter 18 Vascular disease

1. B. Large-volume central PE can present with ischaemic-sounding pain (rather than pleuritic from infarct) and circulatory collapse. Anterior T wave inversion and raised troponin can be seen as a result of right heart strain in PE (as well as myocardial infarction). Ischaemic heart disease/arrhythmia would need to be considered; however, the history of recent surgery and 1 week of unilateral leg swelling/increased breathlessness and hypoxia make subacute DVT/PE with large clot burden the most likely diagnosis. Therefore, urgent CTPA (if remains stable) is most likely to give the diagnosis of PE and demonstrate the size of clot burden, signs of right heart strain and any infarcts (as well as occasionally an undiagnosed malignancy precipitating the episode). If the patient is too unstable for CT, bedside echo is useful if available urgently, as it can demonstrate right heart strain to infer the diagnosis of PE, or may rarely visualize a saddle embolus directly, and can rule out some other causes of collapse (e.g., tamponade). He does not have a STEMI and immediate PCI would not be the first step. Erect and supine BP would not be advisable when the patient is most likely to have a central PE.

2. C. Buttock claudication is generally due to a proximal occlusion in either the abdominal aorta or in the common iliac artery. Given his symptoms are entirely unilateral, the left common iliac artery is more likely the site of stenosis. The other arteries are all more distal – the lateral circumflex femoral artery and profunda femoris artery are branches of the common femoral artery and the peroneal artery is an artery in the calf.

3. C. Inferior mesenteric artery occlusion is most likely given her symptoms, known cardiovascular disease, recent weight loss and elevated lactate. Appendicitis with a caecal tumour would not be expected to cause sudden onset left-sided abdominal pain and would not be expected to cause sudden onset of pain unless associated with perforation (in which case the abdomen is unlikely to be soft). Diverticulitis does not explain the 2-year history of weight loss nor the significantly elevated lactate. It would be unusual for a new diagnosis of inflammatory bowel disease in an 81 year old and this would again not usually be associated with sudden onset of symptoms. A sigmoid flexure mass does not explain sudden onset of symptoms or patient observations and the lactate level.

4. C. This is an accurate description of a positive result from the Buerger test. Arterial ulcers are punched out, sometimes deep ulcers over the lateral malleolus, lateral foot and at pressure areas. Dry gangrene is cool, reddish/black, dry, firm tissue. Superficial thrombophlebitis is firm, tender swelling along the course of a vein. Venous ulcers are shallow sloughy ulcers usually on the 'gaiter area' of the calf.

5. E. This description is of a Stanford Type B aortic dissection (arises distal to the left subclavian artery). These are managed medically in the first instance, with tight control of blood pressure and heart rate. Cardiothoracic surgery or

endovascular repair is later required in some cases of Type B dissection but this is not the most appropriate immediate management, unlike in a Type A dissection (involving the ascending aorta), where immediate surgical repair is indicated. Primary PCI is not indicated; this is not a history of STEMI, although STEMI can complicate some cases of Type A dissection due to involvement of the coronary arteries (classically the right coronary artery). Resuscitative thoracotomy in the emergency department is used for cardiac arrest in trauma when pericardial tamponade is suspected and is not indicated in this case.

6. C. Current National Institute for Health and Care Excellence (NICE) guidance states that people with an abdominal aortic aneurysm (AAA) of 5.5 cm or larger should be referred to the regional vascular service and for them to be seen within 2 weeks. Aneurysm repair should be considered in patients with symptomatic aneurysms, aneurysms of greater than 4.0 cm that have grown more than 1 cm in a year, and aneurysms that are 5.5 cm or larger – this is because these patients are at higher risk of rupture. Ultrasound monitoring alone in the first instance is inappropriate. If she is seen by the vascular service and is felt to be a higher surgical risk (or refuses surgery), she may be followed up with an ultrasound but this would not be the first-line management. There is no indication for immediate emergency department review (there are no features to suggest ruptured/leaking AAA). NICE recommends against offering preoperative beta blockers routinely to those awaiting AAA repair, as it does not provide benefit and may be harmful in some patients (especially if started soon before surgery). Although control of blood pressure and cholesterol is important, this option alone is not appropriate given the size of the patient's aneurysm.

OSCEs and Short Clinical Cases

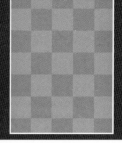

OSCES

OSCE 1 Examination in the breathless patient

Mr White is a 75-year-old gentleman; he has been complaining of shortness of breath on exertion. Please examine his cardio-vascular system:

Checklist

- Introduce yourself, check the patient's details, obtain consent and expose the patient from the waist up.
- Observe the patient from the end of the bed.
- Examine the hands for splinter haemorrhages, clubbing, Osler nodes, Janeway lesions and peripheral cyanosis.
- Palpate the radial pulse and comment on the rate and rhythm. Check for radio-radial delay. Assess for a collapsing pulse by placing the flats of the fingers over the radial artery and raising the patient's arm above their head.
- State that you would like to measure the patient's blood pressure.
- Inspect the eyes, cheeks and mouth.
- Visualize the jugular venous pressure pulse and comment on its height.
- Palpate the carotid pulse and comment on the character and volume of the pulse.
- Inspect the precordium looking for scars, pacemakers and visual impulses.
- Palpate for the apex beat, heaves and thrills over the valve areas.
- Auscultate the four valve areas, the axilla and neck.
- Auscultate for diastolic murmurs: in left lateral position and then sitting forward in held expiration.
- Auscultate the lung bases: feel for sacral oedema and pedal oedema.
- Thank the patient and cover him up.
- To finish your examination, state that you would like to palpate all peripheral pulses, check for radiofemoral delay, perform fundoscopy and order an ECG.

Questions

1. What signs might you find in right heart failure?
   - Peripheral oedema, elevated jugular venous pulse, hepatomegaly, ascites, murmur of tricuspid regurgitation (hepatomegaly may be pulsatile with tricuspid regurgitation).

2. How might you differentiate the jugular venous pulse (JVP) from the carotid pulsation?
   - The JVP is a double pulsation and should not be palpable (whereas the carotid is a single, palpable pulsation). Pressing over the liver should augment the JVP (known as hepatojugular reflux). The height of the JVP varies with respiration and the position of the patient, whereas the carotid pulse does not vary.

3. What signs might you find in left heart failure?
   - Crepitations (particularly bibasally) on auscultation of the chest, evidence of pleural effusion, murmur of mitral regurgitation.

4. What findings might you find on an X-ray in left heart failure?
   - **A**lveolar oedema, Kerley **B** lines, **C**ardiomegaly, upper lobe venous **D**iversion and pleural **E**ffusion (ABCDE can be used to remember these findings).

5. What is the New York Heart Association (NYHA) classification of heart failure?
   - A grading system used to denote the symptoms and functional status of patients with heart failure. Patients are assigned a number (I to IV):
     - I – no limitation of physical activity due to symptoms
     - II – symptoms with ordinary activity
     - III – symptoms with minimal activity
     - IV – symptoms at rest

OSCE 2 Examination in the cyanosed patient

Ms Clark is a 65-year-old lady who has been profoundly cya-nosed for 3 years. She was previously known to have a murmur but never had this investigated. She is not breathless at rest. Please examine her cardiovascular system.

See OSCE 1: Checklist.

Questions

1. How might central and peripheral cyanosis be differentiated clinically?
   - Central cyanosis can be seen in the lips and the tongue. Patients with central cyanosis will generally also be peripherally cyanosed; however, peripheries are normal temperature unless there is also poor peripheral circulation. *Pure* peripheral cyanosis will cause cold, blue hands and feet but no cyanosis centrally, i.e., normal colour lips and tongue.

2. What is the differential diagnosis of central cyanosis and which is most likely in this patient?
   - The most likely diagnosis in this case would be Eisenmenger syndrome, given the history of previous uninvestigated murmur and the fact that she has been cyanosed for the past 3 years (but not previously). Other differentials include:
     - Other conditions that cause a right-to-left cardiac shunt (e.g., cyanotic congenital heart disease).
     - Pulmonary disease of any aetiology sufficient to cause hypoxia.
     - Abnormal haemoglobins, e.g., methaemoglobinaemia (either acquired due to medications, toxins, etc. or rarely congenital causes).
     - Polycythaemia rubra vera (increased chance of cyanosis due to high haemoglobin and therefore greater oxygen requirement to fully oxygenate).
3. What is the aetiology of Eisenmenger syndrome?
   - Eisenmenger syndrome is the end result of a longstanding left-to-right cardiac shunt, generally caused by congenital heart disease (ventricular septal defect, atrial septal defect or sometimes a patent ductus arteriosus), gradually leading to pulmonary hypertension and eventual shunt reversal. The now right-to-left shunt results in deoxygenated blood entering the systemic circulation and the patient becomes cyanosed.
4. How is Eisenmenger syndrome managed?
   - By the time Eisenmenger syndrome develops and the patient becomes cyanosed, there is unfortunately no way to reverse this. Definitive treatment of this condition requires either a heart-lung transplant or a lung transplant with repair of the underlying heart defect. Patients are, however, often managed conservatively, as both these options have high mortality rates.
5. How might the development of Eisenmenger syndrome be prevented?
   - The main way to prevent this condition is through clinical examination and echocardiography to identify congenital heart defects early (before they cause pulmonary hypertension) and treat the underlying condition (e.g., closure of septal defects).

OSCE 3 Examination of the patient with a valve replacement and implantable device

Mr Brown is a 74-year-old gentleman who has previously undergone a valve replacement and insertion of an implantable device. Please examine his cardiovascular system.
See OSCE 1: Checklist.

Questions

1. What are the most common indications for a permanent pacemaker?
   - The most common indications are third-degree (complete) heart block, Mobitz type II second-degree heart block and patients with symptomatic bradycardias, such as in sick sinus syndrome. Other indications include congenital heart disease and patients with certain tachycardias (use of overdrive pacing to suppress abnormal rhythm).
2. In what situations might a biventricular pacemaker be used?
   - Biventricular pacing is also referred to as cardiac resynchronization therapy (CRT) and is generally used in patients with advanced heart failure and left bundle branch block (LBBB). In LBBB, the left ventricle depolarizes after the right ventricle and this results in the dyssynchrony of left and right ventricular contraction. With biventricular pacing, there is a separate lead into each of the ventricles and, generally, also one lead into the right atrium. This allows the pacemaker to deliver electrical impulses to each ventricle such that they contract in a synchronized manner. This hopefully improves the patient's symptoms.
3. What are the most common reasons for a patient to have a median sternotomy scar?
   - Median sternotomy is most commonly used for coronary artery bypass grafting and valve replacements. More rarely, this procedure may be used for transplantation and congenital heart defect repair.
4. How might a metal aortic valve replacement (AVR) be differentiated from a metal mitral valve replacement (MVR) clinically?
   - Patients with metal aortic valve replacements will have a normal S1, an opening click of the prosthetic aortic valve and a metal prosthetic click instead of normal S2.
   - Patients with metal mitral valve replacements will have a metallic S1 (closure of the prosthetic valve), a normal S2 and a metallic opening snap in diastole.
   - Patients with MVR may have had the procedure done via lateral thoracotomy, whereas aortic valve replacement is via median sternotomy.
5. What are the main advantages and disadvantages of a bioprosthetic valve over a metal valve replacement?
   - The main benefit of bioprosthetic valves is that they do not require anticoagulation. However, their lifetime is limited in comparison to mechanical valves – bioprosthetic valves may last, on average, 10 years

(but failure may occur as early as 4 to 5 years or as late as 20 years), whereas mechanical valves may last 25 years or longer (and often may outlast the patient). Bioprosthetic valves are preferable in patients with a contraindication to anticoagulation and the elderly (the valve is expected to outlast the patient), whereas mechanical valves may be preferable in younger patients.

OSCE 4 Incidental murmur (explanation and advice)

Ms Davidson is a 28-year-old lady who attends her GP after being told at a recent hospital visit that she has a murmur. She is asymptomatic but concerned that this may indicate serious pathology. Please explain to her the significance of an incidental murmur, with reference to possible causes and how this might be investigated:

Checklist

- Introduce yourself, check patient's details and assess patient's preexisting knowledge, including their ideas, concerns and expectations.
- Explain that cardiac murmurs are generally the result of turbulent blood flow through the heart and its valves.
- Explain that cardiac murmurs are common and, in the young, often do not represent serious pathology. Some patients may wish to know that murmurs may be the result of a narrowed (stenosed) valve, a leaky (regurgitant) valve or sometimes a hole in the heart muscle (septal defect), whereas other murmurs may occur without any underlying valve defect (functional or so-called 'innocent' murmurs).
- Explain that sometimes murmurs may be the result of increased blood flow through the heart, such as can occur with anaemia and thyroid problems. Explain that these can be investigated with simple blood tests.
- Explain that the definitive investigation of murmurs is mainly through echocardiography. Explain that this involves ultrasound scanning of the heart to look at the heart's valves and chambers and hopefully identify the source of the murmur.
- Ask the patient whether any areas remain unclear or whether she has any questions.

Questions

1. Which common conditions may cause an 'innocent' flow murmur?
   - These murmurs may be seen in any hyperdynamic state, e.g., sepsis, anaemia, hyperthyroidism, exercise and pregnancy.

2. Are systolic murmurs or diastolic murmurs more likely to be pathological?
   - Systolic murmurs can either be functional or secondary to underlying pathology. Diastolic murmurs are always pathological.
3. Ms Davidson later reveals she is concerned because her brother has recently been diagnosed with hypertrophic cardiomyopathy (HCM). What is the usual mode of inheritance of this condition?
   - HCM is autosomal dominant in the vast majority of cases. There have been rare reports of autosomal recessive and X-linked inheritance.
4. HCM used to be called hypertrophic obstructive cardiomyopathy (HOCM). Why was it called this and why is it now commonly referred to as HCM?
   - Some individuals with HCM develop obstruction of the left ventricular outflow tract due to asymmetric septal hypertrophy of the myocardium. This does not occur in all cases, and therefore, the term hypertrophic cardiomyopathy is now used more commonly.
5. How might HCM present?
   - The presentation of HCM varies widely. It may be asymptomatic and identified incidentally following examination/electrocardiography/echocardiography. Symptoms of HCM include exertional chest pain, palpitations, exertional presyncope/syncope and symptoms of pulmonary congestion (e.g., breathlessness, orthopnoea, etc.). HCM may also present with sudden cardiac death.

OSCE 5 Aortic stenosis (explanation and advice)

Mr MacLeod is a 77-year-old gentleman who presents to the cardiologist complaining of exertional chest pain. His GP feels this is likely angina. He is noted to have a murmur. Echocardiography identifies moderate to severe aortic stenosis. He wants some more information about this condition:

Checklist

- Introduce yourself, check patient's details and assess patient's preexisting knowledge, including their ideas, concerns and expectations.
- Explain that the echocardiogram has shown there is a narrowing of one of the heart valves.
- Explain blood leaves the heart through this narrowed valve to enter the main artery (aorta) to be carried to the rest of the body.
- Explain that this generally occurs due to wear and tear (degenerative change), which tends to progress over time.

- Explain that this condition is often asymptomatic initially, but as the valve narrowing progresses, blood flow through the valve is reduced, which can cause certain symptoms, particularly when the body's requirements are higher, e.g., with exercise or illness.
- Explain that the most common symptoms are chest pain, breathlessness and dizziness or fainting (presyncope/syncope).
- Explain there are several possible treatments for this condition but these are not without risk, and additional tests may be helpful to identify the most suitable treatment. If he wants more information, explain that treatment can range from medications alone to heart surgery to replace the valve.
- Ask the patient whether any areas remain unclear or whether he has any questions.

Questions

1. What is the classic triad of symptoms that might present in a patient with aortic stenosis?
   - Chest pain, syncope and breathlessness.
2. What is the significance of a bicuspid aortic valve in the development of aortic stenosis?
   - Congenitally bicuspid valves are more prone to aortic stenosis than tricuspid aortic valves – this results in aortic stenosis presenting earlier.
3. What is meant by the term 'aortic sclerosis'?
   - Aortic sclerosis refers to calcification and thickening of the aortic valve leaflets but without any restriction to valve leaflet movement or obstruction to the left ventricular outflow tract. This can cause an ejection-systolic murmur that classically *does not* radiate to the carotids and is associated with normal pulse pressure and pulse character. Aortic sclerosis is asymptomatic. In some patients, aortic sclerosis is a precursor to later aortic *stenosis.*
4. What are the treatment options in aortic stenosis?
   - There are several different options, including:
     - Medical management
     - Balloon aortic valvuloplasty (BAV)
     - Transcatheter aortic valve implantation (TAVI)
     - Aortic valve replacement (AVR) with either a mechanical valve or a bioprosthetic valve
5. What are the reasons for using a TAVI over a conventional AVR?
   - Aortic valve replacement is a high-risk procedure that frailer patients with multiple comorbidities may not tolerate – it involves median sternotomy, cardiopulmonary bypass and a longer recovery period. TAVI is a percutaneous method of delivering a replacement valve, generally via the femoral artery. This avoids many risks of conventional valve replacement and may allow frailer patients (who would previously have been unfit for treatment) to undergo a procedure that may significantly improve their symptoms and quality of life. In younger, healthier patients, conventional AVR is generally used over TAVI as need for reintervention is lower and long-term TAVI valve durability is unknown (as it is a relatively new procedure).

OSCE 6 Angina explanation and advice

Mr Smith has been suffering from chest pain on exertion for the last 6 months. His GP told him that he has angina and prescribed medication to spray under his tongue when he gets chest pain. Explain to Mr Smith what angina is and the principles of treating it:

Checklist

- Introduce yourself, check patient's details and assess patient's preexisting knowledge, including their ideas, concerns and expectations.
- Angina is a result of inadequate blood supply to the heart when it is working harder, e.g., during exercise.
- It is usually caused by a narrowing of the arteries carrying blood to the heart muscle.
- Management of risk factors, such as hypertension, hyperlipidaemia and diabetes, is important.
- Patients should stop smoking and reduce intake of salt and fatty foods to minimize progression of the disease.
- Medications aim to increase blood flow to the heart and reduce the demand on the heart.
- Coronary artery stenting or bypass surgery can be performed when disease is severe.
- Ask the patient whether any areas remain unclear or whether he has any questions.

Questions

1. Which side effects of glyceryl trinitrate (GTN) is it worth making patients aware of?
   - Palpitations, postural hypotension, light-headedness and other presyncopal symptoms are of particular importance. Rarely, patients may experience syncopal episodes. Patients also often develop an unpleasant throbbing headache.
2. What are the main risk factors for developing coronary artery disease?
   - Male sex, age, smoking, hypertension, hypercholesterolaemia, diabetes, physical inactivity, family history and poor diet.

3. If Mr Smith presented to the emergency department with crushing central chest pain and was noted to have ST segment elevation in leads II, III and aVF, which coronary artery is most likely affected?
   - This situation is an inferior ST-elevation myocardial infarction (STEMI) and the vast majority of the time is due to occlusion of the right coronary artery. Inferior STEMI can infrequently be the result of dominant left circumflex artery occlusion and very rarely due to occlusion of a 'wraparound' left anterior descending artery (anterior ST elevation would also generally be seen in this instance).
4. What clinical signs might you notice in the hypercholesterolaemic patient?
   - Tendon xanthomata, corneal arcus and xanthelasma. Patients with none of these signs may still have elevated cholesterol.
5. In patients who have undergone coronary artery bypass surgery, what signs might be found on clinical examination?
   - The most obvious clinical finding would be a midline sternotomy scar. Other scars may be seen elsewhere due to harvesting of vessels for use as grafts (e.g., scars on the leg from saphenous vein grafting or on the forearm from radial artery grafting).

OSCE 7 Chest pain history

Mrs Anderson has been having episodes of pain in her chest for the past 2 years. Please take a history from her:

Checklist

- Introduce yourself, check her details and obtain consent.
- Fully explore the episodes of pain, e.g., using the SOCRATES method: Site, Onset, Character, Radiation, Associated features, Timing, Exacerbating and relieving factors, Severity. Assess to what extent she is affected by her symptoms.
- Clarify her past medical (and surgical) history. Double check for hypertension, hypercholesterolaemia, diabetes, etc., as they may not always be mentioned.
- Take a drug history; remember allergies!
- Take a social history, including occupation, housing situation (asking about stairs is important), and whether she has any history of smoking, alcohol or other recreational drug use.
- Ask about family history, particularly about ischaemic heart disease (and age of presentation).
- Ask her ideas about what may be causing these episodes of pain and if she has any particular concerns and expectations.
- Summarize findings and clarify whether she thinks there is anything else you need to know.

Questions

1. What is the typical description of angina?
   - Substernal chest discomfort that is of characteristic quality and duration (heavy, 'band-like' pain that lasts for minutes at a time). Pain is provoked by exertion or emotional stress and relieved by rest and/or nitrates within minutes.
2. What would you consider to be a positive family history of cardiovascular disease?
   - A positive family history is generally considered as a diagnosis of cardiovascular disease in a male first-degree relative (father or brother) under the age of 55 or in a female first-degree relative (mother or sister) under the age of 65.
3. If an ECG was performed on Mrs Anderson, what might it show?
   - The ECG is normally unremarkable in patients with angina between episodes. During an attack, there may be evidence of ST segment depression or T wave inversion. There may also be unexpected findings, such as evidence of previous myocardial infarction, left ventricular hypertrophy, etc.
4. What are the main classes of antianginal medications?
   - Main classes of antianginal medications include β-blockers (e.g., bisoprolol), calcium channel antagonists (e.g., amlodipine), and nitrates (e.g., isosorbide mononitrate). Several other medications may be used, including nicorandil, ranolazine and ivabradine.
5. If she has had a previous myocardial infarction, which other medications should she be taking for secondary prevention?
   - In addition to the medications mentioned above, patients should also be on aspirin, a high-intensity statin (e.g., atorvastatin), and an ACE inhibitor (e.g., ramipril) to reduce rates of cardiovascular morbidity and mortality. Medications to control other cardiovascular risk factors (e.g., diabetes) may also be required.

OSCE 8 Hypertrophic cardiomyopathy and counselling

Mr and Mrs Jackson attend the GP. Mrs Jackson was diagnosed with hypertrophic cardiomyopathy (HCM) 3 years ago. They are thinking of starting a family and are concerned the condition may be passed on to their children. Please advise them appropriately:

Checklist

- Introduce yourself, check patient identification and obtain consent.
- Check patient understanding and what information they are seeking.

- Explain that HCM is a genetic condition and may be passed on to their children. Explain that in the vast majority of cases, the risk of a child inheriting the condition is 50%.
- Explain that there may be some benefits to genetic testing in an attempt to identify specific mutation(s) – e.g., it may be useful for prognostic purposes, prenatal or early diagnosis, screening other relatives, etc. It is worth explaining that a particular mutation may not be identified.
- Explain that even if a child is diagnosed with HCM, then the prognosis is difficult to quantify as there is significant variation (even within families with known mutations).
- Clarify if there are any other questions/additional concerns.

Questions

1. What is the mode of inheritance of HCM (if not already stated)?
   - HCM is autosomal dominant in the vast majority of cases (there are a few rarer mutations that may be inherited in an autosomal recessive manner).
2. In individuals with known mutations, in which gene(s) are these found?
   - HCM is the result of mutations in several genes encoding sarcomeric proteins (most commonly in the β-myosin heavy chain gene or the myosin-binding protein C gene).
3. How does HCM generally present?
   - Presentation of HCM varies widely. Patients are often asymptomatic (and diagnosis is incidental). Patients may present with a range of symptoms, including breathlessness, angina, light-headedness, palpitations, syncope or even sudden cardiac death.
4. What clinical signs may be found in HCM?
   - Examination findings may include a 'jerky' peripheral pulse (if obstruction is present), a double apical beat and a systolic murmur (crescendo and decrescendo in nature) with a thrill felt at the lower left sternal edge. The murmur in hypertrophic cardiomyopathy is generally louder with Valsalva manoeuvre or with standing from squatting. Patients may have no signs on clinical examination.
5. What is her risk of complications during pregnancy?
   - Pregnancy is generally well tolerated in individuals with HCM, although she would be at slightly higher risk than a patient without the condition. Patients at higher risk are those who have been symptomatic prior to pregnancy or if there is evidence of severe left ventricular outflow tract obstruction.

OSCE 9 Acute care scenario – acute pulmonary oedema

A 69-year-old patient on the cardiology ward becomes acutely breathless overnight. A nurse practitioner reviews him and arranges a portable chest X-ray. He is concerned the patient has acute pulmonary oedema and requests assistance.

Example assessment template (Note: local guidelines may vary):

	Assessment/Examination	Investigations	Management
A	• Patient position. • Is the patient talking? In full/short sentences? • Any added sounds?	• Nil.	• Sit the patient up – may need adjuncts/airway manoeuvres if reduced Glasgow Coma Scale. • Oxygen 15L via non-rebreathe mask.
B	• Respiratory rate and oxygen saturations. • Work of breathing, any cyanosis? • Trachea – is it central? • Chest expansion – equal and symmetrical? • Percussion. • Chest sounds – reduced air entry, wheeze, focal signs? *History – Ask about cough, respiratory disease and allergies?*	• Chest X-ray - look for ABCDE (**A**lveolar oedema, Kerley **B** lines, **C**ardiomegaly, Upper lobe Venous **D**iversion, **E**ffusions) • Arterial blood gases if patient hypoxic.	• Titrate inspired oxygen to arterial blood gas results if retaining carbon dioxide • Consider nebulisers if wheezy and diagnosis in doubt (i.e., could this be an exacerbation of chronic obstructive pulmonary disease or asthma?).

C	• Heart rate and blood pressure (can be set to auto cycle).
	• Capillary refill and peripheral perfusion.
	• Pulse rhythm and volume.
	• Jugular venous pressure.
	• Heart sounds – normal or additional sounds. Any murmurs?
	• Mucous membranes/peripheral oedema.
	• Urine output.
	History- Any chest pain, previous cardiovascular disease?
		• Continuous cardiac monitoring.
		• ECG – arrhythmia may precipitate heart failure.
		• Blood tests to consider:
		  o Full blood count (for signs of anaemia or infection).
		  o Urea and electrolytes
		  o Troponin (acute coronary syndrome may present with heart failure – note troponin will also be elevated in heart failure itself, therefore history is important).
		  o BNP/NT-proBNP (to differentiate heart failure from other causes of dyspnoea).
		  o Liver function tests (may be deranged in right ventricular failure).
		  o C-reactive protein (if signs of infection).
		  o Glucose.
		  o Venous blood gas (if arterial sample not taken already).
			• Intravenous (IV) Access
			• IV Furosemide – 50mg is a reasonable starting dose; may need repeated. Caution is required as may lower blood pressure.
			• Catheter – useful for monitoring. Also patients may have profound diuresis following IV furosemide and may not be able to manage otherwise.
			• Treat arrhythmia if present (e.g., with DC cardioversion/atropine – heart failure is an adverse feature of arrhythmia and indicates cardiovascular instability).

D	• 'AVPU' (Alert/Responsive to pain/Responsive to Voice/Unresponsive) or GCS (Glasgow Coma Scale). • Pupils/neurological exam if indicated (e.g., neurogenic pulmonary oedema).	• Capillary blood glucose.	• Treat hypoglycaemia if present (e.g., with glucose/glucagon). • Reduced GCS may be a sign of shock/exhaustion.
E	• Temperature. • Brief abdominal exam – e.g., ascites, hepatomegaly. • Review of notes, additional info, etc.	• Will vary depending on clinical picture and any additional pathology/causes of heart failure/co-existing conditions identified.	

CALL FOR HELP early (or as soon as you identify an issue you may not be able to deal with yourself).

REASSESS after interventions made.

Continued

	Assessment/Examination	Investigations	Management
NEXT STEPS	Speak to senior doctor (e.g., medical registrar/cardiology registrar/high dependency/intensive care registrar) as appropriate. May need: • Echocardiogram – Can be done at the bedside to investigate for/exclude mechanical causes (e.g., acquired ventricular septal defect, mitral regurgitation, left ventricular aneurysm, cardiac tamponade). • Higher level care for continuous positive airway pressure (CPAP)/ventilation, insertion of arterial line, central venous line or use of vasoactive drugs e.g., inotropes for cardiogenic shock. Patients may sometimes need intra-aortic balloon counterpulsation or haemofiltration. Return to the beginning and carry out in depth history and examination when appropriate.		
NOTES	Do not routinely offer: • *Morphine – increased risk of respiratory suppression, ICU admission, prolonged hospital stay, death.* • *Glyceryl trinitrate (GTN) – unless under cardiology advice or if there is co-existing evidence of ischaemia e.g., heart failure in context of ongoing myocardial infarction.*		

Questions

1. Why might a patient with previously stable heart failure present with decompensated heart failure?
   - Decompensation of a previously stable heart failure patient may occur for many reasons – as well as treating the heart failure itself, it is equally important to identify and treat any underlying cause of decompensation, e.g., infection, arrhythmia, acute coronary syndrome, valvular disease, nonadherence with medications, etc.

2. What are the main ways in which diuretic medication might be prescribed in the patient with heart failure?
   - Diuretic medication is generally prescribed initially as an intravenous medication in the patient presenting with acute heart failure. Intravenous diuretics may be given as bolus doses (repeated if necessary) or sometimes as an infusion that is delivered at a constant rate over 24 hours.
   - Oral medications may not be absorbed well in the acute setting (due to gastrointestinal oedema) and are generally slower to act. When the patient is stable, intravenous medications should be switched to oral medications before discharge.

3. With a new diagnosis of heart failure, what medications might be started before discharge?
   - Patients with new diagnoses of heart failure should be started on several new medications before discharge, including:
     - All patients should be started on an angiotensin-converting enzyme (ACE) inhibitor or angiotensin II receptor blocker (ARB) – these act to reduce preload, reduce the ventricular remodelling seen in heart failure, reduce afterload on the heart and reduce salt and water retention. This improves the symptoms and prognosis in the patient with heart failure.
     - All patients should be started on a β-blocker – these act to reduce heart rate and as a result, they increase coronary blood flow. They also decrease the metabolic demand of the myocardium. In combination with ACE inhibitors, β-blockers improve survival and reverse ventricular remodelling.
     - Some patients may be started on a mineralocorticoid receptor antagonist (MRA, also known as an aldosterone receptor antagonist), such as spironolactone or eplerenone. These medications improve prognosis; they act to reduce preload by blocking aldosterone receptors in the distal convoluted tubule. Aldosterone promotes sodium retention and potassium excretion; it also has a number of unfavourable extra-renal effects, including promoting fibrosis and adverse remodelling of the heart, sympathetic stimulation, parasympathetic inhibition, and vascular damage and impairment of arterial compliance, all of which adversely affect cardiac function.
     - Sacubitril/valsartan (neprilysin inhibitor/angiotensin receptor blocker combination) may be used in patients with heart failure and reduced ejection fraction (under specialist advice). There is recent evidence to suggest that this combination is more effective than an ACE inhibitor alone.
     - Unless contraindicated (e.g., due to severe renal failure), all patients with reduced ejection fraction should be started on an SGLT2 inhibitor.
     - Most patients will be started on diuretic medications – these provide a symptomatic (but not prognostic) benefit by offloading oedema.
     - There are a number of other medications that may be used in certain situations, for example, if other medications are insufficient or not tolerated. These include digoxin, nitrates, hydralazine and ivabradine.
     - Additional medications dependent on underlying cause of heart failure – e.g., patients may be started on aspirin and a statin if there is evidence of ischaemic heart disease or anticoagulation if heart failure is due to atrial fibrillation.

4. What are the common adverse effects that a patient started on β-blockers may experience?
   - Some patients started on β-blockers may experience adverse effects, including bradycardia and resultant

presyncope/syncope, cold hands/feet, fatigue, impotence and sleep disturbance. β-blockers tend to be avoided in individuals with asthma, as their use may provoke bronchospasm.

5. What information is it important to communicate to patients when starting them on ACE inhibitors?
   • It is important to stress to patients that they will require regular monitoring of blood tests (particularly of electrolytes and renal function), as there is the potential for acute kidney injury and electrolyte abnormalities (especially hyperkalaemia) with ACE inhibitor treatment.
   • It is especially important to advise patients to temporarily withhold ACE inhibitors when they are unwell (especially with conditions prone to causing dehydration, such as diarrhoea or vomiting) and to restart when they are well again – this reduces the risk of acute kidney injury.

OSCE 10 Acute care scenario – collapse

A 72-year-old patient in the acute medical unit has a collapse. A nurse has phoned for immediate review and is carrying out an ECG, as she is concerned that the cardiac monitor shows an arrhythmia.

Example assessment template (Note: local guidelines may vary):

	Assessment/examination	Investigations	Management	
A	• Patient position. • Is the patient talking? Are they confused? • Any audible added sounds?	• Nil.	• If breathless, sit the patient up. • If reduced consciousness, lie flat and consider airway manoeuvres/adjuncts. • Oxygen 15 L via nonre-breathe mask if hypoxic (this could be due to heart failure).	
B	• Respiratory rate, oxygen saturations. • Cyanosis. • Chest sounds – e.g., bibasal crepitations?	• Arterial blood gas (ABG) if hypoxic. • Chest X-ray – look for evidence of heart failure.	• Titrate inspired oxygen to arterial blood gas results if retaining carbon dioxide.	

C	• Heart rate and blood pressure (can be set to auto cycle).
	• Capillary refill time and peripheral perfusion.
	• Pulse rhythm and volume.
	• Jugular venous pressure.
	• Heart sounds- normal or additional sounds. Any murmurs?
	• Mucous membranes/peripheral oedema.
	• Urine output.
	History – Chest pain? Dizziness? Any precipitants – recent events, investigation results? History of heart disease? Allergies?
		• 12-lead ECG – crucial for diagnosis of arrhythmia.
		• Continuous cardiac monitoring – via defibrillator if very fast or unstable.
		• Bloods tests to consider:
		   ○ Full blood count.
		   ○ Urea and electrolytes, magnesium and calcium (electrolyte abnormalities may precipitate arrhythmia).
		   ○ Troponin (if clinical picture is suggestive of arrhythmia due to acute coronary syndrome).
		   ○ Glucose.
		   ○ Venous blood gases (if arterial sample not taken already).
			• Intravenous access.
			• Treatment of arrhythmia depends on particular arrhythmia and whether the patient is stable with this arrhythmia – see **Chapter 14: Arrhythmias** for Tachycardia and Bradycardia algorithms.
			• Remember patient is peri-arrest if life-threatening (or 'adverse') features are present:
			   ○ Shock
			   ○ Syncope
			   ○ Myocardial ischaemia
			   ○ Heart Failure
				CALL FOR HELP early (or as soon as you identify an issue you may not be able to deal with yourself).
				
				REASSESS after interventions made.

D	• 'AVPU' (Alert/Responsive to pain/Responsive to Voice/Unresponsive) or GCS (Glasgow Coma Scale).	• Capillary blood glucose.	• Treat hypoglycaemia if present (glucose/glucagon). • Confusion or reduced GCS may be a sign of brain hypoperfusion.	
E	• Temperature. • Brief abdominal exam – e.g., ascites, hepatomegaly. • Review notes, etc.	Will vary depending on clinical picture and any additional precipitants or coexisting conditions that are identified.		

Continued

	Assessment/examination	Investigations	Management
NEXT STEPS	Speak to senior colleague – e.g., medical registrar/cardiology registrar/high dependency unit (HDU) registrar/intensive care unit (ICU) registrar as appropriate. May require:		

- Higher level care (HDU/ICU/coronary care) for additional monitoring (e.g., continuous cardiac monitoring, central line and arterial line) or organ support (e.g., with inotropes).
- Treatment of any reversible conditions contributing to initiation and maintenance of arrhythmia. Treat ischaemia, hypotension, hypokalaemia and heart failure.
- Additional investigations – e.g., echocardiogram, coronary angiogram or electrophysiological (EP) study to evaluate cause of arrhythmia.
- Medication may be given to prevent arrhythmia or reduce the risk or recurrence if treating the underlying cause is insufficient (e.g., use of amiodarone in ventricular tachycardia).

Patient may go on to require additional procedures such as insertion of permanent pacemaker/implantable cardioverter defibrillator, catheter ablation, etc.

- Return to the beginning and carry out in-depth history and examination when appropriate.

Questions

1. What are the life-threatening (or 'adverse') features of arrhythmia and how might these present clinically?
   - Shock (usually defined as SBP <90 mmHg, symptoms of increased sympathetic activity and decreased cerebral perfusion).
   - Syncope – due to reduced cerebral perfusion.
   - Myocardial ischaemia – either as chest pain, found on 12-lead ECG or from biochemical markers (e.g., elevation of troponin).
   - Severe heart failure – pulmonary oedema (left ventricular failure) either clinically or radiologically +/– raised JVP (right ventricular failure).

2. The patient is awake and responding but is found to have a broad complex tachycardia on the ECG. If life-threatening features were present, then what should the next course of action be?
   - The patient fits the criteria for synchronized DC cardioversion. The patient is also conscious and should be anaesthetized or sedated before this is attempted. Therefore, call early for staff with these skills (e.g., anaesthetist, intensivist, A&E consultant). Another important concern is that some wards may have only automated external defibrillators (AEDs), which cannot always deliver a synchronized shock; it is worth becoming familiar with local equipment.

3. What is the significance of cardioversion in this situation being 'synchronized'? What would happen if a shock was delivered without synchronization?
   - If a patient has an arrhythmia but still has a pulse and a shock is delivered during the ventricular repolarization (during the T wave), this can precipitate ventricular fibrillation and cardiac arrest – the 'R on T' phenomenon. In a synchronized shock, the defibrillator monitors the heart's electrical activity and delivers a shock during the R wave, avoiding this risk.

4. Sometimes supraventricular tachycardia (SVT) with aberrant conduction can mimic ventricular tachycardia (VT). How can these be differentiated?
   - This can be difficult. Several features are pathognomonic of VT:
     - AV dissociation (P waves and QRS complexes at different rates).
     - Capture beats – occur when the sinoatrial node transiently 'captures' the ventricles, in the midst of AV dissociation, to produce a QRS complex of normal duration.
     - Fusion beats – occur when a sinus and ventricular beat coincide to produce a hybrid complex of intermediate morphology.
   - Other features that suggest VT are:
     - Extreme left axis deviation – indeterminate or 'northwest' axis.
     - Very broad QRS complexes (>140 ms).
     - Tachycardia beats identical to ventricular ectopics during sinus rhythm.
     - Positive or negative concordance throughout the chest leads, i.e., leads V1–6 show entirely positive (R) or entirely negative (QS) complexes, with no RS complexes seen.
     - No response to carotid sinus massage or intravenous adenosine.
     - No known typical bundle branch block morphology or evidence of accessory pathway prior to onset of broad complex tachycardia.
     - History of myocardial infarction.

5. There is diagnostic uncertainty as to whether a patient is in VT or SVT with aberrant conduction. What is the safest course of action?
   • If in doubt in this situation, always treat as VT. VT is a life-threatening arrhythmia, whereas SVT generally is not.

OSCE 11 Acute care scenario – chest pain

A 64-year-old man comes into the emergency department with crushing central chest pain for the past hour. The ambulance ECG shows no ST segment elevation. Please assess him appropriately.

Example assessment template (Note: local guidelines may vary):

	Assessment/examination	Investigations	Management	
A	• Patient position. • Is the patient talking? In full/short sentences? • Any added sounds?	• Nil.	• Sit the patient up if poorly positioned. • Oxygen – aim for 94%–98% in the patient without COPD.	
B	• Respiratory rate and oxygen saturations. • Work of breathing. • Cyanosis. • Trachea – is it central? • Chest expansion – equal and symmetrical? • Percussion • Chest sounds – any added sounds?	• Chest X-ray – look for evidence of heart failure – ABCDE (Alveolar oedema, Kerley B lines, Cardiomegaly, Upper lobe venous Diversion, Effusions). • Arterial blood gases if patient hypoxic.	• Consider intravenous furosemide if adequate BP and presence of dyspnoea/hypoxia/wheeze to suggest heart failure (wheeze may be due to pulmonary oedema, especially if patient has no history of asthma/COPD).	

C	• Heart rate and blood pressure (can be set to auto cycle).
	• Capillary refill and peripheral perfusion.
	• Pulse rhythm and volume.
	• Jugular venous pressure.
	• Heart sounds – normal or additional sounds. Any murmurs?
	• Mucous membranes/peripheral oedema.
	• Urine output.
	
	History – Ask about chest pain and heart disease. Any anticoagulation or recent bleeding?
		• 12-lead ECG – vital for diagnosis.
		• Continuous cardiac monitoring.
		• Blood tests:
		  ○ Troponin – vital!
		  ○ Full blood count (patients with anaemia, infection more prone to myocardial infarction).
		  ○ Urea and electrolytes (dehydration may increase thrombotic risk).
		  ○ Liver function tests (as baseline).
		  ○ Lipid profile.
		  ○ Clotting screen.
		  ○ Glucose.
			• Intravenous (IV) access.
			• If not contraindicated, give antiplatelet and anticoagulant therapy – local guidelines may vary but typical regime is:
			  ○ Aspirin 300 mg oral.
			  ○ Ticagrelor 180 mg oral or clopidogrel 300 mg oral.
			  ○ Fondaparinux 2.5 mg subcutaneous.
			  ○ Give vasodilators and analgesia unless contraindicated, e.g., by hypotension:
			  ○ Glyceryl trinitrate, two sprays sublingually.
			  ○ Morphine 1–10 mg IV, titrated to response with prophylactic antiemetic.
			  ○ Consider urinary catheter to monitor urine output.
				CALL FOR HELP early (or as soon as you identify an issue you may not be able to deal with yourself).
				
				REASSESS after interventions made.

D	• 'AVPU' (Alert/Responsive to pain/Responsive to Voice/Unresponsive) or GCS (Glasgow Coma Scale). • Pupils/brief neurological exam if indicated.	• Capillary blood glucose.	• Treat any derangements in blood glucose appropriately. • Reduced GCS may be a sign of cerebral hypoperfusion.	
E	• Temperature. • Brief abdominal exam – e.g., ascites, hepatomegaly. • Review notes, etc.	Will vary depending on clinical picture and any additional precipitants or coexisting conditions that are identified.		

Continued

	Assessment/examination	Investigations	Management
NEXT STEPS	• Speak to senior colleague – e.g., medical registrar/cardiology registrar/high dependency unit (HDU) registrar/intensive care unit (ICU) registrar as appropriate.		
	• Repeat testing of troponin to confirm a rise indicative of myocardial damage. The timing of this repeat test will vary dependent on local guidelines but with high-sensitivity troponins can now be done as early as 3 hours.		
	• Most patients will require inpatient coronary angiography following a non-ST-elevation myocardial infarction. If moderate to high risk, discuss with cardiologist for consideration of *early* coronary angiography with view to percutaneous coronary intervention (PCI) or coronary artery bypass grafting (CABG). Some low-risk patients or patients with multiple comorbidities may be managed medically in the first instance.		
	• Patients may require:		
	o Higher level care (HDU/ICU/coronary care) for additional monitoring (e.g., continuous cardiac monitoring and central line and arterial line) or organ support (e.g., with inotropes).		
	o Additional treatment of any complications of myocardial infarction (pacing, treatment of other arrhythmias or of heart failure, etc.).		
	Return to the beginning and carry out in-depth history and examination when appropriate. Repeat the 12-lead ECG to detect evolving changes that may occur in myocardial infarction.		

Questions

1. What would be the most important thing to do immediately if the patient was stable but the initial ECG showed ST-elevation in the anterior leads?
   - Phone the catheterization laboratory ('cath lab') and cardiologist on call to make them aware of ST-elevation myocardial infarction (STEMI) requiring primary percutaneous coronary intervention (PCI). These patients are often identified by the ambulance crew and taken directly for PCI if available.
2. What is the significance of new left bundle branch block in association with ischaemic sounding chest pain?
   - This should be treated as a STEMI until proven otherwise – the cardiologist on call should be contacted immediately.
3. If you saw ST elevation in leads II, III and aVF, which region of the heart is affected? Occlusion of which coronary artery generally causes this picture?
   - This is an inferior STEMI and in the vast majority of cases, it is the result of occlusion of the right coronary artery. Infrequently, inferior STEMIs can be due to occlusion of a dominant left circumflex artery or rarely due to occlusion of a wraparound left anterior descending artery.
4. What is the significant difference between complete heart block in the context of inferior myocardial infarction and complete heart block in the context of anterior myocardial infarction?
   - When complete heart block occurs in inferior myocardial infarction, it is usually transient; temporary pacing may be required in some instances. Complete heart block in anterior myocardial infarction is generally permanent due to septal infarction and necrosis of the bundle branches; this will require permanent pacing.
5. If a patient came in with sharp chest pain and widespread ST segment elevation across multiple coronary artery territories, what is the most likely diagnosis?
   - This is most likely pericarditis. Patients develop widespread concave ST segment elevation (sometimes with PR segment depression) across multiple leads rather than one coronary artery territory. They often describe pleuritic central chest pain that is worse on lying flat and relieved by sitting forward.

ECG CASES

It is important to be confident in how to assess an ECG, have a good understanding of what normal looks like and know the features of the most common arrhythmias. Asking the student to review an ECG and present the findings is a favourite pastime of examiners in the OSCE situation, so you should develop a system for reviewing them. See Chapter 3 for more details about how to assess an ECG.

You can develop your own system but one way of presenting an ECG is as follows:

- Name, age and sex of the patient.
- Date and time the ECG was taken.
- Rate.
- Rhythm.
- Axis.
  Next, note any abnormalities and in which lead they occur:
- P waves – width and height.
- PR interval.
- QRS complex – width, height and morphology.
- QT interval.
- ST segment – any elevation or depression.
- T waves – negative/positive and height.

If there are abnormalities, look to see whether they are global or territorial. Remember the territories:

- Anterior – V3–V4.
- Septal – V1–V2.
- Inferior – II, III and aVF.

- Lateral – I, aVL, V5–V6.
- Posterior – V7–V9 (may see reciprocal changes in V1–V2).

It is important in the exam to summarize your findings and comment on appropriate investigations/management.

ECG Case 1

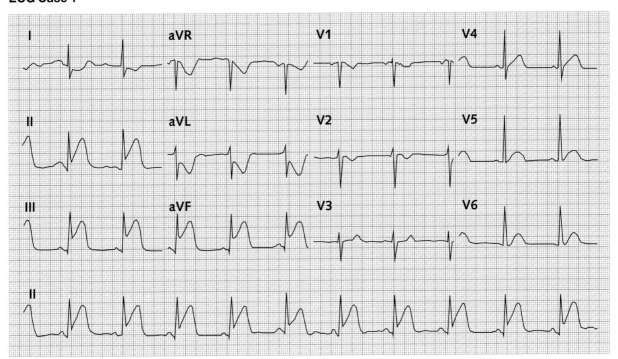

A 56-year-old man admitted with a cellulitis complains of central chest pain. He is nauseated and sweaty. He has a background of hypertension and is a current smoker.

1. Present the findings on his ECG. What is the diagnosis?

2. What is the appropriate management of this patient?
3. What are the risk factors for patients developing this condition?

ECG Case 2

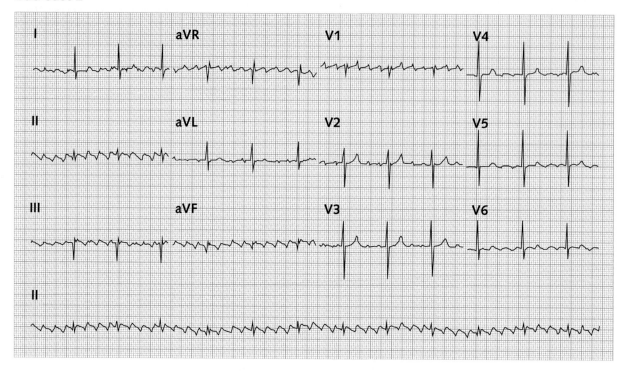

A 71-year-old lady presents with episodes of palpitations and this is her ECG.

1. Present the findings on her ECG. What is the diagnosis?

2. What are the possible complications of this condition?
3. What is the appropriate management of this patient?

ECG Case 3

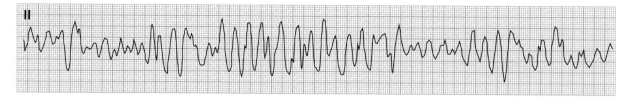

A 68-year-old man collapses in the street and bystanders start CPR. When the ambulance arrives at the scene, this is seen on the cardiac monitor.

1. Present the findings on this rhythm strip. What is the diagnosis?

2. What is the appropriate management of this patient?
3. Can this rhythm be compatible with a cardiac output?

ECG Case 4

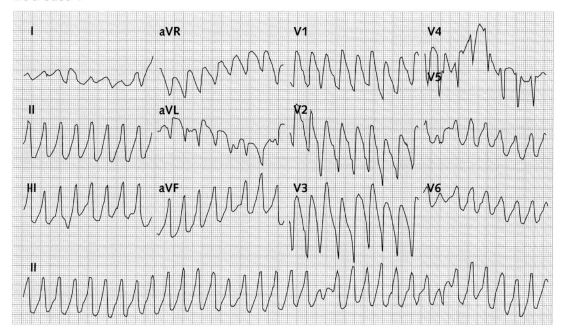

An 81-year-old lady presents with chest pain, light-headedness and a fluttering sensation in her chest. She has a normal ECG documented 1 year ago.

1. Present the findings on her ECG. What is the diagnosis?

2. What is the appropriate management of this patient?
3. What are the life-threatening (or adverse) features you should be aware of in unstable patients with arrhythmias?

ECG Case 5

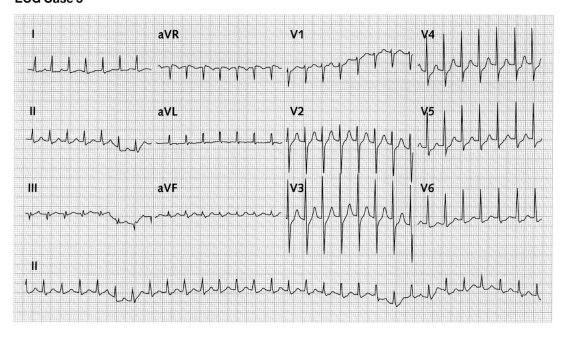

A 32-year-old man presents with a 1-day history of palpitations. He is normally fit and well, without any past medical history.

1. Present the findings on his ECG. What is the diagnosis?

2. What is the appropriate management of this patient?
3. What are the risk factors for developing this heart rhythm?

ECG Case 6

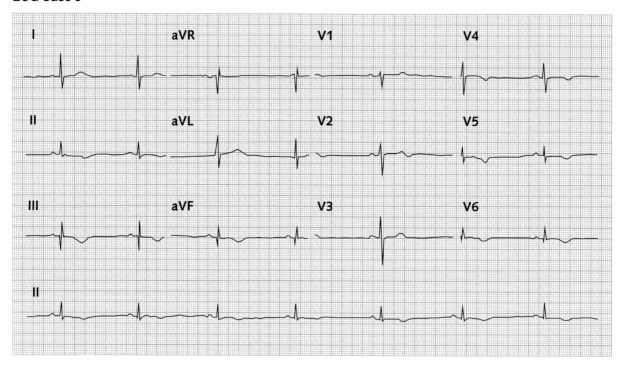

A 64-year-old man presents with lethargy and weight gain.

1. Present the findings on his ECG. What is the diagnosis?
2. What initial investigations may be helpful in this patient?

3. What medications might potentially cause/predispose to this rhythm?

ECG Case 7

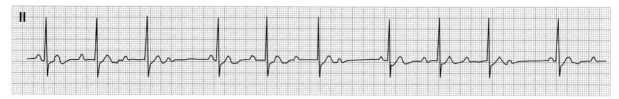

A 32-year-old man presents to the GP with a printout of his heart rhythm from a personal monitoring device. It reports an irregular rhythm and says 'possible atrial fibrillation'. He is asymptomatic and otherwise well – he is an amateur triathlete and has a very good exercise tolerance.

1. Present the findings on his ECG. What is the diagnosis?
2. What is the appropriate management of this patient?
3. What is the electrophysiological mechanism behind this arrhythmia?

ECG Case 8

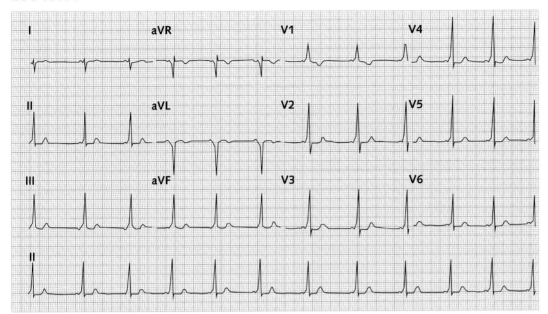

A 43-year-old lady is referred to the cardiology clinic following multiple episodes of very rapid palpitations and associated presyncopal episodes. This is her ECG when asymptomatic.

1. Present the findings on her ECG. What is the diagnosis?

2. What is the appropriate management of this patient?
3. If this ECG was carried out as part of a private medical assessment and patient had no previous symptoms, what would the appropriate management be?

ECG Case 9

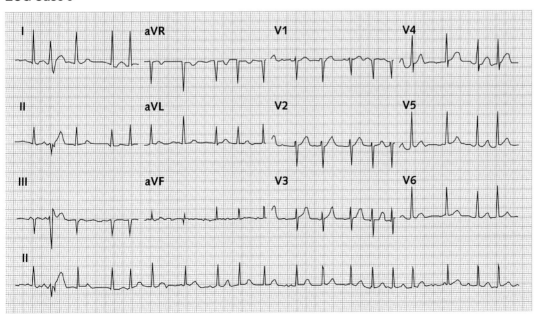

293

A 71-year-old woman presents with a 3-month history of worsening palpitations. She has a history of hypertension but otherwise is well.

1. Present the findings on her ECG. What is the diagnosis?

2. What is the most appropriate management?
3. What potential triggers may cause a patient in sinus rhythm to develop this arrhythmia acutely?

ECG Case 10

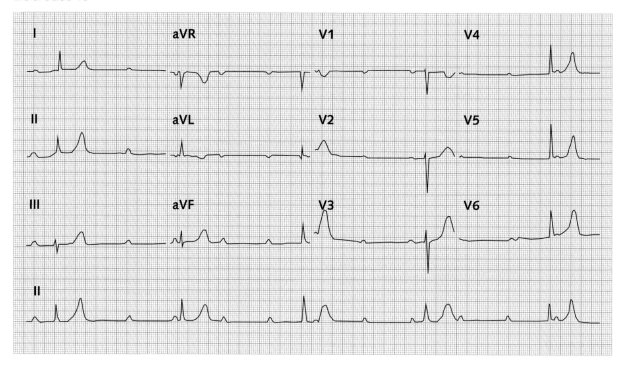

A 64-year-old man presents with breathlessness, dizziness and lethargy.

1. Present the findings on his ECG. What is the diagnosis?
2. What is the most appropriate management?

3. Would you be more concerned seeing this rhythm after an anterior or inferior myocardial infarction, and why?

ANSWERS

Case 1

1. Summary of the ECG:
   - Patient/ECG details: 56-year-old man with chest pain. Give the date and time of the ECG if provided.
   - Rate: Approximately 60 bpm.
   - Rhythm: Regular/sinus rhythm.
   - Axis: Normal.
   - Abnormalities in individual components of the ECG trace:
     - ST elevation with hyperacute T waves in leads II, III and aVF (inferior leads).
     - Reciprocal ST depression in aVL and, to a lesser extent, I.
     - Otherwise normal.
   - Summary/diagnosis: Inferior ST-elevation myocardial infarction (STEMI).

   In an OSCE, an example answer might be:

   'This is a 12-lead ECG of a 56-year-old man presenting with chest pain. His ECG shows sinus rhythm at a rate of approximately 60 beats per minute. The most striking abnormality is ST elevation across the inferior leads (leads II, III and aVF), with reciprocal ST depression in aVL and I. In summary, this patient has presented with an inferior ST-elevation myocardial infarction'.

2. The patient requires urgent primary percutaneous coronary intervention (PCI), antiplatelets and anticoagulation, and symptomatic treatment (morphine and antiemetics). Assuming he is treated successfully, he should be started on appropriate secondary prevention medications (see Chapter 12) and smoking cessation should be discussed.

3. The risk factors for developing an ST-elevation myocardial infarction are mostly the risk factors for atherosclerosis, including:
   - Hypertension
   - Hypercholesterolaemia
   - Smoking history
   - Family history
   - Male gender
   - Age
   - Diabetes

   Other factors may also predispose/lead to STEMI, including:
   - Cocaine use.
   - Other medical conditions including: chronic kidney disease, rheumatoid arthritis, etc.
   - Arterial dissection (either aortic dissection involving the coronary arteries or primary dissection of the coronary arteries).

Case 2

1. Summary of the ECG:
   - Patient/ECG details: 71-year-old lady with palpitations.
   - Rate: Ventricular depolarization at a rate of approximately 75 bpm. Atrial depolarization at a rate of approximately 300 bpm.
   - Rhythm: Regular.
   - Axis: Normal (More difficult than Case 1 as leads aVF and II close to isoelectric but axis is between 0 and −30 degrees; the vector method can be used if you are uncertain).
   - Abnormalities in individual components of the ECG trace:
     - 'Sawtooth' appearance of the P waves which are rapid, at approximately 300 bpm. Only 1 in 4 of these are associated with QRS complexes.
   - Summary/diagnosis: Atrial flutter with 4:1 conduction.

2. Complications of atrial flutter are the same as that for atrial fibrillation:
   - Complications relating to rapid heart rate – prolonged periods of rapid heart rate may lead to heart failure; rapid heart rate in patients with coronary artery disease may lead to myocardial ischaemia (with symptoms of angina) and, in some cases, myocardial infarction.
   - Thromboembolic complications – including stroke and other arterial embolization.

3. Management of atrial flutter includes:
   - Management of any underlying predisposing condition, e.g., thyrotoxicosis.
   - Ablation – catheter ablation is considered first-line treatment to ablate the reentrant circuit. This is very often successful (90%–95%) and has few complications.
   - Synchronized DC cardioversion – this will require an anaesthetist or other doctor trained in safe sedation. It is more likely to be successful in atrial flutter than with atrial fibrillation.
   - Pharmacological control:
     - Rhythm control (chemical cardioversion) – several medications can be used for this purpose, including amiodarone, β-blockers, certain calcium channel blockers (verapamil and diltiazem), digoxin or class 1A/1C antiarrhythmics.
     - Rate control – with many of the same agents as for rhythm control (β-blockers, calcium channel blockers, digoxin, amiodarone). However, rate control is more difficult in atrial flutter than with atrial fibrillation and less likely to be successful.
   - Anticoagulation – to reduce risk of thromboembolic events. Before electrical or chemical cardioversion, anticoagulation is required if the rhythm has been

ongoing for more than 48 hours. In chronic atrial flutter, patients should be assessed using the CHA_2DS_2-VASc scoring system for risk of these and the ORBIT or HAS-BLED scoring system for risk of bleeding with anticoagulation. This means most patients with atrial flutter should be treated appropriately with direct oral anticoagulants (DOACS) or warfarin.

Case 3

1. Summary of the ECG:
   - Patient/ECG details: Rhythm strip from a 68-year-old man who has collapsed in the street and is undergoing CPR.
   - Rate: Fibrillation – no regular QRS complexes.
   - Rhythm: Irregularly irregular.
   - Axis: Unable to assess.
   - Abnormalities in individual components of the ECG trace:
     - Disorganized cardiac electrical activity.
   - Summary/diagnosis: Ventricular fibrillation.
2. This patient is in cardiac arrest. Management is with cardiopulmonary resuscitation as per the 'shockable' rhythms arm of the Resuscitation Council's ALS algorithm. Defibrillation as soon as it is available will improve patient outcomes.
3. Ventricular fibrillation (VF) is never associated with a cardiac output, as there are no coordinated ventricular contractions to generate a pulse. This is in contrast to ventricular tachycardia (VT) that can be seen either with a pulse or pulseless.

Case 4

1. Summary of the ECG:
   - Patient/ECG details: 81-year-old lady presents with chest pain, light-headedness and fluttering sensation in her chest.
   - Rate: Approximately 200 bpm.
   - Rhythm: Regular.
   - Axis: Difficult to assess.
   - Abnormalities in individual components of the ECG trace:
     - Broad complex QRS complexes throughout.
   - Summary/diagnosis: Ventricular tachycardia. Less likely to be SVT with aberrant conduction because of:
     - Age of the patient – VT is more common in older patients, especially if they have a history of heart disease.
     - Complex morphology – suggests VT (see Table 14.7 and look up the Brugada criteria for additional reading – this will help differentiate VT from SVT with aberrancy). There is absence of RS complexes

across the precordial leads (all leads are monomorphic R or S waves), concordance of complexes across the precordial leads (depolarization is all in the same direction), and some variety in complex morphology.
   If in doubt, it is always safer to treat as VT rather than SVT with aberrancy.
2. The treatment of VT is determined by whether the patient has a pulse. Presumably in this case, she does but it is important to assess the patient fully if you see this on an ECG. Pulseless ventricular tachycardia (pVT) is one of the shockable rhythms that may be seen in patients in cardiac arrest. Ventricular tachycardia with a pulse should be treated as per Resuscitation Council's Adult Tachycardia protocol (2021 Guidelines). If there are life-threatening or 'adverse' features, then patient should initially be treated with synchronized DC shocks (up to 3 attempts) – remember appropriate sedation will be required if the patient is conscious. If none of these features, then patient should initially be treated with amiodarone 300 mg IV over 10 to 60 minutes.
3. The life-threatening or adverse features of arrhythmia include:
   - Shock – hypotension (e.g., systolic blood pressure of less than 90 mmHg), symptoms of increased sympathetic activity and decreased cerebral perfusion.
   - Syncope – due to reduced cerebral perfusion.
   - Myocardial ischaemia – either as chest pain, finding on 12-lead ECG or from biochemical markers (e.g., elevation of troponin).
   - Severe heart failure – pulmonary oedema (left ventricular failure) +/– raised JVP (right ventricular failure).

Case 5

1. Summary of the ECG:
   - Patient/ECG details: 32-year-old man with palpitations
   - Rate: Approximately 180 bpm.
   - Rhythm: Regular
   - Axis: Normal
   - Abnormalities in individual components of the ECG trace:
     - No definite P waves
     - Otherwise normal
   - Summary/diagnosis: AV nodal reentrant tachycardia (AVNRT). This is often also referred to as supraventricular tachycardia (SVT), although it is worth noting that SVT is an umbrella term that may also refer to other rhythms of supraventricular origin.
2. Management of AVNRT includes:
   - If life-threatening features of arrhythmia (shock, syncope, myocardial ischaemia or severe heart failure)

are present, then synchronized DC cardioversion should be carried out.
- If patient is stable, the following can be attempted:
  - Vagal stimulation (Valsalva manoeuvres, stimulating diving reflex by applying icy water/flannel to the face, carotid sinus massage).
  - Rapid IV injection of adenosine followed by saline flush (initially at a dose of 6mg but can be repeated at 12 mg and then 18 mg if no response to the lower dose).
3. Risk factors for AVNRT include:
   - Anything that increases risk of ectopic beats, including:
     - Alcohol
     - Caffeine
     - Anxiety
     - Exercise
     - Anaemia
   - Female sex
   - Presence of an accessory conduction pathway, e.g., in Wolff-Parkinson-White syndrome

Case 6

1. Summary of the ECG:
   - Patient/ECG details: 64-year-old man with lethargy and weight gain.
   - Rate: Approximately 42 bpm.
   - Rhythm: Regular/sinus rhythm.
   - Axis: Normal.
   - Abnormalities in individual components of the ECG trace:
     - T wave inversion in the inferior (II, III, aVF) and in the lateral chest leads (V4 – V6).
     - QT interval is approximately 520 ms (13 small squares of 40 ms each). QT interval is affected by heart rate. Calculating the corrected QT interval (QTc) using the Bazett formula ($QTc = QT/\sqrt{RR}$) gives a result of 435 ms, within normal limits.
   - Summary/diagnosis: Sinus bradycardia (with possible inferolateral ischaemic change).
2. The symptoms that the patient presented with (lethargy and weight gain) plus the bradycardia might suggest hypothyroidism so thyroid function tests will be important. It would also be worth checking other electrolytes, including calcium and magnesium.
3. Medications that might cause/predispose to sinus bradycardia include β-blockers, certain calcium channel blockers (including verapamil and diltiazem), digoxin and amiodarone. For patients presenting with bradycardia, their medication history should be carefully assessed for possible causative agents.

Case 7

1. Summary of the ECG:
   - Patient/ECG details: 32-year-old man with incidental finding of irregular heartbeat on a rhythm strip from a personal ECG monitoring device.
   - Rate: Approximately 60 bpm.
   - Rhythm: Regularly irregular.
   - Axis: Not possible to assess on single lead.
   - Abnormalities in individual components of the ECG trace:
     - Progressive elongation of PR interval with successive beats until a QRS complex is dropped (with this process then repeating).
   - Summary/diagnosis: Wenckebach phenomenon/ second-degree atrioventricular block, Mobitz type I.
2. If the patient is asymptomatic, then this rhythm doesn't require any treatment. The patient's monitor has presumably flagged up this rhythm due to the irregular heart rate. However, this is usually a benign rhythm with little clinical significance. Very rarely patients may progress to complete heart block. It may be seen in young, healthy individuals (especially athletes) but may also be seen in association with certain medications (e.g., β-blockers, digoxin) or following inferior MI.
3. The Wenckebach phenomenon is thought to be due to progressive fatigue of the atrioventricular nodal cells until an impulse fails to conduct, resulting in a dropped QRS complex. This cycle then repeats. In athletes, this process is thought to be related to high vagal tone.

Case 8

1. Summary of the ECG:
   - Patient/ECG details: 43-year-old lady with episodes of very rapid palpitations and associated presyncopal episodes.
   - Rate: Approximately 65 bpm.
   - Rhythm: Regular.
   - Axis: Right axis deviation.
   - Abnormalities in individual components of the ECG trace:
     - Short PR interval (approximately 80 ms – 2 small squares).
     - Slurred upstroke of the QRS complex (a delta wave).
   - Summary/diagnosis: Evidence of an accessory pathway and ventricular preexcitation – Wolff-Parkinson-White syndrome.
2. This patient has evidence of an accessory pathway, with a short PR interval and slurred upstroke of the QRS complex. Although she is in sinus rhythm at the moment, given that she has had multiple episodes of palpitations associated

with presyncope, it should be assumed that she is having paroxysmal tachyarrhythmias.

It would be helpful to have documented ECG evidence of these tachyarrhythmias, which might be achievable using ambulatory monitoring e.g., a 24-hour ECG; however, these tests may not capture an arrhythmia if they are occurring less frequently.

An electrophysiological (EP) study is likely to be useful for investigation but is also the first line treatment in Wolff-Parkinson-White syndrome. An EP study is an invasive investigation using catheters to assess the heart's electrical activity and can be used to assess the accessory pathway, induce arrhythmia (to identify origin and nature of the pathway) and ultimately to definitively treat the accessory pathway by catheter ablation.

It is worth remembering that in Wolff-Parkinson-White (WPW) syndrome, there is a small risk of sudden cardiac death. This may occur due to rapid conduction of atrial fibrillation through the accessory pathway (which may not have the same refractory period the AV node has) with resultant ventricular fibrillation.

Do not give digoxin to a patient with AF and WPW syndrome, as this may slow conduction through the AV node but not through the accessory pathway, resulting in an increased risk of conduction through the accessory pathway, which may potentially be fatal.

3. If this patient is asymptomatic and evidence of accessory pathway/ventricular preexcitation is an incidental finding, then the patient may just need intermittent review rather than any specific treatment. Properties of accessory pathways vary widely and some may not be prone to rapid conduction and resultant tachyarrhythmia. If these asymptomatic patients later go on to have evidence of tachyarrhythmia, then they can be investigated/managed at that time.

Case 9

1. Summary of the ECG:
   - Patient/ECG details: 71-year-old woman with 3-month history of worsening palpitations.
   - Rate: Approximately 115 bpm.
   - Rhythm: Irregularly irregular.
   - Axis: Normal.
   - Abnormalities in individual components of the ECG trace:
     o No convincing P waves.
     o Irregular R-R interval.
     o Incidental premature ventricular complex (PVC; a ventricular ectopic beat) – second QRS complex in leads I, II, III (and rhythm strip).
   - Summary/diagnosis: Atrial fibrillation (AF).

2. Management of AF includes:
   - Management of medical conditions that may be driving AF, e.g., sepsis, thyrotoxicosis.
   - Pharmacological control – rhythm control is more likely to be successful in younger patients with recent onset AF without ongoing factors predisposing to AF and may improve quality of life for patients with symptomatic AF.
     o Rhythm control (chemical cardioversion) – medications from group IC (e.g., flecainide) if there is no structural heart disease or group III (e.g., amiodarone). These may cardiovert and maintain sinus rhythm.
     o Rate control – Either β-blockers or rate-limiting calcium channel blockers can be used, but not both together due to the risk of complete heart block. Digoxin may be particularly useful if heart failure is present.
   - Anticoagulation – to reduce risk of thromboembolic events. Before electrical or chemical cardioversion, anticoagulation is required if the rhythm has been ongoing for more than 48 hours. In chronic AF, patients should be assessed using the CHA2DS2-VASc scoring system for risk of these and the ORBIT or HAS-BLED scoring system for risk of bleeding with anticoagulation. This means most patients with atrial flutter should be treated appropriately with direct oral anticoagulants (DOACS) or warfarin.
   - Synchronized DC cardioversion (DCCV) – This may be used acutely if the patient has life-threatening (or 'adverse') features; however, the patient is not likely to remain in sinus rhythm after cardioversion if there are ongoing predisposing factors for AF, e.g., acute illness, dilated left atrium. In a noncompromised patient, synchronized DCCV is an alternative to chemical cardioversion and is more effective but requires sedation, and recurrent AF may occur with either.
   - Ablation – This involves isolating the pulmonary veins to try to prevent future episodes of AF. This is less successful than ablation for atrial flutter.

3. Potential triggers for a patient previously in sinus rhythm developing atrial fibrillation acutely include:
   - Alcohol
   - Caffeine
   - Infection
   - Stress
   - Recreational drugs – including cocaine and amphetamines in particular
   - Electrolyte disturbances
   - Pulmonary embolus

Many conditions increase a patient's risk of AF including:
- Hypertension
- Obesity

- Smoking history
- Coronary artery disease
- Valvular disease – especially mitral stenosis
- Cardiomyopathy – e.g., dilated cardiomyopathy and hypertrophic cardiomyopathy
- Thyroid disease

Case 10

1. Summary of the ECG:
    - Patient/ECG details: 64-year-old man with breathlessness, dizziness and lethargy.
    - Rate: Ventricular rate (QRS complexes) of approximately 25 to 30 bpm, atrial rate (P waves) of approximately 70 bpm.
    - Rhythm: Regular.
    - Axis: Normal.
    - Abnormalities in individual components of the ECG trace:
        o No relationship between P waves and QRS complexes.
        o QRS complexes are narrow – implies the ventricular escape rhythm is high, close to the AV node.
    - Summary/diagnosis: Complete heart block.
2. The management of complete heart block varies dependent on the clinical setting:
    - Given the very slow rate in this case, atropine, isoprenaline infusion or temporary pacing may be required.

- If on any medications that may potentially cause complete heart block (β-blockers, digoxin and certain calcium channel blockers), these should be first discontinued and patient should be monitored for a few days to see if normal conduction returns.
- If recent inferior/anterior MI, then complete heart block may complicate this – prognosis and requirement for permanent pacing varies dependent on type of MI (see answer to question 3).
- Other conditions may also lead to complete heart block, e.g., hypothyroidism, infectious endocarditis, post aortic valve surgery.
- If there is no obvious reversible cause, then patient will require definitive treatment with insertion of a permanent pacemaker.

3. Complete heart block is more concerning after an anterior MI than an inferior MI. If it occurs following inferior MI, then heart block is usually a temporary phenomenon that may require temporary external pacing but then would usually be expected to resolve. If complete heart block occurs following anterior MI, then this is usually due to septal necrosis and necrosis of the conduction system – this would not be expected to resolve and requires permanent pacing.

Glossary

Abscess a collection of pus within a cavity.

Accessory pathway an abnormal connection between atrium and ventricle that is capable of propagating a cardiac impulse.

Acute coronary syndrome (ACS) a range of clinical presentations that includes myocardial infarction and unstable angina.

Afterload the pressure that the left ventricle must produce to eject blood out of the heart.

Ambulatory blood pressure monitoring (ABPM) monitoring of blood pressure during the day and night as the patient goes about their normal activities.

Anticoagulation treatment intended to prevent blood clotting.

Angina pectoris commonly known as angina, it is chest pain due to ischaemia (a lack of blood and hence oxygen supply) of the heart muscle, generally due to obstruction of one or more coronary artery/arteries.

Angiogram a technique where blood-filled structures, including arteries, veins and the heart chambers, are imaged, usually following the injection of a contrast medium.

Angioplasty see **Percutaneous coronary intervention**.

Apex beat the most inferior and lateral position on the chest wall where the cardiac impulse is palpable.

Arrhythmia a disturbance of cardiac rhythm.

Asystole absence of contraction. Asystole is when the heart has stopped beating. It is different from ventricular fibrillation where the heart is still contracting but not in a coordinated manner.

Atheroma an accumulation and swelling in artery walls consisting of cells (or cell debris) containing lipids (cholesterol and fatty acids), calcium and a variable amount of fibrous connective tissue.

Atrial fibrillation (AF) irregular uncoordinated contraction of the atria resulting from disorganized electrical activity, typically resulting in an irregularly irregular pulse.

Atrioventricular (AV) node region of specialized conducting tissue between the atria and ventricles that functions to regulate electrical conduction.

Atrium one of the two (upper) collecting chambers of the heart.

Bradycardia a heart rate < 60 beats per minute.

Brain natriuretic peptide (BNP) a peptide released by ventricular cardiomyocytes in response to stretching; a clinical marker that can be used in the diagnosis of heart failure.

Bundle branch block failure of either the left (LBBB) or right (RBBB) bundle branches.

Cardiac catheterization an invasive procedure to access the coronary and pulmonary circulation and chambers of the heart using a catheter. It can be used for both diagnosis and treatment.

Cardiac failure (also known as **heart failure**) a reduction in cardiac pump function such that there is inadequate perfusion to metabolizing tissues. Patients may have left ventricular failure (**LVF**), right ventricular failure (**RVF**) or, more frequently, a combination of both.

Cardiac output (CO) the amount of blood pumped out by the heart every minute; the product of stroke volume (SV) and heart rate (HR), i.e., CO = SV × HR.

Cardiac tamponade compression of the heart as a result of accumulation of fluid in the pericardial space. This results in reduced cardiac output and can be fatal if untreated.

Cardiomyopathy disease of the myocardium (heart muscle).

Cardioversion reverting the heart to a normal rhythm, either electrically (with a DC shock) or using drugs (pharmacological or chemical cardioversion).

Central venous pressure (CVP) the pressure of blood in the great veins as they enter the right atrium.

Coarctation of the aorta a congenital defect characterized by an abnormal narrowing of part of the aorta.

Contractility the strength with which the myocardium contracts.

Cyanosis bluish discolouration of the skin due to the presence of deoxygenated haemoglobin.

Defibrillation the definitive treatment for the life-threatening cardiac arrhythmia of ventricular fibrillation. Defibrillation consists of delivering a therapeutic dose of electrical energy to the heart with a device called a defibrillator.

Defibrillator can be external, transvenous or implanted, depending on the type of device used.

Dehiscence reopening at the site of a surgical closure of apposition.

Diastole part of the cardiac cycle where the ventricles are relaxed and filling.

Echocardiogram an ultrasound scan of the heart used to image two-dimensional slices of the heart.

Ectopic an event occurring at a place other than its normal location. For example, ventricular ectopic beats originate from the ventricles, not the sinoatrial node.

Electrocardiogram (ECG) a graphical representation of the electrical activity of the heart over time.

Electrophysiological (EP) study an invasive test used to assess the heart's electrical pathways, and allow accurate diagnosis (and potentially treatment) of arrhythmia.

End-diastolic pressure (EDP) the amount of pressure in the ventricle at the end of diastole.

End-diastolic volume (EDV) the amount of blood in the ventricle at the end of diastole; the greatest amount of blood found in the ventricle throughout the whole cardiac cycle.

Ejection fraction the proportion of the EDV which is ejected by contraction.

Glyceryl trinitrate (GTN) a vasodilator often used in patients with angina.

Heart block also called atrioventricular block, this is abnormal slowing or failure of conduction from the atria to the ventricles.

Holter monitor ambulatory ECG, usually attached to the patient for 24–48 hours.

Home blood pressure monitoring (HBPM) the patient monitors their own blood pressure in their own home.

Hypertension high blood pressure.

Hypertrophy increase in the size of a tissue or organ resulting from an increase in cell size.

Hypertrophic cardiomyopathy (HCM) an inherited disease of the heart muscle where the myocardium is hypertrophied (enlarged). HCM used to be called HOCM (hypertrophic obstructive cardiomyopathy) but has been renamed as obstruction occurs in a minority of cases.

Hypotension low blood pressure.

Hypoxia low oxygen levels.

Implantable cardioverter defibrillator (ICD) a device set up to detect an arrhythmia, delivering a shock to the patient as necessary.

Infective endocarditis infection of the endothelial surface of the heart or the heart valves by a microorganism.

Ischaemia lack of blood supply to a tissue.

Infarction tissue death caused by inadequate perfusion.

Jugular venous pressure (JVP) the visible pulsation of the internal jugular vein, seen in the neck.

Mean arterial pressure (MAP) the average pressure in the arterial system at any point in time, approximated as the diastolic pressure + (1/3 × pulse pressure).

Myocardial infarction death of heart muscle due to interruption of the blood supply, most commonly due to thrombosis of a ruptured atheromatous plaque in a coronary artery.

Myocarditis inflammation of the heart muscle.

Non-ST elevation myocardial infarction (NSTEMI) myocardial infarction without elevation of the ST segment on the ECG.

Pacemaker an area or device that generates cardiac electrical activity; this may be natural (such as the sinoatrial node) or artificial (such as a permanent pacemaker).

Percutaneous coronary intervention (PCI) commonly known as coronary angioplasty (or simply angioplasty); a therapeutic procedure to treat the stenotic (narrowed) coronary arteries of the heart found in coronary heart disease.

Perfusion movement of blood through an organ or tissue.

Pericarditis inflammation of the pericardium (the fibrous sac surrounding the heart).

Permanent pacemaker (PPM) an implantable device used to control the electrical activity of the heart.

Precordium the surface of the lower anterior chest wall.

Preload the degree of ventricular myocyte stretch before contraction; it is determined by the end-diastolic volume.

Pulse pressure the difference between systolic and diastolic blood pressure readings.

Radiofrequency ablation (RFA) the use of radiofrequency energy to create a therapeutic burn intended to treat cardiac arrhythmia.

Septal defect a hole in the wall dividing the chambers of the heart; this may be between the ventricles (a VSD, or ventricular septal defect) or between the atria (an ASD, or atrial septal defect).

Shunt flow of blood through an abnormal communication between cardiac chambers or blood vessels (e.g., due to a septal defect). This may allow blood to flow between the pulmonary and systemic circulations.

Shock a situation where insufficient blood flow is reaching the body's tissues; causes commonly described as hypovolaemic, cardiogenic, distributive (e.g., anaphylactic, septic, etc.), or obstructive (e.g., due to tamponade, pulmonary embolism).

Sinoatrial (SA) node the impulse-generating (pacemaker) tissue located in the roof of the right atrium.

Sinus rhythm the 'normal' heart rhythm under direct control from the sinoatrial node.

Sphygmomanometer a device used for measuring blood pressure.

Starling's Law a phenomenon whereby the heart increases its output by increasing its strength of contraction when the fibres of the myocardium are stretched.

ST elevation myocardial infarction (STEMI) myocardial infarction with elevation of the ST segment on the ECG.

Stenosis an abnormal narrowing in a blood vessel or other tubular organ/structure.

Stent a tubular metal cage that is inserted to counteract a localized obstruction to flow. Often used in the coronary arteries during percutaneous coronary intervention (PCI).

Stroke volume (SV) the amount of blood ejected from the left ventricle with each beat.

Stroke work (SW) the amount of external energy expended in one ventricular contraction. Stroke work is the arterial pressure multiplied by stroke volume.

Supraventricular literally above the ventricle, i.e., originating from the atria or AV node.

Syncope temporary loss of consciousness as the result of reduced blood flow to the brain.

Systemic vascular resistance (SVR) the resistance to blood flow offered by all of the systemic vasculature (not including the pulmonary vasculature). It is calculated as (mean arterial pressure – right atrial pressure) / cardiac output.

Systole the part of the cardiac cycle where the ventricles are contracting.

Tachycardia a heart rate > 100 beats per minute.

Tetralogy of Fallot a congenital heart condition characterized by four defects: ventricular septal defect, pulmonary stenosis, right ventricular hypertrophy and an overriding aorta (the aorta is positioned over the septal defect).

Torsades de pointes literally means 'twisting of the points'; a polymorphic ventricular tachycardia (i.e., ventricular complexes have variable shapes).

Total peripheral resistance (TPR) the resistance to the flow of blood in the whole system. It is calculated as arterial pressure / cardiac output.

Transposition of the great arteries (TGA) a congenital heart defect where the aorta and the pulmonary artery are switched, i.e., the aorta arises from the anatomical right ventricle and the pulmonary artery arises from the anatomical left ventricle.

Troponin a complex of proteins that is integral to muscle contraction in skeletal and cardiac muscle (but not smooth muscle). Damage to cardiomyocytes leads to an elevation in cardiac specific troponin levels in the plasma.

Unstable angina angina with at least one of the following: occurring at rest or minimal exertion and usually lasting >20 minutes; being severe and of new onset; occurring in a crescendo pattern. May have ECG changes indicative of ischaemia but not elevation in troponin; if troponin is elevated, this is myocardial infarction.

Vasodilatation increase in the calibre of a blood vessel.

Vegetation a mass (generally consisting of fibrin, platelets and microorganisms) seen in infective endocarditis; they are generally associated with the valves of the heart.

Ventricular relating to the heart's ventricles.

Ventricular fibrillation (VF) irregular uncoordinated contraction of the ventricles that is fatal if untreated.

Index